Alternative Medicine Resource Guide

Francine Feuerman

and

Marsha J. Handel

Medical Library Association
and
The Scarecrow Press, Inc.
Lanham, Md., & London

DISCLAIMER: This book is intended as a reference work only. It is not intended as a recommendation for any form of medical or self-treatment.

SCARECROW PRESS, INC.

Published in the United States of America
by Scarecrow Press, Inc.
4720 Boston Way
Lanham, Maryland 20706

4 Pleydell Gardens, Folkestone
Kent CT20 2DN, England

British Library Cataloguing in Publication Information Available

Library of Congress Cataloging-in-Publication Data

Feurman, Francine.
Alternative medicine resource guide / Francine Feurman and Marsha J. Handel.
p. cm.
Includes bibliographical references and index.
ISBN 0–8108–3284–4 (cloth: alk. paper)
1. Alternative medicine—Information resources. 2. Alternative medicine—Bibliography. I. Handel, Marsha J. II. Title.
R733.F48 1997
615.5—dc21 96–49534

ISBN 0–8108–3284–4 (cloth : alk. paper)

∞™ The paper used in this publication meets the minimum requirements of American National Standard for Information Sciences—Permanence of Paper for Printed Library Materials, ANSI Z39.48–1984.
Manufactured in the United States of America.

CONTENTS

PREFACE

Interest in alternative medicine has increased dramatically in recent years with an attendant increase in the need for information in this area. Although there is an abundance of material available on various aspects of alternative medicine, there is no one source to which a user can turn for information on publications, organizations, educational and treatment programs, and products. Information on these resources is scattered, incomplete, and often of questionable authority. With respect to books and journals, users face a vast number of materials on these subjects which vary widely in quality, appropriateness, authority and readability.

This book is intended for public and medical librarians, health care professionals and the lay public. It can be used by librarians as a collection development tool in building consumer health and patient education collections, and as a reference source. Health care professionals increasingly need information on alternative medicine to respond to inquiries from patients, for patient education, and to pursue their own interests in this field. The general public seeks information on alternative medicine in order to maximize choices, make informed decisions, and be active participants in their health care management. In response to this wide range of health-related needs, the authors have developed a single guide to resources and publications which provides authoritative, reliable and balanced information on alternative medicine.

The scope of this guide is limited to print sources. The authors recognize the usefulness of online resources for current information, especially in the rapidly evolving field of alternative medicine. Readers are encouraged to seek out CD-ROM products such as The Interactive BodyMind Information System, available from Alchemical Medicine Research and Teaching Association (AMR'TA), 800-627-6871, and Health Reference Center Gold, a full-text and database product available from Information Access Company, 800-228-8431; Internet resources such as altmed-res@virginia.edu, homeopathy@dungeon.com, parcelsus@teleport.com; and Internet news groups such as alt.health.ayurveda, alt.hypnosis and alt.meditation.

The selective nature of this guide required selection decisions related to modalities covered and, within those modalities, selection decisions regarding which organizations, programs, suppliers and print materials to include. Criteria used for the choice of modalities included: historical significance; likelihood of public or professional knowledge and interest; availability of practitioners, products or information in most geographic areas; ability to substantiate the reliability of practitioners through educational or certification programs; and, purported benefits of the approach.

Specific organizations, educational programs, treatment centers and suppliers within the modalities were selected based on their reliability, authority and contributions to the field. A variety of criteria were considered, including the age of the organization; qualifications of the practitioners, instructors or administrators; national or state certification or licensure; reputation of the institution in the alternative medicine community; connections with established institutions and practitioners; geographic balance; usefulness of services for the lay public and the professional audience; and, the significance of the mission, function and accomplishments of the organization. Resources which met the appropriate criteria were included for each modality. While this may appear to have resulted in an imbalance of coverage, it is simply an outcome of the development of each therapeutic approach. This seeming imbalance is not a statement about the validity of an approach but rather a reflection of its established presence at this time.

Criteria applied to the selection of books for the bibliography included author qualifications, significance of the topic and quality of treatment, quality of writing style, ease of use, accuracy, currency and reliability of information, and physical characteristics. Only English language materials published in the United States were included. Variations in the extent of coverage of modalities reflect the availability of the literature meeting the above criteria. Journals and newsletters were chosen based on substantive content, authority of the editorial board and contributing writers, and quality of writing style. Newsletters primarily reporting on the activities of the publishing or sponsoring organization were not included. Some publications available only through membership in an organization were included, but only if they met the criteria noted above. Some general health newsletters and journals not exclusively devoted to alternative medicine were reviewed because they periodically have interesting, pertinent, and informative articles relating to this field.

Resources evaluated for inclusion in this guide were obtained from a variety of sources. These include the *Encyclopedia of Associations;* DIRLINE, an online database of the National Library of Medicine; the professional monographic and journal literature; recommendations from individual professionals, organizations, educational programs and treatment centers in the field of alternative medicine; resource lists provided by organizations and other published resource guides; existing consumer health collections in libraries and bookstores; consumer health databases; RLIN (Research Libraries Information Network); publishers' catalogs and vendor lists; book reviews from the professional and library journal literature; and the personal knowledge of the authors. All organizations, treatment centers, educational programs, and suppliers were contacted directly in order to verify the accuracy of location information and the services provided. Review copies of books and journals were obtained from many publishers and organizations. We would like to thank everyone who cooperated in this endeavor.

This book is organized into two main sections: a resource guide and a selective bibliography of books, journals and newsletters. Each section is intended to address different needs of the reader. The resource guide is designed to provide reference information on the specific products and services available to the lay public and the professional audience by the organizations and the companies covered. The bibliography serves the educational and informational needs of the audience and provides a guide for librarians in building a collection in alternative medicine.

The work is designed to lead the reader to authoritative, reliable and balanced sources of alternative medicine information and services. While there are other points of view regarding alternative medicine in general as well as the particular modalities covered, no attempt has been made to include literature that refutes this perspective or any particular practice. Although there is ample literature available which provides a more critical look at the field, it was not considered in the scope of this book.

INTRODUCTION

Health care delivery in the United States is moving toward a health-oriented system rather than a disease-treatment system. The high cost of technology-based medicine, new discoveries in immunology and behavioral medicine, and increased consumer interest in self-care and participation in health care decisions are influencing this new direction. This shift from treating disease to promoting wellness has occasioned a heightened awareness of alternative, complementary, or holistic medicine practices. These approaches focus on the whole individual, how a person thinks, feels, lives, eats, moves and handles stress. Many alternative medicine modalities emphasize personal responsibility and empowerment, interest in the physical, mental, emotional and spiritual aspects of a person, and use of the natural healing powers within the individual facilitated by a practitioner through a variety of methods. Some of these methods are new and emerge from a blend of science and medicine; many are ancient, based on practices developed by various cultures thousands of years ago. Most share a conceptualization of the human body as an energy system striving toward balance, openness, and self-regulation.

This book contains information on resources and publications in the general field of alternative medicine and thirty-two specific modalities. Listings for nutrition, exercise, and alternative treatments for specific diseases are not included. The book is organized into two main sections: a resource guide and a selective bibliography of books, journals and newsletters. Each section is intended to address different needs of the reader. The resource guide provides reference information on the specific services and products available to the lay public and professional audience by the organizations and companies included. The bibliography serves the educational and informational needs of the audience and provides a guide for librarians in building a collection in alternative medicine.

Part I, the resource guide, contains information on U.S.-based organizations, schools and educational programs, treatment centers and product suppliers. Several of the resources listed provide services that span multiple categories. Where those services require substantial explanation, the resource is listed in the appropriate categories with "See also" references. In instances where those services are not a significant component of an organization's program, those resources have been listed in the appropriate categories with "See" references directing the reader to the primary program category. Entries include address, telephone and Fax numbers, and other pertinent contact information; a complete description of services and programs offered for the professional and for the lay public; and organizational publications where appropriate. In those instances where a distinction has not been made between services for the public and for the professional, they have been grouped together under the heading "Services." For those modalities that have no treatment centers listed, the reader is encouraged to contact the major organizations or educational institutions for referral to individual practitioners.

While not comprehensive, every effort has been made to include most of the national resources, many of which serve as referral sources to regional and local programs and services. In addition, many of the more prominent regional organizations, schools and institutions are also listed and described.

Part II is a selective, evaluative, annotated bibliography of over 150 books and more than seventy journals and newsletters covering the field of alternative medicine. As in the resource guide, this section begins with the general category of alternative medicine and is followed by separate sections covering specific therapeutic modalities. Works appropriate to the lay public, the health professional, or both have been included in order to serve the diverse needs of the intended audience. No attempt has been made to be comprehensive, but rather to offer representative authoritative works which provide varying perspectives on the field. Only English language books published in the United States since 1988 are included; exceptions have been made for works considered classic or definitive in their fields. As of June, 1995, all of these works were currently in print. An appendix lists book publishers in the field of alternative medicine with addresses, telephone and Fax numbers where available.

PART I: RESOURCES

CHAPTER 1: GENERAL RESOURCES

The basic underlying assumptions that characterize an alternative or complementary medicine approach to health are reflected in the terms that are used to describe this field. Holistic health implies attention to the condition of the whole person: body, mind and spirit. Mind/body medicine indicates the belief in the oneness of the mind and body, an integration on the deepest levels of the psychophysiological aspects of the human being. This point of view focuses on what constitutes health, rather that what causes disease. In fact, disease is reconceptualized as dis-ease (a lack of ease) rather than a pathological condition to be cured by external means. The term *allopathy,* used to describe the philosophy behind the generally accepted form of medical practice in the United States, comes from the Greek word *allopatheia* (subjection to external influences) and indicates treatment based on the application of remedies that produce opposite effects to those produced by the disease. In contrast, the work of alternative medicine therapies is to enhance those processes within the body/mind that lead to an ongoing renewal of energetic, chemical, structural, emotional and spiritual balance, ease and flow. The emphasis is on prevention, and wellness is seen as a continual process of internal balance rather than a fixed state of either health or illness. This approach calls for participation and self-awareness, a willingness to understand, practice and learn from the process of healing.

Organizations

1. The Alliance/Foundation for Alternative Medicine (A/FAM)
160 N.W. Widmer Place, Albany, OR 97321
Telephone: 503-926-1626; Fax: 503-684-9605
Contact: Marge Jacob, co-founder, secretary/treasurer

The alliance represents organizations, physicians and other medical professionals, as well as alternative therapy practitioners. The foundation is comprised of patients and the lay public who support alternative therapies. A primary goal is to encourage open and free communication and exchange of information between the government, the alternative medicine field and the lay public.

Services for the professional: Serves as an international networking organization; sponsors special public events; engages in political action advocacy for the field of alternative medicine.

Services for the public: Provides an information sheet on treatment guidebooks and research services, informational videotapes, books, audiotapes, magazines and newspapers, and congressional hearings and government reports related to the field of alternative therapy.

2. Alliance for Alternatives in Healthcare, Inc. (AAH)

Post Office Box 6279, Thousand Oaks, CA 91359-6279
Telephone: 805-494-7818; Fax: 805-494-8528
Contact: Steve Gorman, president; Sherry Gorman, executive vice president

Part of a health care purchasing coalition called the Alternative Health Group.

Services for the professional: Providers of natural, complementary, and alternative health care services can participate in the Holistic Health Network and gain exposure to many prospective patients or clients.

Services for the public: The health care purchasing coalition offers group health plans that include benefits for conventional medical care as well as a wide range of complementary alternative health care modalities including acupuncture, Ayurvedic Medicine, biofeedback, bodywork and massage therapy, chelation therapy, chiropractic, colon therapy, and midwives and alternative birthing centers.

3. Alternative Medicine Connection (ARxC)

Post Office Box 683, Herndon, VA 22070
Telephone: 703-471-4734
Contact: Arline Brecher, system operator

An online information service devoted totally to the networking of individuals, organizations, associations, and societies representing health care professionals and the public interested in alternative medicine and freedom of choice in medical care. Addresses the political and scientific interests of the holistic health community through interactive networking twenty-four hours a day, seven days a week. Dial 703-471-8465. A free dial-up disk can be obtained by calling ARxC.

4. American College for Advancement in Medicine (ACAM)
23121 Verdugo Drive, Suite 204, Laguna Hills, CA 92653
Telephone: 714-583-7666, 800-532-3688; Fax: 714-455-9679
Contact: Edward A. Shaw, Ph.D., executive director

A nonprofit medical society dedicated to promoting innovative therapies in preventive/nutritional medicine through professional education of its membership, research, publication, and cooperation with other medical organizations with similar objectives worldwide.

Services for the professional: Provides patient referrals to doctors listed in the ACAM Membership Roster; provides research opportunities; conducts special workshops; offers legislative and political support through the American Preventive Medical Association, ACAM's sister organization (see entry no. 9 below); sponsors biannual programs for continuing medical education credit; sells books, tapes and slides; publishes a journal and newsletter.

Services for the public: Provides a patient packet with a national listing of membership doctors, a book/articles list, and an informational pamphlet about chelation therapy. (Send a self-addressed, stamped envelope to: ACAM, Post Office Box 3427, Laguna Hills, CA 32654.)

Publications: Journal of Advancement in Medicine, quarterly, free to members, $62.00 (subscription), (reviewed under General—Journals and Newsletters).

5. American Holistic Health Association (AHHA)
Post Office Box 17400, Anaheim, CA 92817-7400
Telephone: 714-779-6152

An educational, nonprofit corporation serving as an information resource for the general public.

Services for the public: Prepares self-help literature on health and wellness-related topics; provides referrals to national organizations representing various therapeutic modalities and to AHHA practitioner members; publishes a list of organizations that research information and treatment on various diseases and conditions as well as a booklet entitled *Wellness from Within: The First Step*; sponsors a monthly lecture series in Irvine, CA.

Publications: AhHa!, quarterly newsletter, free to members.

6. American Holistic Medical Association (AHMA)
4101 Lake Boone Trail, Suite 201, Raleigh, NC 27607
Telephone: 919-787-5181; Fax: 919-787-4916
Contact: Susan Kruse, executive director

A professional organization for medical doctors, doctors of osteopathy, and medical students who practice holistic medicine. Associate membership is available to health care practitioners certified, registered or licensed in the state in which they practice. Supports practitioners in their continuing personal and professional development and promotes holistic medicine.

Services for the professional: Offers networking and continuing education opportunities through the National Practitioners Support Network; conducts an annual scientific conference, regional meeting and local support groups; publishes a membership directory.

Services for the public: Provides referrals to holistic practitioners by geographic area through the AHMA referral list.

Publications: AHMA National Referral Directory, updated annually, $8.00; *Holistic Medicine,* quarterly journal, free to members, $30.00 (subscription) (reviewed under General—Journals and Newsletters); various patient information publications about holistic medicine.

7. American Holistic Nurses' Association (AHNA)

4101 Lake Boone Trail, Suite 201, Raleigh, NC 27607
Telephone: 919-787-5181; 800-278-2462; Fax: 919-787-4916

A nonprofit membership organization open to nurses, other health care professionals and the public, dedicated to education in the concepts of holistic health care, research, networking with other health-related organizations and the promotion of new directions of health care, especially within the practice of nursing.

Services for the professional: Maintains a networking list of members by region or state; offers scholarships and certificate programs; conducts AHNA seminars and conferences; offers resources and publications including journal and newsletter.

Publications: Journal of Holistic Nursing, quarterly, $68.00 (institutional subscription), $36.00 (individual subscription), free to members; *Beginnings,* newsletter, ten times a year, $16.00 (subscription).

8. American Holistic Veterinary Medical Association (AHVMA)

2214 Old Emmorton Road, Bel Air, MD 21015
Telephone: 410-569-0795; Fax: 410-515-7774
Contact: Carvel G. Tiekert, D.V.M., executive director

A professional organization for the study and exploration of alternative modalities of health care, other than acupuncture, in veterinary medicine.

Services for the professional: Conducts an annual conference and half-day meeting within larger conferences; publishes *Book Shelf* (list of books available through the association); publishes a journal, conference tapes and proceedings.

Services for the public: Provides a referral list to holistic veterinarians; offers *Book Shelf* (see above).

Publications: Journal of the AHVMA, quarterly, free with membership.

9. American Preventive Medical Association (APMA)
459 Walker Road, Great Falls, VA 22066
Telephone: 703-759-0662; Fax: 703-759-6711
Contact: Candace Campbell, executive director

A public advocacy membership organization for health care professionals, the health care industry and the lay public which works toward assuring freedom of practice for health care professionals using complementary therapies and freedom of choice for patients.

Services for the professional: Tracks federal and state legislation on health-related issues; lobbies Congress for legislation; supports court actions on behalf of consumers, health care practitioners, supplement manufacturers and distributors; provides information to the media and members of Congress on complementary medicine; maintains a library of informational materials, books, studies and articles available to the media and legislators; offers group insurance programs covering legal defense expenses; operates a Fax Network at least twice monthly informing members of legal and legislative developments including bills moving through Congress, FDA activities, grassroots efforts, physician harassment and other events (sent by mail to those without a Fax machine).

Services for the public: Provides doctor referrals to complementary physicians.

10. Archaeus Project (AP)
Post Office Box 7079, Kamuela, HI 96743
Telephone: 808-885-6773; Fax: 808-885-9863
Contact: Dennis Stillings, director

A nonprofit public educational foundation dedicated to exploring new ideas related to the prevention and treatment of disease, especially as they relate to self-regulation and consciousness, including biofeedback, hypnosis, music therapy, imagery, psychoneuroimmunology, meditation, and other alternative therapies.

Services: Provides information and networking on health care issues, alternative medicine, and anomalies; sells audiotapes and videotapes; conducts colloquia, monthly meetings, special events and congresses; publishes books, informational booklets, and journal.

Publications: Healing Island, occasional journal, $20.00 (donation); some back issues of former journals *Artifax* and *Archaeus* are available.

11. Association for Research and Enlightenment, Inc. (ARE)
Post Office Box 595, Virginia Beach, VA 23451-0595
Telephone: 800-333-4499; 804-428-3588 (in Virginia); Fax: 804-422-4631
Contact: Kevin J. Todeschi, director of communications

An international, nonprofit membership organization founded in 1931 to preserve, organize and make available for research and study the psychic readings of Edgar Cayce. Readings deal substantially with maintaining health and treating illness from a natural and holistic therapeutic perspective.

Services for the professional: Offers a 600-hour certified massage therapist training course at the Harold J. Reilly School of Massotherapy (see chapter 4: Massage —Schools); offers a master's degree program in Transpersonal Psychology (accredited) in affiliation with Atlantic University; conducts medical research by physicians, chiropractors and osteopaths based on the Cayce medical readings.

Services for the public: Conducts conferences, workshops, and seminars; offers home-study courses on mind/body health, dreamwork, meditation, psychic development, near-death experiences, and death and dying; maintains circulating files of Cayce Readings; supports local study groups; runs ARE camp; provides monthly extracts from Cayce Readings; sells books; conducts international tours; publishes bimonthly magazine and newsletter.

Publications: Venture Inward, bimonthly magazine, free with membership; *A.R.E. Community,* bimonthly newsletter, free with membership.

12. Association of Holistic Healing Centers (AHHC)
109 Holly Crescent, Suite 201, Virginia Beach, VA 23451
Telephone: 804-422-9033; Fax: 804-422-8132
Contact: Margaret W. Irby, Ph.D., director; Theresa A. Lungwitz, R.N., director

A nonprofit membership organization for individuals and organizations involved in the healing arts. Encourages a multidisciplinary approach to health care by actively supporting the development and operation of holistic healing centers; fosters the development and research of a metatheory of body/mind/spirit integration (holistic healing); encourages the formation of integrated diagnostic and treatment programs for illness and wellness.

Services for the professional: Maintains an AHHC membership roster; provides descriptive summaries of member centers' services and activities; sponsors conferences and workshops; provides consultations; maintains a listing of members' publications; awards an annual research grant and three Best Article Awards; publishes a newsletter.

Publications: The AHHC Newsletter, quarterly, free with membership.

13. Citizens for Health (CH)

Post Office Box 1195, Tacoma, WA 98401
Telephone: 206-922-2457; 800-357-2211; Fax: 206-922-7583
Contact: Wendy Boehmler, membership services director

A community-based, nonprofit health advocacy organization with 165 chapters worldwide. Works to protect alternative and natural therapy practitioners from government overregulation and protect the public's right to make informed health care choices. Supports research, education and legislative advocacy toward a new vision of health care emphasizing wellness and prevention.

Services for the professional: Participates in legislative activism; offers support for individuals and organizations who practice effective and safe preventive medicine and natural therapy approaches to health care.

Services for the public: State and local chapters hold public forums, organize public rallies, and involve citizens in political activism and lobbying training.

Publications: Citizens for Health Digest, bimonthly newsletter, $15.95 (subscription); *Citizens for Health Report,* bimonthly, free with membership (reviewed under General—Journals and Newsletters); *Action Alerts,* periodic.

14. Committee for Freedom of Choice in Medicine, Inc. (CFCM)

1180 Walnut Avenue, Chula Vista, CA 91911
Telephone: 619-429-8200; 800-227-4458; Fax: 619-429-8004
Contact: Michael L. Culbert, D. Sc., chairman emeritus/editor

A nonprofit organization fighting for freedom of choice with informed consent for physician and patient.

Services for the professional: Offers referrals for metabolic/integrative therapists nationally and internationally; sells monographs published by The Bradford Research Institute, C & C Communications and the Committee.

Services for the public: Maintains a doctor-patient referral service nationally and internationally; actively lobbies and provides political statements and position papers for legislative bodies; publishes a quarterly magazine.

Publications: The Choice, quarterly magazine, $16 (subscription, included with membership) (reviewed under General—Journals and Newsletters).

15. The Fetzer Institute (FI)
9292 W. KL Avenue, Kalamazoo, MI 49009-9398
Telephone: 616-375-2000; Fax: 616-372-2163

A nonprofit educational organization dedicated to furthering research in health care based on the principles of the mind/body connection in order to develop scientifically based health care approaches that expand standard medical practices and offer individuals greater control over their own health. The institute works in the area of research in collaboration with other organizations and institutions, and in the area of education to develop curricula in schools and disseminate reliable information on effective mind/body/spirit therapeutic approaches to health.

Services: Conducts symposia, seminars and conferences; offers a fellowship program for researchers and educators; conducts research programs in mind/body/spirit health; provides educational programs for health professionals, teachers and the public; conducts studies in the nature of consciousness and spirit; publishes a journal.

Publications: Advances: The Journal of Mind-Body Health, quarterly journal, $39.00 (individual subscription), $79.00 (institutional subscription) (reviewed under General—Journals and Newsletters); *Overview of Legislative Developments Concerning Alternative Health Care in the United States,* an Occasional Study, possibly the first legislative overview of existing statutory law in the United States concerning the alternative health care field as a whole.

16. Foundation for the Advancement of Innovative Medicine (FAIM)
2 Executive Boulevard, Suite 204, Suffern, NY 10901
Telephone: 914-368-9797; Fax: 914-357-8803
Contact: Dr. Howard Hindi, treasurer

An educational and activist organization on the state and federal level working to promote freedom of choice in health care and a greater acceptance of complementary medicine.

Services for the professional: Supports networking among professionals, researchers and lobbyists; holds a yearly health care symposia; maintains a library of audiotapes and videotapes.

Services for the public: Guides patients through small claims court actions to recover insurance reimbursement; provides referrals to member practitioners.

Publications: Innovations, quarterly health letter, for members only.

17. Health Horizons (HH)
Post Office Box 278205, Sacramento, CA 95827
Telephone: 800-769-9355; Fax: 916-791-8394
Contact: Tom Long, M.D.

A health information service providing up-to-date information on both traditional and alternative medical treatments.

Services: Provides research on various approaches to diseases and their treatment programs for both professionals and the lay public, including Chinese medicine, homeopathy, herbology, vibrational therapies and more; provides disease synopsis information on any disease or condition from literature searches of conventional medical databases; supplies article summaries or reprints of articles from the international medical literature on any disease or condition; provides information on drug side effects and interactions, and complete travel medical advice.

18. The Health Resource, Inc. (HR)
564 Locust Street, Conway, AR 72032
Telephone: 501-329-5272; 800-949-0090; Fax: 501-329-9489
Contact: Janice Guthrie, director

A medical information service providing clients with individualized, in-depth research reports on their specific medical problems. Reports contain information on the latest treatment options, both conventional and alternative, including their advantages and disadvantages, and on nutrition, self-help measures, specialists, and resource organizations. A list of books and glossary of medical terms is also included. Research is done through medical school, university and public libraries as well as database searching on computers to locate the most current medical information worldwide. Reports are completed within three to five days with fees ranging from $195.00 to $295.00 for a fifty- to 200-page report.

19. Institute of Noetic Sciences (ION)
475 Gate Five Road, Suite 300, Sausalito, CA 94965-0909
Telephone: 415-331-5650; Fax: 415-331-5673
Contact: Willis W. Harman, president

A research foundation, educational institution and international membership organization promoting an interdisciplinary study of mind/body health, meditation and consciousness, and a vision of societal transformation based on the full development of human potential.

Services for the professional: Conducts research activities including small seed contracts for scientific and scholarly research, in-house research and scholarly exchange through conferences; sponsors lectures and conferences; publishes books, research reports, and educational materials and a biannual membership directory.

Services for the public: Sponsors conferences, lectures, local groups and special events; provides an annotated catalog of books, audiotapes and videotapes; offers a travel program; encourages participation in member research projects; publishes books, educational materials and a biannual membership directory.

Publications: Noetic Sciences Bulletin, quarterly journal, free with membership; *Noetic Sciences Review,* quarterly journal, free with membership (reviewed under General—Journals and Newsletters); *Healing Ourselves: A Resource Guide to Mind-Body Health,* free with membership.

20. The International Academy of Nutrition and Preventive Medicine (IANPM)

Post Office Box 18433, Asheville, NC 28814-0433
Telephone: 704-258-3243; Fax: 704-253-7781
Contact: Elizabeth Pavka, M.S., executive director

A membership organization of health care professionals and the interested lay public (Friends of IANPM) working to advance the goals of health and preventive medicine among health professionals and the public. IANPM encourages research, disseminates knowledge about health and disease prevention, and encourages a focus on nutrition and preventive medicine in medical education and the professional practice of physicians, dentists, optometrists, chiropractors, nutritionists, researchers, teachers and other health professionals. All effective therapies are supported, and the organization works actively with groups seeking to expand the acceptance of nontraditional, complementary health care.

Services for the professional: Lists prevention-oriented health care professionals for referral purposes; publishes journal and newsletter.

Services for the public: Offers a referral service to complementary physicians and health care providers nationally and internationally (directory of professional members, $15.00 to nonmembers); publishes a newsletter offering current information on nutrition and preventive medicine.

Publications: The Journal of Applied Nutrition, quarterly, $75.00 (individual and institutional subscriptions), $40.00 (student subscription); *Your Health,* bimonthly newsletter, free to members.

21. The Mankind Research Foundation (MRF)

1315 Apple Avenue, Silver Spring, MD 20910
Telephone: 301-587-8686; Fax: 301-585-8959
Contact: Dr. Carl Schleicher, president

A nonprofit scientific, educational and charitable organization seeking innovative solutions to major social and medical problems in the United States. Research programs are underway in various areas that encompass the sphere of holistic medicine, including prevention and treatment of specific conditions by biofeedback, color and light therapy, music therapy, stress management, acupuncture, yoga, meditation and homeopathy.

Services: Provides innovative treatments, medical devices and natural products targeted primarily to cancer, HIV, neuromuscular disorders and degenerative diseases. Availability of any treatments and location information are provided upon request.

22. Monterey Institute for the Study of Alternative Healing Arts (MISAHA)

400 Virgin Avenue, Monterey, CA 93940
Telephone: 408-646-0339; Fax: 408-646-8019
Contact: Savely L. Savva, M.S., founder and executive director

A nonprofit scientific research center for the study of alternative healing practices in order to scientifically validate these practices and facilitate their acceptance and use in medical and scientific communities. Emphasis is given to psi-healing, seeking unequivocal statistical data based on the results of clinical trials on the healing effects of the most talented individual healers internationally, and presenting results of these studies to the international scientific community through publication in scientific journals. MISAHA works with over 300 institutions in the U.S. and abroad that are involved in the study of alternative medicine and psi-phenomena, including the Office of Alternative Medicine of the National Institutes of Health. Their quarterly newsletter discusses these current and future research projects as well as findings, events and developments in the field.

Publications: MISAHA Newsletter, quarterly, $20.00 donation.

23. National Animal Health Alliance, Inc. (NAHA)

Post Office Box 351, Trilby, FL 33593-0351
Telephone: 904-583-2770; Fax: 904-583-4667
Contact: Charlene Smith, editor-in-chief, *Natural Pet Magazine;* Howard Peiper, marketing director

A not-for-profit research and educational organization focusing on all aspects of holistic pet care, especially alternative approaches to companion animal care.

Services: Conducts research and provides information on the use of vitamins, minerals and herbs in animal care; provides public speakers; publishes a journal.

Publications: NaturalPet, magazine, six times a year, $5.00/sample issue, $20.00 (subscription) (reviewed under General—Journals and Newsletters).

24. National Health Federation (NHF)

212 West Foothill Boulevard, Monrovia, CA 91016
Telephone: 818-357-2181; Fax: 818-303-0642
Contact: Patrick Von Mauck, financial officer

A nonprofit consumer organization dedicated to protecting the public's freedom to choose a health practitioner, therapy or approach. Monitors, analyzes and reports on legislation. Works for passage of health and freedom legislation on a local, state and national level. Advocates against dangerous practices such as toxic chemicals and fluoridation.

Services for the professional: Provides education in the newest alternative treatments; conducts continuing education programs; provides a referral list; maintains a speakers' bureau.

Services for the public: Supports natural health education through its convention and magazine; maintains a 25,000-volume indexed alternative health library; sells current books on alternative health; provides doctor referral by geographic area ($10 donation requested).

Publications: Health Freedom News, ten issues/year, $36 (subscription) (reviewed under General—Journals and Newsletters).

25. National Wellness Institute (NWI)

1045 Clark Street, Suite 210, Post Office Box 827, Stevens Point, WI 54481-0827
Telephone: 715-342-2969; Fax: 715-342-2979
Contact: Linda R. Chapin, D.D.S., M.S., executive director

A nonprofit resource center for health promotion and wellness professionals and organizations, dedicated to achieving a broader understanding of the factors that contribute to health and expand the traditional practice of health care worldwide. Various categories of membership are available for professionals working in all areas of health promotion and wellness.

Services for the professional: Provides information and resource referrals; supports networking, continuing education and professional growth through the Annual National Wellness Conference and the National Wellness Association, the membership division of NWI; prepares Wellness Assessments in print questionnaire and software formats for health promotion programs.

Publications: Presentation Resource Manual, annual conference proceedings, $34.95; *Wellness Resource Directory,* annual, $29.95; *Health Issues UP-*

DATE, newsletter, quarterly, free to NWA professional members; *Wellness Management,* newsletter, quarterly, free to NWA associate and professional members; *NWA Membership Directory,* annual, free to NWA associate and professional members.

26. Office of Alternative Medicine of the National Institutes of Health (OAM/NIH) Information Center

9000 Rockville Pike, Building 31, Room 5B-38, Mail Stop 2182, Bethseda, MD 20892
Telephone: 301-402-2466; Fax: 301-402-4741

Established by an act of the United States Congress in 1992 to "facilitate the evaluation of alternative medical treatment modalities" to determine their effectiveness and help integrate effective treatments into conventional medical practice.

Activities: Sponsors research in alternative health therapies; conducts workshops on the grant-writing process; provides technical support for field investigations in alternative medical practices; currently developing a comprehensive networked electronic information resource for practitioners and the public seeking information; sponsors conferences and workshops; conducts an international program to coordinate, standardize and make available information from other countries on alternative medicine; coordinates efforts with other government agencies for collaboration on research; evaluates current rules and regulations governing devices, herb and homeopathic drug research and use.

Publications: A.M. (renamed: *Complementary and Alternative Medcine at the NIH),* bimonthly newsletter, free (reviewed under General—Journals and Newsletters); *Alternative Medicine: Expanding Medical Horizons,* report to the NIH, $25.00.

27. Planetree Health Resource Center (PHRC) at California Pacific Medical Center

2040 Webster Street, San Francisco, CA 94115
Telephone: 415-923-3680

A nonprofit consumer health organization offering a variety of health information services that support consumer participation in health care decisions and promote personal responsibility for health.

Services for the professional: Planetree of Good Samaritan Health System in San Jose, California, offers multipage information fact sheets on over 150 medical conditions, tests and procedures, and medications, including some titles in Spanish and Vietnamese. These are available to libraries, hospitals, clinics or agencies. Call 408-977-4549.

Services for the public: Maintains a health and medical library free to the general public that includes professional medical literature, popular health publications and alternative therapy resources. Also available are directories of support groups, health practitioners and health organizations, a CD-ROM database of medical literature, and health-related audiotapes and videotapes. Books and tapes are available for sale at Planetree and through their catalog. Planetree also offers a health information service providing information by mail for a fee. These include in-depth, personalized health information packets consisting of current medical and consumer health literature and computer printouts on specific health concerns ($100.00 per topic); a computer-generated listing of medical articles on a particular topic ($35.00 per topic); and a basic packet of about twenty pages of general health information on a common health topic ($20.00 per topic).

28. The Rosenthal Center for Complementary and Alternative Medicine
Columbia University, College of Physicians and Surgeins, 630 West 168th Street, New York, NY 10032
Telephone: 212-305-4755; Fax: 212-305-1495

An educational and research initiative, The Rosenthal Center for Complementary and Alternative Medicine was established by Columbia University's College of Physicians and Surgeons through a grant from the Richard and Hinda Rosenthal Foundation. The first such resource located at an American university medical school, it is one of ten specialty research centers funded by the Office of Alternative Medicine, National Institutes of Health. The primary objectives of The Rosenthal Center include fostering and conducting research to determine the efficacy and safety of alternative and complementary practices, to develop curriculum and training programs that promote knowledge and understanding of these practices, and to provide information to health practitioners, researchers and the public internationally on alternative and complementary therapies.

Services: Conducts symposia; develops, tests and evaluates research methodologies; offers public lectures, workshops and seminars; partially supports alternative medicine research conducted by Columbia faculty.

29. Wellness Referral Network, Inc. (WRN)
5307 East Mockingbird Lane, Suite 404, Dallas, TX 75206
Telephone: 214-827-9355, 800-520-WELL; Fax: 214-828-4064
Contact: Connie Dye, president/chief executive officer

A telephone referral service providing information on available treatment options and referrals to holistic health care providers.

Services for the professional: Serves as a marketing resource for licensed or certified practitioners who use an holistic approach or alternative therapies in their practice.

Services for the public: Provides a free telephone referral and information service for holistic and natural health care and referrals to practitioners of alternative and complementary health care modalities.

30. World Research Foundation (WRF)

15300 Ventura Boulevard, Suite 405, Sherman Oaks, CA 91403
Telephone: 818-907-5483; Fax: 818-907-6044
Contact: LaVerne Ross, vice president/founder; Steven Ross, president/founder

A nonprofit health and environmental information research network providing information on both traditional and alternative medicine therapies from around the world to support informed decisions about health care options. Maintains an extensive library collection of books and periodicals as well as a link to over 500 computer databases providing access to medical, scientific and environmental information worldwide. Services are provided to the public, health professionals, government agencies and the media.

Services: Three types of research are available: the library is open five days a week for patrons to conduct their own research; library searches are performed by staff on complementary, nontraditional approaches to specific health issues (basic fee $50.00); computer searches on conventional medicine from over 5000 international medical journals are available (basic fee $50.00). The foundation sponsors the International Health Congresses on innovative medical breakthroughs for major diseases; audiotapes and videotapes of the congresses are available.

Publications: World Research News, quarterly newsletter, $15.00 (subscription) (reviewed under General—Journals and Newsletters).

Schools

31. California Institute of Integral Studies (CIIS)

765 Ashbury Street, San Francisco, CA 94117
Telephone: 415-753-6100, x270; Fax: 415-753-1169
Contact: LaVera Draisin, M.D., program director; Tina York, program coordinator

The institute, a graduate school which integrates the intellectual and spiritual aspects of western and eastern traditions in study and practice, offers a seventy-six unit program leading to a master of arts in health education. This program trains graduate health education students to apply principles, values and knowledge of integral health to the field of health education, and is particularly appropriate for individuals with a background in health sciences. Students may also integrate the institute's herbal studies curriculum (see below) into their health education curriculum. Graduates are eligible to take the National Certifying Examination for Health Educators. Also offered is a twenty-seven unit certificate in Integral Health Studies which provides an integral health framework and enables health professionals to cultivate knowledge of multicultural approaches (i.e., Asian, western and indigenous practices), holistic health and systems theory into a viable philosophy and practice. This program is open to all health professionals, healing practitioners and graduates of healing arts programs. In addition, the institute has recently developed a twenty-seven unit Herbal Studies certificate program which is designed to enhance the professional's understanding of modern herbalism. The program is primarily designed for herbal practitioners desiring advanced training, ethnobotanists, practitioners or students of other therapeutic modalities, and those involved in the manufacture or sale of herbal products. Several doctoral programs are also available for students who wish to focus on integral health studies. The institute is accredited by the Western Association of Schools and Colleges.

32. Center for Mind-Body Medicine (CMBM)

5225 Connecticut Avenue N.W., #414, Washington, D.C. 20015
Telephone: 202-966-7338; Fax: 202-966-2589
Contact: James S. Gordon, M.D., director; Carol B. Goldberg, M.A., M.S.W., assistant director

Educates both health care professionals and the general public about the principles of mind/body medicine through a variety of programs and activities including: The Comprehensive Program of Mind-Body Studies at the Georgetown University Medical School, in which medical students and residents examine the scientific evidence for the mind's ability to affect the body; The Community Health Education Program, in which trained CMBM volunteers bring the mind/body approach to community health organizations serving the working poor, the indigent and the chronically ill; a Public Workshop Series, conducted by leaders in the field of mind/body health, including Herbert Benson, M.D., Joan Borysenko, Ph.D., Larry Dossey, M.D., and Dean Ornish, M.D.; educational and support groups for people with chronic illness or cancer and for those who care for them; internship programs for high school, college, graduate and medical students; a professional training program, currently being developed, which will provide instruction to healing professionals who wish to incorporate mind/body approaches into their work.

33. Esalen Institute (EI)

Highway One, Big Sur, CA 93920
Telephone: 408-667-3061; Fax: 408-667-2724
Contact: Mary Mooney, general manager

Among the many courses given by the institute, workshops are offered on biofeedback, hypnosis, health and healing, and somatics. Some programs qualify for continuing education credits with the California Board of Registered Nursing. Some scholarship assistance is available through the institute in exchange for a work commitment (usually in housekeeping).

34. Heritage Holistic Center

314 Laskin Road (Street Address), Virginia Beach, VA 23451; Post Office Box 444 (Mailing Address), Virginia Beach, VA 23458
Telephone: 804-428-0100; Fax: 804-428-3632
See General—Product Suppliers.

35. Institute for Holistic Healing Studies (IHHS)

San Francisco State University, 1600 Holloway Avenue, San Francisco, CA 94132
Telephone: 415-338-1200; Fax: 415-338-0573
Contact: Dr. George Araki, director

Offers a twenty-eight credit Holistic Health minor to matriculating students and a Holistic Health Certificate program to nondegree candidates. The program includes courses on biofeedback and Chinese healing, as well as general holistic health courses. Both programs are the same, and all courses are eligible for continuing education credits for nurses.

36. Maharishi International University (MIU)

1000 North 4th Street - DB 1028, Fairfield, IA 52557-1028
Telephone: 515-472-7000; Fax: 515-472-1189
Contact: John W. Salerno, Center for Health and Aging Studies

Programs at MIU integrate traditional academic course work with daily practice of transcendental meditation, the study and development of the self. Undergraduate and graduate programs are offered in Fine Arts, Sciences, Business, Government, as well as such subjects as Maharishi Ayur Veda and the Science of Creative Intelligence, and lead to bachelor's, master's and doctoral degrees. Financial aid is available.

37. The Naropa Institute (NI)

2130 Arapahoe Avenue, Boulder, CO 80302
Telephone: 303-444-0202; Fax: 303-444-0410
Contact: Ina Russell, publicity director

Offers year-round, nondegree classes and workshops that address health issues through meditation practice, art therapy, and the like. Tuition discounts are offered to senior citizens on a space-available basis. Undergraduate and graduate degrees are offered in a range of subjects including Psychology of Health and Healing, Art Therapy and Music Therapy. The institute is a fully-accredited, Buddhist-inspired, nonsectarian liberal arts college. A wide range of financial aid programs is available to students enrolled in the institute's programs.

38. The New Center for Wholistic Health Education & Research (NCWHER)

6801 Jericho Turnpike, Syosset, NY 11791
Telephone: 516-364-0808; Fax: 516-364-0989
Contact: Steven Schenkman, director

Offers a 30-month, 652-hour wholistic nursing program, providing nurses with a course of study in wholistic health care. The program is accredited by the Accrediting Council for Continuing Education and Training and approved for continuing education credits. For the lay public, the center offers community education programs including free lecture series in wholistic health and wholistic dentistry, as well as classes in T'ai Chi and yoga. Also offers Diploma programs in Acupuncture and Oriental Herbal Medicine (see also chapter 2: Chinese Medicine/Acupuncture—Schools) and Massage (see also chapter 4: Massage—Schools).

39. New York Open Center (NYOC)

83 Spring Street, New York, NY 10012
Telephone: 212-219-2527; Fax: 212-219-1347
Contact: Steven Schubert, managing director

A holistic learning center offering courses and workshops on a variety of subjects including alternative health and body work. Certification programs are offered in polarity therapy, focusing on hands-on learning and in-depth exploration of the mind/body connection, and reflexology. Tuition discounts are available to seniors, full-time students, and faculty; some scholarship assistance is also available.

40. Oasis Center (OC)

"New Horizons for Mind, Body & Spirit"
7463 North Sheridan Road, Chicago, IL 60626
Telephone: 312-274-6777; Fax: 312-274-0097
Contact: DeLacy Sarantos, executive director

Offers a variety of programs and weekend workshops dealing with the mind, body and/or spirit, including training programs in mind/body medicine, energy healing, and movement therapy. Workshops are given by well-known professionals in these fields such as Dr. Bernie Siegel, Dr. Deepak Chopra, Jeanne Achterberg and Helen Bonny. Some courses are accepted for continuing education credits by various professional associations. Partial scholarships are available on a limited basis.

41. Omega Institute for Holistic Studies (OIHS)

260 Lake Drive, Rhinebeck, NY 12572-3212
Telephone: 914-266-4444; Fax: 914-266-4828
Contact: Kathleen Jesperson, marketing projects coordinator

A holistic education center offering workshops and conferences every summer and fall on a wide variety of subjects relating to personal and professional development. Holistic health-related workshops are offered on topics such as Ayurveda, QiGong, energy healing, and color and light therapy; practitioner training is offered in areas such as mind/body medicine and Chinese medicine. Many workshops are led by well-known individuals such as Jon Kabat-Zinn, Bernie Siegel and Don Campbell. Work/study options and some partial scholarship assistance are available. The institute has a wellness center on campus where workshop and conference participants may avail themselves of massage and bodywork and other holistic health therapies.

42. University of Colorado Health Sciences Center (UCHSC)

School of Nursing/Center for Human Caring
4200 East 9th Avenue, Campus Box C288-08, Denver, CO 80262
Telephone: 303-270-4331; Fax: 303-270-8660
Contact: Karen Holland, program administrator

Offers a Professional Development Certificate in Caring Praxis, consisting of 150 hours of required courses on topics such as Theory of Human Caring in Action, Foundations of Healing Praxis, and Mind-Body-Spirit Medicine, and forty-five hours of electives in such subjects as Massage Therapy, Therapeutic Touch and Health of the Human Spirit. For those not interested in pursuing a certificate, courses may be taken individually. The program is appropriate for nurses, social workers and other healing and health care professionals. Also offers an Advanced Postgraduate Study Program in Caring and Healing, and a Visiting Fellows Program. Visa and MasterCard accepted for payment of fees.

Treatment Centers/Referrals

See General—Organizations for referrals to individual practitioners.

43. Georgetown University Medical Center (GUMC)
Behavioral Medicine Programs
3800 Reservoir Road N.W., Washington, DC 20007-2197
Telephone: 202-687-8770; Fax: 202-687-6658
Contact: Rebecca E. Chen, coordinator specialty programs

This program focuses on the role of the individual in disease prevention and health maintenance via behavioral change. A wide variety of conditions are addressed, including gastrointestinal disturbances, sleep problems, pain, stress, anxiety, cardiovascular and pulmonary disorders, rheumatological conditions, temporomandibular joint problems, headaches, and hypertension. There are several specialty programs within the department using biofeedback training as a treatment modality. These include the Biofeedback Lab, Cardiac Rehabilitation Program, and the Behavioral Medicine Pain Program.

44. The Institute of Preventive Medicine (IPM)
95 East Main Street, Denville, NJ 07834
Telephone: 201-586-4111

320 Belleville Avenue, Bloomfield, NJ 07003
Telephone: 201-743-1151

230 Silver Lake Road, Blairstown, NJ 07825
Telephone: 908-362-8446
Contact: Majid Ali, M.D.

Institute programs focus on the reversal of chronic diseases without drugs and the promotion of health through patient education, stress management and self-regulation. Natural healing methods, including relaxation and stress control, are used to treat such conditions as allergies, stress-related diseases, the Dis-Ease Syndrome, and nutritional diseases. All diagnosis and treatments are carried out by M.D. physicians. Various treatment programs are available using nutrition, stress management, allergy desensitization, vitamin therapy and fitness. In addition, the institute offers workshops, laboratory sessions and patient support groups as well as books and tapes on most of the common chronic health disorders of our time. Also publishes a newsletter entitled *Lifespanner,* monthly, $1.25 (single issue), $12.00 (subscription).

45. Life Transition Therapy, Inc. (LTT)
100 Delgado Compound, Suite A, Santa Fe, NM 87501
Telephone: 505-982-4183

This private clinic uses various therapeutic treatment modalities for pain and stress, emotional disorders, physical dysfunction, and grief and bereavement. The clinic offers a free weekly meditation group, Swedish and connective tissue massage, a blend of eastern and western psychotherapy, Rolfing, and yoga. The Stress Reduction and Relaxation Program is a thirty- to forty-hour, two-month program that includes psychotherapy, somatotherapy, yoga instruction, pre- and post-testing, guided meditation, educational literature and a six hour retreat. It is based on the mindfulness meditation program used at the University of Massachusetts Medical Center, and is used to treat a wide range of medical problems such as heart disease, back pain, headaches, anxiety, depression, AIDS and others. Individual stress and pain management sessions are also offered.

46. Livingston Foundation Medical Center (LFMC)
3232 Duke Street, San Diego, CA 92110
Telephone: 619-224-3515; Fax: 619-224-6253

The center was established in 1971 by the late Dr. Virginia C. Livingston, a physician, teacher and medical researcher specializing in the study of the body's immune system and its relation to disease. Two outpatient immunological programs are designed to enhance the body's immune system as a treatment for severe life-threatening illness, for other conditions such as allergies and stress-related syndromes, and as a preventive health strategy. The first is a complete ten-day clinical immunotherapy program for patients with an advanced debilitating illness such as lupus, arthritis or cancer. The program includes an initial interview, comprehensive medical history, and physical examination with the use of conventional diagnostic testing to evaluate the immune system and identify any underlying infection. If the immune system is inadequate, a multifaceted immune enhancement program may be instituted including use of broad spectrum vaccines, specific antibodies, antibiotics, stimulation and restoration of liver function, detoxification, and use of vitamins and dietary supplements. A counseling program teaches visualization and stress reduction techniques to help patients manage their conditions and feel more powerful in relation to their health. The second program is a two-day diagnostic immune system evaluation to ascertain the body's ability to detect and fight off disease and illness.

47. The New Center for Wholistic Health Education & Research (NCWHER)

6801 Jericho Turnpike, Syosset, NY 11791-4413
Telephone: 516-496-7766; Fax: 516-364-0989

With the goal of treating the whole person, not just the symptoms and illness, the center provides a wide range of services including acupuncture, AMMA Therapy® (a therapy developed by one of the founders of the center, which promotes and restores patients' well-being), biofeedback, Chinese herbalism, chiropractic, nutritional counseling, yoga and other therapies.

48 Planetree (P)

621 Sansome Street, San Francisco, CA 94111
Telephone: 415-956-4215; Fax: 415-956-6503

This nonprofit consumer health care organization was founded in 1978 to humanize the health care system for patients through nursing, family involvement, patient education and architectural design of hospital units. The Planetree approach has been implemented in a variety of hospital settings with the intention of creating a new kind of hospital focused on patient and family-centered care. Planetree offers a variety of services: consultation services including on-site presentations for medical and nursing staff, administration, Board of Directors and department heads; speaking engagements at conferences, workshops and events; tours of Planetree sites; and Planetree Assessment and Program Development consisting of focus groups, review of current operations, a written implementation plan and report, and direct help in developing and implementing specific programs. The following hospitals currently have Planetree Model Units: California Pacific Medical Center, San Francisco, CA; San Jose Medical Center, San Jose, CA; Beth Israel Medical Center, New York, NY; Mid-Columbia Medical Center, The Dalles, OR; Delano Regional Medical Center, Delano, CA. In addition there are fifteen Planetree Affiliate Hospitals in the United States. Contact the Planetree National Office for complete information on these facilities.

49. Preventive Medicine Research Institute (PMRI)

900 Bridgeway, Suite 1, Sausalito, CA 94965
Telephone: 415-332-2525; Fax: 415-332-5730

These one-week residential retreats present Dr. Dean Ornish's Program for Reversing Heart Disease, and are designed for people with or without heart disease. They provide the most current scientific information on the power of comprehensive lifestyle changes on health and offer Dr. Ornish's complete program, including stress management techniques, exercise, diet, nutrition and group support. The retreats are led by the same group of health professionals who have worked with Dr. Ornish on previous studies, with a staff-to-participant ratio of one to two. Staff includes physicians and other medical personnel, trained group support leaders, nutritionists, past participants and nationally known chefs demonstrating gourmet low fat, low cholesterol cooking. Dr. Ornish attends each retreat, lecturing and answering questions about his program, with other nationally known guest lecturers featured as well. The institute also makes available audiotapes, books and videotapes on various aspects of the mind/body approach to health.

50. Shealy Institute for Comprehensive Health Care (SICHC)
1328 East Evergreen, Springfield, MO 65803
Telephone: 417-865-5940; Fax: 417-865-6111

This rehabilitation facility provides a multidisciplinary program in alternative and holistic medicine for patients with chronic pain, stress and depression. The institute is involved in clinical research, education and treatment of patients. Special treatment programs include the Headache Center of the Ozarks, the Backache Center of the Ozarks, the Shealy Health-Wise Assurance Program consisting of a two-day health evaluation and three-day lifestyle training, the Shealy Regenesis Program for depression, and the Comprehensive Outpatient Rehabilitation Program for Chronic Pain and Stress Management. The institute's involvement in education consists of in-service programs, educational activities for the public, an annual seminar for health professionals, weekly radio broadcasts, workshops locally, nationally and abroad, and educational programs for health care professionals at the institute. The Shealy Institute is known worldwide for its clinical research, testing and evaluation of a wide range of alternative health-related treatments and therapies. A separate clinical research department investigates migraines, hypertension, cardiovascular diseases, depression, back pain, and myofascial and rheumatoid arthritis pain. Treatment modalities offered by the institute include biofeedback, relaxation training, acupuncture, massage, homeopathy, meditation, music therapy and more.

Product Suppliers

51. Heritage Holistic Center

314 Laskin Road (Street Address), Virginia Beach, VA 23451; Post Office Box 444 (Mailing Address), Virginia Beach, VA 23458
Telephone: 804-428-0100; Fax: 804-428-3632
Credit Cards: Visa, MasterCard, Discover

Based upon formulas from the Edgar Cayce readings, the center sells herbal tonics and herbal products, massage formulas and equipment, aromatherapy essential oils and general remedies, as well as other related products. Volume discounts available. Also offered are a wide variety of evening programs and classes. Contact Robert O. Clapp, the center's director, for information on classes.

52. Holistic Animal Health Care

3150 North Lodge, Tucson, AZ 85715
Telephone: 602-886-1727; 800-497-5665
Credit Cards: None

Offers natural animal care products and programs to support animals' natural healing. Discounts available for large orders.

CHAPTER 2: SYSTEMS OF ALTERNATIVE MEDICINE

Ayurvedic Medicine

Ayurveda is a Sanskrit word that roughly translates to "the science of life." This 5,000-year-old system of Indian medicine is based on the concept of restoring and maintaining balance of the body, mind and spirit. In essence, Ayurveda focuses on the person as a whole and prescribes dietary, herbal and lifestyle regimens for achieving and maintaining optimal health including purification, rejuvenation, exercise and meditation. Remedies include herbal wines and supplements, jellies, resins and pills, and various mineral preparations; treatments include steam therapy and oil massage. Ayurveda places a strong emphasis on preventive care and may be used to treat digestive disorders, obesity, hypertension, anemia, respiratory ailments and many other conditions.

Organizations

53. The Ayurvedic Institute (AI)

11311 Menaul N.E. (Street Address), Albuquerque, NM 87112; Post Office Box 23445 (Mailing Address), Albuquerque, NM 87192-1445
Telephone: 505-291-9698; Fax: 505-294-7572

An educational nonprofit corporation promoting the traditional knowledge of Ayurveda. Dr. Vasant Lad, well-known Ayurvedic physician and teacher, is the director of the institute.

Services: Offers an Ayurvedic Studies Program and Ayurvedic correspondence course by Dr. Robert E. Svoboda; introductory, weekend and intensive seminars (see Ayurvedic Medicine—Schools); private consultations by Dr. Lad, Dr. Svoboda and others; sells herbs, audiotapes, videotapes and other products; publishes Dr. Lad's books and articles and other Ayurvedic works as well as a quarterly journal.

Publications: *Ayurveda Today,* quarterly journal, free to members (reviewed under Ayurvedic Medicine—Journals and Newsletters).

Schools

54. Ayurveda Holistic Center (AHC)

82A Bayville Avenue, Bayville, NY 11709
Telephone: 516-628-8200; Fax: 516-628-8200 "Press 'START'"
Contact: Swami Sada Shiva Tirtha

Offers Ayurvedic practitioner certification program both on-site and as a correspondence course. The program is comprised of theoretical course work and internships, each of which is 108 hours in length. Therapies discussed include herbology, aromatherapy, meditation, yoga, color therapy, and Ayurvedic massage. Also sells Ayurvedic products. (See Ayurvedic Medicine—Product Suppliers.)

55. The Ayurvedic Institute (AI)

11311 Menaul N.E. (Street Address), Albuquerque, NM 87112; Post Office Box 23445 (Mailing Address), Albuquerque, NM 87192-1445
Telephone: 505-291-9698; Fax: 505-294-7572
Contact: Wynn Werner, administrator

Led by the well-known Ayurvedic physician and author Dr. Vasant Lad, the institute teaches the principles of the traditional Ayurvedic health care system. Two years of Ayurvedic studies are offered. The first year Ayurvedic studies program provides a general overview of the science of Ayurveda and is appropriate for both health care professionals and members of the lay public. The second year Ayurvedic studies program, with the first year program as a prerequisite, is intended for health care professionals and those planning a career in the health care field. Weekend seminars and intensives are available for those who cannot or do not want to take the Ayurvedic studies program. A limited work/study program is available. The institute also offers a one-year correspondence course consisting of twelve individual lessons, including two tapes of lectures and a tape of Sanskrit pronunciations, leading to a certificate of completion.

56. Maharishi International University (MIU)

1000 North 4th Street - DB 1028, Fairfield, IA 52557-1028
Telephone: 515-472-7000; Fax: 515-472-1189
Contact: John W. Salerno, Center for Health and Aging Studies
See chapter 1: General—Schools.

57. Sharp Institute for Human Potential and Mind Body Medicine (SIHPMBM)

1450 Frazee Road, Suite 609, San Diego, CA 92108

Telephone: 800-827-4277; Fax: 619-686-5522
Contact: Deepak Chopra, executive director; David Simon, medical director

Offers a five-day program, "Training in Mind Body Medicine and Ayurveda," which explores natural and holistic approaches to health and their use in conjunction with western modalities. The program is appropriate for health care professionals and those interested in learning more about mind/body medicine and Ayurveda. Visa and MasterCard accepted for payment of tuition.

Treatment Centers/Referrals

58. The Ayurvedic Institute (AI)
11311 Menaul N.E. (Street Address), Albuquerque, NM 87112; Post Office Box 23445 (Mailing Address), Albuquerque, NM 87192-1445
Telephone: 505-291-9698; Fax: 505-294-7572

Offers private consultations with Dr. Vasant Lad, director of the institute and well-known Ayurvedic physician and teacher, Dr. Robert E. Svoboda, faculty Ayurvedic physician, and other qualified persons both at the institute and by telephone.

59. Center for Mind Body Medicine (CMBM)
Post Office Box 2022, Rancho Santa Fe, CA 92067
Telephone: 619-794-2425

Developed by Dr. Deepak Chopra and Dr. David Simon, the program focuses on correcting imbalances which lead to disease rather than treating specific diseases. The main goal is to provide the education and tools to incorporate mind/body principles into daily life. Programs and education in mind/body medicine include: 1) a seven-day residential treatment and education program consisting of a comprehensive evaluation and follow-up visit with a center physician, private consultations with a nurse educator, and therapeutic recommendations based on assessment of mind/body type and specific areas of physiological imbalances. Includes diet, exercise, breathing, relaxation, massage, rejuvenating and purifying treatments such as aromatherapy, sound therapy, and herbal massage. Also emphasizes the educational aspects of health promotion through instruction in primordial sound meditation, yoga and mind/body integration classes as well as daily programs and lectures on various topics such as natural vision improvement, Ayurvedic herbs, nutrition and more; 2) an eight-session education course developed by Drs. Simon and Chopra entitled "The Magic of Healing" on the components of life that create health and well being; 3) Primordial Sound Meditation instruction, four sessions over a three-day period. The center also provides a physician referral list of health professionals that have completed a basic training program in Ayurvedic medicine.

60. Maharishi Ayur-Veda Medical Center (MA-VMC)

4910 Massachusetts Avenue, N.W., Suite 315, Washington, D.C. 20016
Telephone: 202-244-2700; Fax: 202-244-7695

10801 Main Street, Fairfax, VA 22030
Telephone: 703-273-6631; Fax: 703-273-4410

This treatment center utilizes Maharishi Ayur-Ved to prevent disease, maintain health, and promote longevity. It employs the development of consciousness, specific diets, exercise programs, a variety of massage, internal purification, herbal supplements and treatments, and personalized daily and seasonal routines. Various health disorders are treated, such as high blood pressure, headaches, anxiety, premenstrual syndrome, asthma and other chronic diseases. All treatment is supervised by physicians with extensive training in Maharishi Ayur-Ved. Initial three-part evaluation with a licensed physician or nurse practitioner consists of diagnosis of a person's Ayur-Vedic body type and specific health problems through pulse diagnosis, medical history and necessary laboratory tests; an individual health care program is prescribed, and patient education is provided on key principles of Maharishi Ayur-Ved.

61. The Raj (R)

Maharishi Ayur Veda Health Center
Jasmine Avenue, Fairfield, Iowa 52556
Telephone: 800-248-9050; 515-472-9580 (in Iowa)

The center offers rejuvenation programs, purification treatments, diet and exercise, and stress reduction techniques based on the Maharishi Ayur Veda system of natural health care to prevent disease and promote health. Three-day, five-day and seven-day in-residence packages include consultation and evaluation with an Ayurvedic physician, two hours of Panchakarma (rejuvenation) treatments per day, health enhancement education courses including diet and yoga, guest lecturers, vegetarian meals and meditation practice. Individualized programs to address the effects of stress and strengthen the body are available. A simple home program is also offered.

Product Suppliers

62. Auromere Ayurvedic Imports
1291 Weber Street, Pomona, CA 91768
Telephone: 909-629-0108; 800-735-4691; Fax: 909-623-9877

2621 West Highway 12, Lodi, CA 92540
Credit Cards: None

Sells Ayurvedic oils, an herbal toothpaste compatible with homeopathic remedies, and related products. Wholesale only.

63. Ayurveda Holistic Center
82A Bayville Avenue, Bayville, NY 11709
Telephone: 516-628-8200; Fax: 516-628-8200 "Press 'START'"
Credit Cards: Visa, MasterCard, Discover

Sells herbal products at both the wholesale and retail levels. A minimum order of fifteen products is needed to qualify for wholesale prices. Also sells books on Ayurveda, yoga and natural healing.

64. The Ayurvedic Institute (AI)
11311 Menaul N.E. (Street Address), Albuquerque, NM 87112; Post Office Box 23445 (Mailing Address), Albuquerque, NM 87192-1445
Telephone: 505-291-9698; Fax: 505-294-7572
See Ayurvedic Medicine—Organizations.

65. Frontier Cooperative Herbs
3021 78th Street, Post Office Box 118, Norway, IA 52318-0118
Telephone: 800-786-1388
See Herbal Medicine—Product Suppliers.

66. Maharishi Ayur-Ved Products International, Inc.
Post Office Box 49667, Colorado Springs, CO 80949-9667
Telephone: 800-255-8332 (Orders Only); 800-345-8332 (Customer Service); 719-260-5500 (International Orders); Fax: 719-260-7400
Credit Cards: Visa, MasterCard, Discover

Sells a variety of Ayurvedic products including antioxidants, herbal formulas, aromatherapy and massage oils, books, audiotapes, compact disks and videotapes.

67. Quantum Publications, Inc.
Post Office Box 598, South Lancaster, MA 01561
Telephone: 800-858-1808; Fax: 508-368-1809
Credit Cards: Visa, MasterCard

Owned by the well-known Ayurvedic physician Dr. Deepak Chopra and his family, this company sells Dr. Chopra's books, audiotapes and videotapes, and programs, as well as herbal food supplements, Ayurvedic herbs and oils.

Chinese Medicine/Acupuncture

Chinese medicine is an ancient system of healing which incorporates the use of acupressure, acupuncture, herbal medicine, massage, moxibustion, nutrition and various physical exercises. Theories of Chinese medicine are based on the concept of Qi (or Chi), the life force which flows through the energy pathways (also known as meridians) of the body. This life force has two polarities, yin and yang, and disease is viewed as a disruption in the balance of these polarities. Treatment seeks to restore balance by removing obstructions and reestablishing the free flow of energy through the system. In the past several decades, Chinese medicine in general and acupuncture in particular have gained growing acceptance and have become viable health care options in the United States. Numerous schools of traditional Chinese medicine have opened, many with rigorous programs of training leading to masters' degrees in acupuncture and/or oriental medicine.

Organizations

68. American Association for Acupuncture and Oriental Medicine (AAAOM)
433 Front Street, Catasauqua, PA 18032
Telephone: 610-433-2448; Fax: 610-264-2768
Contact: Joy Ostrander, executive communications manager

A national membership organization dedicated to the advancement of oriental medicine in the United States, AAAOM works toward licensing acupuncturists in every state as independent health care providers and as covered providers under all insurance policies. The association is involved in educating the public, insurance companies and legislators on the benefits of acupuncture; conducting research; and maintaining high educational standards for acupuncture practitioners.

Services for the professional: Provides a referral service; actively advocates and monitors national and state legislation; offers insurance coverage;

conducts educational programs; offers seminars and supplies; provides OSHA testing; maintains mailing lists; publishes a journal, newsletter, membership directory, office brochures and educational materials.

Services for the public: Offers a referral service; provides information about schools, licensure, acupuncture in general, and detoxification.

Publications: *American Acupuncturist,* biannual journal, for members only; *Update,* monthly newsletter, for members only; *Educational Options in Oriental Medicine,* $10.00.

69. American Foundation of Traditional Chinese Medicine (AFTCM)

505 Beach Street, San Francisco, CA 94133
Telephone: 415-776-0502; Fax: 415-776-9053

A nonprofit organization providing education and information services for clinics and hospitals, health care professionals, teachers, students and the general public. Its goal is to create an international health center bringing together eastern and western medicine and to develop a new comprehensive health care system offering broader treatment options at reduced costs.

Services for the professional: Acts as clinical consultants to hospitals, clinics and schools on developing an effective acupuncture clinical program; provides resources and information through a national network of acupuncturists and referrals to practitioners and clinics with substance abuse programs; provides technical assistance with funding proposals; maintains a speakers' bureau of scientists, researchers and practitioners on alternative medicine, disease prevention and detoxification; offers continuing education opportunities.

Services for the public: Provides information and referrals to practitioners, clinics and substance abuse programs using traditional Chinese medicine; offers classes in QiGong, a health maintenance program.

70. Council of Colleges of Acupuncture and Oriental Medicine (CCAOM)

8403 Colesville Road, Suite 370, Silver Spring, MD 20910
Telephone: 301-608-9175

The membership organization for colleges of acupuncture and oriental medicine, CCAOM is dedicated to advancing the status of acupuncture and oriental medicine in the United States. Formerly known as the National Council of Acupuncture Schools and Colleges, the council is concerned with the quality of the educational system and works toward higher standards of training for the profession. Currently twenty-four schools and colleges are members of CCAOM.

Services for the professional: Provides educational information and a listing of member schools.

Services for the public: Provides listing of member schools.

Publications: *CCAOM News*, biannual newsletter, free to members.

71. Institute for Traditional Medicine and Preventive Health Care (ITMPHC)

2017 S.E. Hawthorne, Portland, OR 97214
Telephone: 503-233-4907; 800-544-7504; Fax: 503-233-1017

A nonprofit research and educational organization with a focus on Chinese herbs, ITMPHC works to provide instruction in the history, practice and application of traditional medical systems, conducts and coordinates scientific research, and fosters public interest in traditional medicine including western, Chinese and Tibetan systems of natural healing.

Services for the professional: Provides literature and video programs on the use of Chinese herbs and other aspects of natural healing; sponsors lectures and seminars; provides consultations by phone, fax and letter; maintains a library of technical books and journals (Library of East Asian Medical Arts and Sciences); provides referral listings; publishes books and other materials.

Services for the public: Provides a referral list of approximately 250 practitioners by geographic area; offers free resource guides of books and journals, schools and institutes.

Publications: Free resource guides listing herb suppliers, schools and institutes, books and journals; various books on Chinese medicine and herbology; a looseleaf subscription service, consisting of quarterly mailings about traditional and modern formulas and their applications.

72. National Accreditation Commission for Schools and Colleges of Acupuncture and Oriental Medicine (NACSCAOM)

8403 Colesville Road, Suite 370, Silver Spring, MD 20910
Telephone: 301-608-9680; Fax: 301-608-9576
Contact: Dolores Llanso, director of administrative services

NACSCAOM is a not-for-profit corporation dedicated to fostering excellence in acupuncture and oriental medicine education. It reviews and accredits educational programs at the first professional master's degree level and professional master's level certificate and diploma programs in acupuncture, and first professional master's degree and professional master's level certificate and diploma programs in oriental medicine with a concentration in both acupuncture and herbal therapies. It is currently developing standards for doctoral level programs.

Services for the professional: Provides a current list of accredited and candidate programs and information about the accreditation process and standards; conducts workshops for acupuncture and oriental medicine programs; holds commission meetings.

Services for the public: Provides a list of accredited and candidate programs; provides recognition that the quality of education by an accredited institution or program meets or exceeds the educational standards for practice of acupuncture and oriental medicine; holds commission meetings open to the public during public sessions.

Publications: Accredited and Candidate Programs, twice a year, free; *Accreditation Handbook,* annual, $20.00; *Accreditation: Toward Excellence in Acupuncture and Oriental Medicine Education,* annual, free brochure.

73. National Acupuncture and Oriental Medicine Alliance (National Alliance) (NAOMA)

638 Prospect Avenue, Hartford, CT 06105
Telephone: 203-586-7509; Fax: 203-586-7550
Contact: M. Suzanne C. Berry, executive director; Maria A. Clayton, association administrator

A nonprofit organization devoted to the promotion of acupuncture and oriental medicine, the alliance encourages communication among practitioners and collaborates with like-minded organizations. It assists membership on licensure, regulation and health care issues, and supports consumer education, action and access to freedom of choice in health care. Other goals include promoting research, working toward the integration of acupuncture and oriental medicine into state and national health care systems, and supporting educational and professional standards.

Services for the professional: Sponsors an annual conference; publishes newsletter informing members of pending state and federal issues.

Services for the public: Works to foster broader consumer access to acupuncture and oriental medicine.

Publications: The National Alliance Forum, quarterly newsletter, free to members.

74. QiGong Institute (QI)

East West Academy of Healing Arts
450 Sutter Street, #2104, San Francisco, CA 94108
Telephone: 415-788-2227; Fax: 415-788-2242
Contact: Effie Poy Yew Chow, president; Kenneth M. Sancier, co-president

This nonprofit organization, a subsidiary of the East West Academy of Healing Arts, focuses on the promotion of health, healing and peak performance through education, research and clinical work. QiGong is a part of traditional Chinese medicine that includes acupuncture, herbs, nutrition, movement and massage.

Services for the professional: 110-hour, 200-hour and 300-hour training courses in Chow Integrated Healing System; organizes conferences, such as the first International Congress on QiGong and the fifth International Congress of Chinese Medicine at the University of California at Berkeley; maintains a QiGong computerized database; holds monthly QiGong science forum for scientists; conducts clinical and experimental research on QiGong and healing.

Services for the public: Offers monthly lectures on QiGong; sponsors QiGong classes in San Francisco and Palo Alto; publishes a bimonthly newsletter.

Publications: Proceedings of the International QiGong Conferences, with over 600 abstracts of research studies, $23.00; *Miracle Healing from China—QiGong,* by Charles McGee, M.D., and Effie Chow, $19.45; Computerized Database of QiGong for Macintosh based on titles, authors and institutions from proceedings of the international conferences, 1987 version 1.0 is $25.00, 1993 version 1.5 is $75.00; videotapes of QiGong meetings, $23.00 each (37 are available); *450 Sutter,* bimonthly newsletter, free with membership; many other materials available for purchase.

75. QiGong Research Society (QRS)

104 London Lane, Mt. Laurel, NJ 08054
Telephone: 609-234-3056; Fax: 609-727-1233
Contact: Debra LeBlan, programs director; Rochelle Fleishman, research director

This organization is dedicated to introducing QiGong to the general public through classes, workshops, demonstrations, lectures and written materials; raising public awareness of the benefits of QiGong practices through educational programs; and supporting clinical research on QiGong. The society was founded in 1992 by Master Hou, a fifth generation Master of Medical QiGong and traditional Chinese medicine.

Services for the professional: Provides programs in applied QiGong therapy for health professionals and body workers, including massage therapists, acupuncturists, physicians, nurses, physical therapists and others.

Services for the public: Teaches a QiGong healing program for nonhealth professionals consisting of classes and workshops for self-healing and health maintenance.

Schools

76. Academy of Chinese Culture and Health Sciences (ACCHS)
1601 Clay Street, Oakland, CA 94612
Telephone: 510-763-7787; Fax: 510-834-8646
Contact: Dr. Wei Tsuei, president

Offers a professional graduate program leading to a master of science degree in traditional Chinese medicine, preparing the student for licensure as a primary health care provider. Total curriculum consists of 146.5 units. The program is accredited by the National Accreditation Commission for Schools and Colleges of Acupuncture and Oriental Medicine. It is also approved by the California Acupuncture Committee as a continuing education provider for licensed acupuncturists, and by the California Board of Registered Nursing as a continuing education provider for registered nurses. Low-interest private bank loans available to qualified students.

77. Acupressure-Acupuncture Institute (AAI)
9835 Sunset Drive, Suite 206, Miami, FL 33176
Telephone: 305-595-9500; Fax: 305-274-0675
Contact: Nancy Browne, administrative director

Offers a twenty-four-month, 1,684-hour program and a twenty-seven-month, 1,784-hour program, both leading to an acupuncture physician diploma. The twenty-four-month program qualifies graduates to sit for the Florida state exams. Because this examination is currently written by the National Commission for the Certification of Acupuncturists, those who pass the exam can apply for and receive their national diplomate. The twenty-seven-month program is intended for those who do not plan to be licensed in the state of Florida. Successful completion of this program qualifies students to take the national examination directly. The institute also offers a one-year postgraduate program in Chinese herbology and homeopathy, which consists of advanced course work in these subjects. (See also chapter 4: Acupressure/Shiatsu—Schools.)

78. Bastyr University (BU)
144 N.E. 54th Street, Seattle, WA 98105-9916
Telephone: 206-523-9585; Fax: 206-527-4763
Contact: Stephen E. Bangs, director, marketing and admissions

Offers a 226-credit program leading to a master of science in acupuncture and oriental medicine, a 171.5-credit program leading to a master of science in acupuncture, and a ninety-one-credit program leading to a bachelor of science in oriental medicine. The acupuncture and oriental medicine programs are candidates for professional accreditation by the National Accreditation Commission for Schools and Colleges of Acupuncture and Oriental Medicine. Also offered is a certificate program in Chinese herbal medicine, which includes extensive study in traditional Chinese medicine and is appropriate for acupuncturists, naturopathic doctors, and individuals with equivalent backgrounds. (See also Naturopathic Medicine—Schools for information on the university's naturopathic medicine program.)

79. Beijing School of Acupuncture and Oriental Medicine (BSAOM)
2901 Montgomery Street, Fort Worth, TX 76107
Telephone: 817-737-7401; Fax: 817-737-9079
Contact: Professor Hadi Kareem, president

Offers a 1,845-hour, 123-credit program in acupuncture and oriental medicine, consisting of classroom instruction and clinical internship, leading to a professional acupuncture certificate. A very limited number of scholarships and work/study positions are available.

80. Colorado School of Traditional Chinese Medicine (CSTCM)
1441 York Street, Suite 202, Denver, CO 80206-2127
Telephone: 303-329-6355
Contact: Christine Harrison, executive administrator

Offers a three-year, 1,800-hour program, consisting of classroom instruction and clinical training, leading to a diploma in traditional Chinese medicine. Part-time pursuit of the degree is also an option. Graduates are eligible to take the National Commission for the Certification of Acupuncturists examination in acupuncture or Chinese herbal medicine. Opportunities for advanced study in China are available for continuing education credits. The school also offers a 750-hour doctoral program which emphasizes Chinese herbal medicine, advanced Chinese, Oriental and Asian theory, and specialized techniques.

81. Emperor's College of Traditional Chinese Medicine (ECTCM)
1807-B Wilshire Boulevard, Santa Monica, CA 90403
Telephone: 310-453-8300; Fax: 310-829-3838
Contact: Kathryn White, academic dean

Offers a 2,490-hour program of academic instruction and clinical practice, including training in acupuncture, oriental medicine, herbology and western diagnosis, and leading to the degree of master of traditional

Oriental medicine. Graduates are eligible to take the national certification examination administered by the National Commission for the Certification of Acupuncturists. Part-time study is available for those not seeking a degree or professional licensing. The college also has a postgraduate study program which gives students the opportunity to observe and practice oriental medicine at the Heilongjiang College of Traditional Chinese Medicine in China. The program is accredited by the National Accreditation Commission for Schools and Colleges of Acupuncture and Oriental Medicine. Federal financial aid programs are available for full-time students. In addition, the college offers a 250-hour acupressure certificate program (see also chapter 4: Acupressure/Shiatsu—Schools) and a 272-hour acupuncture orthopedics program.

82. Five Branches Institute (FBI)
200 7th Avenue, Santa Cruz, CA 95062
Telephone: 408-476-9424; Fax: 408-476-8928
Contact: Sue Hansen, executive director; Kaz Wegmuller, registrar

Offers a three-and-one-half year, 150-credit master's degree program in traditional Chinese medicine. The program consists of course work and clinical training in traditional Chinese medicine theory and diagnosis, acupuncture, Chinese herbal medicine, dietetics, QiGong energetics and massage. Completion of the degree allows graduates to sit for the National Commission for the Certification of Acupuncturists examination and California State Acupuncture Licensing examinations. The institute also accepts "limited status applicants" who are not pursuing a degree in Chinese medicine but who require specific courses in pursuit of some other defined educational objective. The institute is accredited by the National Association for Schools and Colleges of Acupuncture and Oriental Medicine.

83. Florida Institute of Traditional Chinese Medicine (FITCM)
5335 66th Street North, St. Petersburg, FL 33709
Telephone: 813-546-6565; Fax: 813-547-0703
Contact: Su Liang Ku, director; Don Baker, administrator; Linda Nash Stevenson, admissions

Offers a three-year, six-semester, 2,882-hour accredited program in traditional Chinese medicine, consisting of courses in acupuncture, herbology and tui na Chinese massage. Upon graduation, students are eligible for national certification and to apply for admission to various state licensing examinations. Financial aid available.

84. Institute of Chinese Herbology (ICH)
3871 Piedmont Avenue, #363, Oakland, CA 74611
Telephone: 510-428-2061
Contact: Kenneth Morris, director

Founded in 1986, this home-study program consists of audiotapes, coordinated notes, study guides and exercises and, for most classes, herb samples. Two levels of training are offered, both of which are appropriate for professionals and the lay public: comprehensive herbalist training provides the fundamentals of practicing Chinese herbology (no previous background in herbology or Chinese medicine is required); advanced certified herbalist training is offered to students who have completed comprehensive herbalist training. The institute awards certificates to students who successfully complete each program.

85. International Institute of Chinese Medicine (IICM)
Post Office Box 4991, Santa Fe, NM 87502
Telephone: 505-473-5233; Fax: 505-471-5551
Contact: Nancy Sanghara, administrator

Offers a four-year, 2,400-hour program of classroom instruction and clinical practice leading to the degree of master of oriental medicine. The degree may also be pursued on a part-time basis, to be completed in no more than eight years. The program is approved by the New Mexico State Board of Acupuncture and the Medical Board of California Acupuncture Committee, and is accredited by the National Accreditation Commission of Schools and Colleges of Acupuncture and Oriental Medicine. The institute also offers a continuing education certificate in advanced Chinese herbology and oriental medical studies. This certificate program, appropriate for acupuncturists, oriental medicine doctors, current students and graduates of the institute, is expected to develop into a degree program which will award the doctor of oriental medicine degree. Students of the master of oriental medicine program and the continuing education program may also participate in the yearly organized tour to China or arrange individual study in China to take intensive classes and clinical training in Chinese colleges and hospitals.

86. Minnesota Institute of Acupuncture and Herbal Studies (MIAHS)
1821 University Avenue West, Suite 278-S, Saint Paul, MN 55104
Telephone: 612-603-0994; Fax: 612-603-0995
Contact: Janice Olson, administrative director

Offers a four-year, 2,400-hour oriental medicine program including acupuncture and Chinese herbal therapy. Graduates are eligible to take the National Commission for the Certification of Acupuncturists examination in both acupuncture and herbs. Also offers a three-year, 1,800-hour program in acupuncture without herbs, and a 352-hour acupressure certificate program. A supervised student clinic offers oriental medical health care to the community. The institute has been approved for candidacy status by the National Accreditation Commission for Schools and Colleges of Acupuncture and Oriental Medicine. Financial aid available.

87. The New Center for Wholistic Health Education & Research (NCWHER)

6801 Jericho Turnpike, Syosset, NY 11791
Telephone: 516-364-0808; Fax: 516-364-0989
Contact: Barbara Lawrence

Offers a three-year, 2,700-hour program in oriental herbal medicine, consisting of theoretical studies and clinical training. Completion of the program leads to a diploma in oriental herbal medicine and a National Commission for the Certification of Acupuncturists diplomate in Chinese herbology. Also offers a three-year, 2,700-hour diploma program in acupuncture, consisting of academic course work and clinical training. In addition, the center offers a four-year program in oriental medicine that integrates the coursework and training of the acupuncture and oriental herbal medicine programs. These latter two programs currently hold candidacy status and anticipate receiving accreditation from the National Accreditation Commission for Schools and Colleges of Acupuncture and Oriental Medicine by the end of 1996. Both programs are approved by the Accrediting Council for Continuing Education and Training. Financial aid is available through a variety of grant and loan programs. The center also offers a diploma program in massage (see also chapter 4: Massage—Schools) and a program in wholistic nursing (see also chapter 1: General—Schools).

88. New England School of Acupuncture (NESA)

30 Common Street, Watertown, MA 02172
Telephone: 617-926-1788; Fax: 617-924-4167
Contact: Doris A. McAleavey, office manager

A founding member of both the American Association of Acupuncture and Oriental Medicine and the National Council of Schools and Colleges of Acupuncture and Oriental Medicine, the school offers a three-year, 2,000-hour master's level program in acupuncture and Chinese medicine consisting of a combination of classroom instruction and clinical training. In rare instances, students may be approved for part-time study, which must be completed within six years. Also offers a twenty-seven month, 465-hour program in traditional Chinese herbal medicine which may be taken concurrently with the acupuncture program. The school is accredited by the National Accreditation Commission for Schools and Colleges of Acupuncture and Oriental Medicine. Federal financial aid programs are available.

89. Northwest Institute of Acupuncture and Oriental Medicine (NIAOM)
1307 North 45th Street, Seattle, WA 98103
Telephone: 206-633-2419; Fax: 206-633-5578
Contact: Frederick O. Lanphear, president

Offers a three-year program in acupuncture and oriental medicine leading to a master of acupuncture degree. The program consists of one year of academic studies in western and traditional Chinese medicine followed by two years of clinical science and supervised clinical practice. A three-month China internship program is available following the academic studies. Two general continuing education programs are sponsored by the institute: one in oriental medicine and one in herbal studies, featuring seminars, demonstrations and visiting lecturers. The master's program is accredited by the National Accreditation Commission for Schools and Colleges of Acupuncture and Oriental Medicine.

90. Oregon College of Oriental Medicine (OCOM)
10525 S.E. Cherry Blossom Drive, Portland, OR 97216
Telephone: 503-253-3443; Fax: 503-253-2701
Contact: Elizabeth Goldblatt, president; Jim Eddy, dean of institutional services

This three-year professional program in acupuncture and oriental medicine leads to a master of acupuncture and oriental medicine degree (M.Ac.O.M.). The program consists of a total of 2,890.5 hours, for which 204.25 credits are awarded. Clinical observation and internship comprise approximately one-third of the program. An on-campus clinic affiliated with the college provides access for the public to oriental medical services and public education programs (see entry no. 117 below). A collaborative program with the National College of Naturopathic Medicine (NCNM) (see Naturopathy—Schools) allows OCOM students to simultaneously enroll in NCNM's homeopathy certificate program or their doctoral program in naturopathic medicine. OCOM is accredited by the Council of Colleges of Acupuncture and Oriental Medicine and by the National Accreditation

Commission for Schools and Colleges of Acupuncture and Oriental Medicine. The college offers a limited number of work-study positions, and students are eligible to apply for certain portions of the Federal Family Education Loan Program.

91. Oriental Medical Institute of Hawaii (OMIH)
181 South Kukui Street, Suite 206, Honolulu, HI 96813
Telephone: 808-536-3611; 808-537-3873; Fax: 808-537-5821
Contact: Kathy Low, office manager

Provides training in the diagnosis and treatment of health problems through the use of traditional Chinese medicine. The institute offers a 1,700-hour program, consisting of 800 classroom hours and 900 clinic hours. Students who complete the program are eligible to take the National Commission for the Certification of Acupuncturists examination. A 450-hour herbal program is offered for individuals who are interested in herbal studies. The institute also offers continuing education courses for health care practitioners and introductory courses for the general public.

92. Pacific College of Oriental Medicine (PCOM)
7445 Mission Valley Road, Suite 105, San Diego, CA 92108
Telephone: 619-574-6909; 800-729-0941; Fax: 619-574-6641
Contact: David Orman, admissions counselor

Offers a master of traditional oriental medicine degree upon completion of the 2,807-hour program. The program is accredited by the National Accreditation Commission of Schools and Colleges of Acupuncture and Oriental Medicine and approved by the California Acupuncture Committee, a division of the state medical board. Graduates of the program are eligible to take the California acupuncture licensing examination and the national certification examination given by the National Commission for the Certification of Acupuncturists. Financial aid is available through various state and federal programs.

93. Pacific Institute of Oriental Medicine (PIOM)
915 Broadway, 3rd Floor, New York, NY 10010
Telephone: 212-982-3456; Fax: 212-982-6514
Contact: Jayne Bliss, director of communications and media relations.

This east-coast campus of the Pacific College of Oriental Medicine offers two master's-level programs, both of which are accredited by the National Accreditation Commission of Schools and Colleges of Acupuncture and Oriental Medicine: a 2,807-hour diploma program in traditional oriental

Medicine and a 2,198-hour diploma program in Acupuncture. Completion of either program allows the student to take the National Certification Examination given by the National Commission for the Certification of Acupuncturists or any acupuncture licensing examination required in New York State. The institute is approved by the New York State Board of Regents. Federal and state financial aid programs are available.

94. QiGong Institute (QI)

East West Academy of Healing Arts
450 Sutter Street, Suite 2104, San Francisco, CA 94108
Telephone: 415-788-2227; Fax: 415-788-2242
Contact: Effie Chow, president

Offers 110-hour, 200-hour and 300-hour training courses in the Chow Integrated Healing System. Also offers lecture/demonstrations and classes in QiGong, a part of traditional Chinese medicine which achieves therapeutic balancing by combining meditation with certain physical exercises, and on the Chow Integrated Healing System, a blend of modern western practices and ancient eastern healing arts. Maintains a computerized QiGong database which allows individuals to search for information on QiGong in the areas of clinical work, experimental research, and integration with western medical care.

95. QiGong Research Society (QRS)

104 London Lane, Mt. Laurel, NJ 08054
Telephone: 609-234-3056; Fax: 609-727-1233
Contact: Debra LeBlanc, programs director

Offers the following ongoing QiGong classes and workshops: twelve- to fifteen-hour introductory and foundation classes and workshops teach a series of breathing, concentration and body movement exercises appropriate for students of all ages and physical conditions, no previous experience necessary; continuing hour-long classes and workshops add new and more advanced exercises, theories and techniques, previous experience minimum of ten class hours; applied QiGong therapy workshops for health professionals or anyone with a background in traditional Chinese medicine and applied healing arts teaches the more medical aspects of QiGong including the meridian system, five element and yin and yang theories, acupoints and QiGong therapy techniques. Weekend workshops are also available. Programs are also offered in Los Angeles (310-440-0103), San Francisco and Fresno, CA (209-243-0545) at specific times of the year. Preregistration for all classes and workshops is required. In addition, private appointments with Master Hou are available in the South Jersey and Philadelphia areas (609-234-3056) and in Los Angeles (310-440-0103).

96. Samra University of Oriental Medicine (SUOM)
600 St. Paul Avenue, Los Angeles, CA 90017
Telephone: 213-482-8448; Fax: 213-482-9020
Contact: Richard Scaffidi, director of admissions; Denise Neumark-Reimer, academic dean

Offers a twelve-quarter, 2,502-hour master's program in oriental medicine, consisting of academic course work and clinical practice. Study emphasizes acupuncture, herbology, nutrition, massage and exercise therapy. The program is accredited by the National Accreditation Commission for Schools and Colleges of Acupuncture and Oriental Medicine. A variety of federal financial aid programs and a limited number of scholarships are available. Following successful completion of the program, graduates are eligible to take the California state licensing examination. Through its affiliation with schools of traditional Chinese medicine in China, the university offers its graduates the opportunity to continue their studies in China.

97. Santa Barbara College of Oriental Medicine (SBCOM)
1919 State Street, Suite 204, Santa Barbara, CA 93101
Telephone: 805-682-9594; Fax: 805-682-1864
Contact: Lark Batteau Bailey, registrar

Offers a 2,368-hour program of classroom instruction and clinical training leading to a master's degree in acupuncture and oriental medicine. Thorough training in Chinese herbs is included in the program. Graduates are eligible to take the California state licensing examination. An eight-month Shiatsu practitioner program is also offered for the lay public. The college is accredited by the National Accreditation Commission of Schools and Colleges of Acupuncture and Oriental Medicine.

98. Sarasota School of Natural Healing Arts (SSNHA)
8216 South Tamiami Trail, Sarasota, FL 34238
Telephone: 800-966-7117; Fax: 813-966-4414
Contact: Isabelle Dunkeson, director
See chapter 4: Massage—Schools.

99. Seattle Institute of Oriental Medicine (SIOM)
7106 Woodlawn Avenue N.E., Seattle, WA 98115
Telephone: 206-517-4541

Contact: Paul Karsten, director

Offers a three-year, clinically based program designed to train students in the use of acupuncture, Chinese herbs, and other modalities frequently used in oriental medicine. The program consists of 1,260 hours of clinical instruction and 1,170 hours of academic course work, leading to a diploma in acupuncture and oriental medicine. A program of Chinese language and thought prepares the graduate to access Chinese medical literature.

100. South Baylo University (SBU)
School of Oriental Medicine, Acupuncture and Herbology
1126 North Brookhurst Street, Anaheim, CA 92801
Telephone: 714-533-1495; Fax: 714-533-6040
Contact: Xochitl Mannriquez, public relations

Offers a twelve-quarter, 230-credit program of academic course work and clinical experience in oriental medicine, acupuncture and herbology, leading to a master's degree in acupuncture and oriental medicine. The school is approved by the California Board of Medical Quality Assurance, which administers an examination for California state licensing as an acupuncturist. Financial aid is available.

101. Southwest Acupuncture College (SAC)
325 Paseo de Peralta, Suite 500, Santa Fe, NM 87501
Telephone: 505-988-3538; Fax: 505-988-5438

4308 Carlisle N.E., Suites 203, 204, 205, Albuquerque, NM 87107
Telephone: 505-888-8898
Contact: Dr. Skya Gardner-Abbate, chairman, department of clinical medicine

This school has two campuses, one in Santa Fe and one in Albuquerque. Both schools offer the same 2,400-hour program of course work and clinical training in traditional Chinese medicine, with emphasis on the study and practice of acupuncture and herbal medicine. The program at the Santa Fe campus is taught on an accelerated basis; full-time students can complete the program in as little as twenty-eight months. Part-time study must be completed within seven years. The program at the Albuquerque campus is structured to allow for some flexibility in the students' schedule. The full-time program can be completed in thirty-four months. The program is accredited by the National Accreditation Commission for Schools and Colleges of Acupuncture and Oriental Medicine. Graduates from both campuses are eligible to take the national certification examination as well as the New Mexico state examination. The college also runs a continuing education program consisting of seminars with international authorities, advanced summer classes and foreign study opportunities. Advanced clinical training programs in acupuncture and herbal medicine are held annually at the International Training Center for the Academy of Traditional Chinese Medicine in Beijing. These programs are open to interested members of the public, graduates, and licensed professionals, provided they have the required level of training for any given course. Federal loans and privately sponsored scholarship and grant programs provide financial aid to students.

102. Tai Hsuan Foundation College of Acupuncture and Herbal Medicine (THFCAHM)

2600 South King Street, Suite 206, Honolulu, HI 96826
Telephone: 808-947-4788; Fax: 808-947-1152
Contact: Dr. Gayle Todoki; Dr. Eric Ono

Offers a three-year master of acupuncture program consisting of classroom studies and clinical training. The program is accredited by the National Accreditation Commission of Schools and Colleges of Acupuncture and Oriental Medicine. Some financial assistance is available.

103. Texas Institute of Traditional Chinese Medicine (TITCM)

4005 Manchaca Road, Suite 200, Austin, TX 78704
Telephone: 512-346-3336; 512-444-4082; Fax: 512-346-0987
Contact: Jimmie L. Coombes, administrator; David A. Nelson, assistant administrator

Sister school of Heilongjiang College of Traditional Chinese Medicine in the Peoples Republic of China, the institute focuses on the traditional and classical understanding and practice of Chinese medicine. This three-year, 120-credit program in oriental medicine meets the educational requirements of all states where acupuncture is licensed.

104. Tri-State Institute of Traditional Chinese Acupuncture (TSITCM)

80 Eighth Avenue, 4th Floor, New York, NY 10011
Telephone: 212-332-0787
Contact: Dr. Mark Seem, executive director

The oldest school of acupuncture training in the New York area, the institute offers a three-year, 91-credit master's level diploma program in meridian acupuncture. Program components include classroom studies, internships and a student clinic which provides students the opportunity to practice their skills in an urban clinical setting. The program is targeted to health professionals and others interested in obtaining classical training in acupuncture, and is accredited by the National Accreditation Commission for Schools and Colleges of Acupuncture and Oriental Medicine. Postgraduate programs in advanced acupuncture, related oriental healing arts, and herbology are offered for professionals in all health fields. For doctors and dentists, the professional enrichment series offers a 300-hour program leading to New York State certification. Financial aid through federal student loan programs is available.

105. The Worsley Institute of Classical Acupuncture (WICA)
6175 N.W. 153rd Street, Tao House - Suite 324, Miami Lakes, FL 33014
Telephone: 305-823-7270; Fax: 305-823-6603
Contact: Betty Bailey, R.N., M.N., school director

Affiliated with The College of Traditional Acupuncture in England, the institute offers a 2,976-hour acupuncture training program, including academic course work and supervised clinical work, leading to a licentiate in acupuncture. Also offered are continuing education seminars, post-graduate workshops and, for the lay public, lectures on "Acupuncture: Is It For You?"

Treatment Centers/Referrals

See Chinese Medicine/Acupuncture—Organizations for referrals to individual practitioners.

106. Academy of Chinese Culture and Health Sciences
1601 Clay Street, Oakland, CA 94612
Telephone: 510-763-7787; Fax: 510-834-8646

At the teaching clinic, students work with patients at four levels from observer to intern under the supervision of clinic supervisors and clinic managers. Diagnosis, treatment, prescription of herbs, tui na acupressure, acupuncture, moxa, cupping, etc. are offered.

107. Acupressure-Acupuncture Institute
9835 Sunset Drive, Suite 206, Miami, FL 33176
Telephone: 305-595-9500; Fax: 305-274-0675

The institute maintains a clinic in acupuncture where second year interns become involved with history taking, diagnosis and treatment of patients under the supervision of the clinical staff.

108. The American Foundation of Traditional Chinese Medicine
505 Beach Street, San Francisco, CA 94133
Telephone: 415-776-0502; Fax: 415-776-9053

A nonprofit organization which operates as an outpatient traditional Chinese medicine (TCM) clinic. Practitioners are licensed in TCM and specialize in a variety of applications including general and sports medicine, allergies, digestive, gynecological, dermatological, cardiovascular and respiratory disorders, stress and pain management, substance abuse, asthma, and others. Treatment includes Chinese diagnosis, acupuncture, acupressure, massage therapy, breathing exercises (QiGong), diet, nutrition and herbal prescriptions.

109. Chinese Medicine Works
1201 Noe Street, San Francisco, CA 94114
Telephone: 415-285-0931

The company operates a clinic and Chinese herbal pharmacy offering acupuncture, herbal medicine and dietary counseling.

110. East West Academy of Healing Arts
450 Sutter Street, Suite 210, San Francisco, CA 94108
Telephone: 415-788-2227

The academy offers a range of services including sports medicine and rehabilitation, clinical treatments for private clients, stress management, corporate health, and others. Directed by Dr. Effie Poy Yew Chow, the academy uses the Chow Integrated Healing System, combining western medical practices and eastern healing arts. These include acupuncture and acupressure, meditation, deep breathing, stretching and aerobics, T'ai Chi Chuan, QiGong, herbal medicine, massage and bodywork, visualization, touch therapy, counseling, nutrition and other techniques.

111. Emperor's College of Traditional Oriental Medicine
1807-B Wilshire Boulevard, Santa Monica, CA 90403
Telephone: 310-453-8300; Fax: 310-829-3838

The college maintains a teaching clinic with treatment rooms, a lab and an extensive herb pharmacy containing over 450 herbs. Clinical interns under the supervision of licensed acupuncturists diagnose, evaluate, treat and offer follow-up care. Low-cost treatment includes acupuncture, acupressure and massage therapy for pain management, arthritis, headaches, back pain, premenstrual syndrome, and more. Stop smoking programs and weight reduction programs are also offered.

112. Five Branches Institute
200 7th Avenue, Santa Cruz, CA 95062
Telephone: 408-476-9424; Fax: 408-476-8928

The institute provides low-cost treatment through the internship program, a part of the students' clinical training. Students work under licensed acupuncturists who teach and practice through the school clinic, and are supervised in diagnosis, treatment plan, treatment and herbal application.

113. International Institute of Chinese Medicine
Post Office Box 4991, Santa Fe, NM 87502
Telephone: 505-473-5233; Fax: 505-471-5551

An advanced student clinic is open to the public. After the second year/second semester of study, students give acupuncture treatments and herbal remedies, products and formulas under the supervision of licensed qualified faculty members. IICM has one of the largest herbal pharmacies in the Southwest.

114. Minnesota Institute of Acupuncture and Herbal Studies
1821 University Avenue West, Saint Paul, MN 55104
Telephone: 612-603-0996

A student clinic is open to the public, offering a sliding fee scale. Students are supervised by faculty for all treatment services.

115. The Natural Health Clinic
Bastyr University (BU)
144 N.E. 54th Street, Seattle, WA 98105-9916
Telephone: 206-523-9585; Fax: 206-527-4763
See Naturopathy—Treatment Centers/Referrals.

116. Northwest Institute of Acupuncture and Oriental Medicine
1307 North 45th Street, Seattle, WA 98103
Telephone: 206-633-2419; Fax: 206-633-5578

The institute maintains a community teaching clinic for low-cost acupuncture. Students perform patient intakes, formulate diagnosis and treatment plans, and treat patients under the supervision of clinic instructors and senior interns.

117. Oregon College of Oriental Medicine
10525 S.E. Cherry Blossom Drive, Portland, OR 97216
Telephone: 503-253-3443; Fax: 503-253-2701

Maintains an on-campus full service clinic and traditional herbal dispensary offering oriental medical services under the supervision of senior clinical supervisors and instructors on the clinical faculty.

118. Pacific Institute of Oriental Medicine
915 Broadway, 3rd Floor, New York, NY 10010
Telephone: 212-982-3456; Fax: 212-982-6514

Offers low-cost acupuncture, herbal consultation and tui na to the public through its community clinic, Pacific Health Services. All treatment is given by a New York State-licensed acupuncturist assisted by advanced students.

119. Samra University of Oriental Medicine
600 St. Paul Avenue, Los Angeles, CA 90017
Telephone: 213-482-8448; Fax: 213-482-9020

The Samra University clinic offers low-cost treatment services to the community in acupuncture, herbology and traditional Chinese medical therapies. All students are supervised by the clinical staff.

120. Santa Cruz Traditional Chinese Medicine Clinic
200 7th Avenue, Santa Cruz, CA 95062
Telephone: 408-476-8211; Fax: 408-476-8273

The clinic, which is affiliated with the Five Branches Institute, offers low-cost acupuncture and herbal treatments to the public. Patients may see student interns in supervised practice, or may see licensed acupuncturists who teach and practice through the clinic.

121. Shealy Institute for Comprehensive Health Care
1328 East Evergreen, Springfield, MO 65803
Telephone: 417-865-5940; Fax: 417-865-6111
See chapter 1: General—Treatment Centers/Referrals.

122. Southwest Acupuncture College and Chinese Medicine Clinic
325 Paseo de Peralta, Suite 500, Santa Fe, NM 87501
Telephone: 505-988-3538; Fax: 505-988-5438

4308 Carlisle N.E., Suites 203, 204, 205, Albuquerque, NM 87107
Telephone: 505-888-8898

The college maintains a year-round clinic where students offer treatment in oriental medicine supervised by American and Asian practitioners with an average of ten years clinical experience. The clinic provides the community with low-cost medical health care, with treatment by students ranging from free to $18.00. Reduced cost and free treatments are offered to segments of the population such as the elderly, handicapped, battered women, drug abusers and patients with AIDS or cancer. At least one-third of the treatments are free of charge. In addition, within the college facilities, clinical faculty conduct their private practices. This clinic operates approximately twenty hours per week and uses a sliding scale. A full range of services are offered, including acupuncture, Chinese herbal medicine, exercise, diet and nutritional counseling.

123. Tai Hsuan Foundation College of Acupuncture and Herbal Medicine
2600 South King Street, Suite 206, Honolulu, HI 96826
Telephone: 808-947-4788; Fax: 808-947-1152

The school operates an on-site clinic for acupuncture, herbal therapy, tui na and Chi Kung. It is open seven days a week.

124. Texas Institute of Traditional Chinese Medicine
4005 Manchaca Road, Suite 200, Austin, TX 78704
Telephone: 512-346-3336; 512-444-4082; Fax: 512-346-0987

The institute operates a clinic staffed by certified acupuncturists, interns and assistants offering no-fee acupuncture treatments sixteen hours per week.

125. Tri-State Institute of Traditional Chinese Acupuncture
80 Eighth Avenue, 4th Floor, New York, NY 10011
Telephone: 212-332-0787

The institute offers three types of low-cost clinic services. The school clinic, staffed by senior student-interns under expert faculty supervision, specializes in acute and chronic pain in performing artists and repetitive strain and overuse injuries. Stress disorders, performance anxieties, gastrointestinal complaints and reproductive disorders are treated as well. The Pain Management Clinic, under the direction of Mark Seem, Ph.D., uses acupuncture and myofascial release trigger points to treat pain. All treatments are done by Dr. Seem and assisted by student-interns. Other clinical services include private practitioner treatments in acupuncture and oriental medicine, including herbology. The institute manages the acupuncture services of the Institute for Urban Family Health in New York City, specializing in complex immune disorders and chronic pain.

Product Suppliers

126. Chinese Medicine Works

1201 Noe Street, San Francisco, CA 94114
Telephone: 415-285-0931; Fax: 415-821-7804

For the professional, distributes a line of Chinese herbal formulas called Chinese Modular Solutions, available through K'an Herb Company (see below). For the lay public, distributes a line of herbal products called Heaven and Earth Formulas through Frontier Cooperative Herbs (see Herbology—Resources).

127. Digital Health, Inc.

1770 East Fort Union Boulevard, #101, Salt Lake City, UT 84121
Telephone: 801-944-4070; Fax: 801-944-4067
Credit Cards: Visa, MasterCard

In order to make the principles of acupuncture more accessible to western health care professionals, this company has created a computer database, "Clinical Acupuncture Essentials," which consists of the most widely read acupuncture information. The program is available on CD-ROM or 3.5-inch floppy disk for Windows or Mac.

128. Dragon River Herbals

Post Office Box 74, Ojo Caliente, NM 87549
Telephone: 505-583-2118
Credit Cards: Visa, MasterCard

Produces and sells a line of Chinese medicine single herbs and combination formulas. Discounts available for bulk orders. Customized formulas prepared upon request.

129. Elixir Farm Botanicals

Elixir Farm, Brixey, MO 65618
Telephone: 417-261-2393
Credit Cards: Visa, MasterCard

Sells Chinese herb seeds, indigenous medicinal seeds, and some nursery plants, most grown and harvested on the farm. Medicinal information is included on plants' historical, medicinal and therapeutic lineage. The company does not make recommendations on usage. Some books and herbal products are also available.

130. Great China Herb Company
857 Washington Street, San Francisco, CA 94108
Telephone: 415-982-2195; Fax: 415-982-5138
Credit Cards: None

Sells a wide variety of Chinese herbs by the pound, as well as other animal and mineral products.

131. HerbCare
Post Office Box 60279, Sacramento, CA 95860
Telephone: 916-487-9044; 800-888-9044; Fax: 916-487-3828
Credit Cards: Visa, MasterCard

Sells single herbs and combination formulas at the wholesale and retail levels. The catalog is cross-referenced by several different names of traditional Chinese medicine formulas and herbs and also incorporates Chinese characters in the cross-references.

132. Institute for Traditional Medicine and Preventive Health Care
2017 S.E. Hawthorne, Portland, OR 97214
Telephone: 503-233-4907; 800-544-7504; Fax: 503-233-1017

Sells a limited number of herbal products directly, and provides a resource list of suppliers of herbs, dried extracts, acupuncture needles and related products.

133. K'an Herb Company
6001 Butler Lane, Scotts Valley, CA 95066
Telephone: 408-438-9450; 800-543-5233; Fax: 408-438-9457
Credit Cards: Visa, MasterCard

Offers K'an Herbals, medicines in tablet and liquid extract form, and Chinese Modular Solutions, basic Chinese herbal formulas created by the well-known acupuncturists, Chinese herbalists and authors Efrem Korngold and Harriet Beinfeld. Also sells other Chinese herbal formulas, acupuncture needles and selected books. Products are sold only to health care professionals. Volume discounts are available.

134. Mayway Corp.
1338 Cypress Street, Oakland, CA 94607
Telephone: 510-208-3113; Fax: 510-208-3069; 800-909-2828 (Orders only)
Credit cards: Visa, MasterCard

Sells a wide variety of Chinese herbal extracts, concentrated powders and formulas made under Mayway's own label, Plum Flower, and through an exclusive arrangement with Lanzhou Pharmaceutical Works, a prestigious manufacturer of herbal patents in China.

Herbal Medicine

Herbal medicine is a system of medicine that has been in use for thousands of years. It is only in the last hundred years that this treatment has experienced a decline in popularity in western countries, as the rise of the pharmaceutical industry increased the availability of antibiotics and other prescription drugs. Herbal therapy can be used to cleanse the body of impurities, regulate and tone the body's organs, provide nourishment, raise the body's energy level, and stimulate the body's natural healing systems. Herbs may be used internally or externally, and can be prepared in a variety of ways such as infusions, capsules, decoctions, poultices and plasters. Several sources of herbal products are listed under "Suppliers," some of which state that their products are "certified organically grown" or "wildcrafted." "Certified organically grown" means that the herbs are grown without the use of chemicals, fumigants, or other synthetic products and that the farm on which the herbs are grown is periodically inspected and certified organic by an independent third party agent. "Wildcrafted" refers to the manner in which the herbs are harvested: gathered by hand from the herb's natural environment.

Organizations

135. American Botanical Council (ABC)
Post Office Box 201660, Austin, TX 78720-1660
Telephone: 512-331-8868; Fax: 512-331-1924
Contact: Mark Blumenthal, executive director; Margaret Wright, circulation manager

A nonprofit organization dedicated to educating the public and professionals on beneficial herbs and plants.

Services: Maintains an involvement with federal herbal regulatory development; conducts a radio news education program; provides information and materials to writers, journalists and editors; translates and publishes the English version of the German Commission E Monographs, authoritative works that provide scientific information on the use of herbs and phytomedicine; hosts ethnobotanical ecotours; offers scholarships for botany graduate students; sells scientifically based, difficult to find medicinal plant books; publishes a journal, original monographs and articles, botanical booklets, conference proceedings of herb-related conferences and classical botanical reprints from technical and academic journals (three volumes).

Publications: *HerbalGram*, quarterly journal, $25.00 (subscription) (reviewed under Herbal Medicine—Journals and Newsletters); *Classical Botanical Reprints*, $29.00 per volume or $2.00-$5.00 per article; Botanical Booklet Series, $1.00/ individual booklet, $9.95/ set of twelve.

136. American Herb Association (AHA)

Post Office Box 1673, Nevada City, CA 95959
Telephone: 916-265-9552; Fax: 916-274-3140
Contact: Kathi Keville, director

An education and research organization of medical herbalists and the public interested in increasing the public's knowledge of herbs and herbal products and promoting their use for health and pleasure.

Services for the professional: Conducts research on all aspects of herbs; offers educational programs; publishes a newsletter.

Services for the public: Publishes an herb education directory listing over forty herb schools, correspondence courses and herb classes; publishes an herb products directory with over 100 listings of herb products, supplies, fresh and dried herbs, essential oils, books, etc.; publishes a recommended herb book list.

Publications: The American Herb Association Quarterly (*AHA Quarterly*), newsletter, free to members, $20.00 (subscription) (reviewed under Herbal Medicine—Journals and Newsletters); *The Herb Education Directory*, biannual, $3.50, $2.50 to members; *The Herb Products Directory*, $4.00, $3.50 members; *Recommended Herb Book List*, $2.50, $2.00 members.

137. American Herbalists Guild (AHG)

Post Office Box 1683, Soquel, CA 95073
Telephone: 408-464-2441; Fax: 408-464-2441
Contact: Roy Upton, president

A nonprofit national, peer-reviewed membership organization representing professional medical herbalists. AHG is dedicated to increasing educational opportunities, providing comprehensive educational guidelines, and developing standards of practice and codes of ethics for the profession. It works to strengthen communication between herbalists, other health care providers and professional associations and regulatory agencies, and to support research and the integration of herbalism into community health care.

Services for the professional: Conducts an annual herb symposium and other AHG-sponsored events; maintains a referral service for practicing herbalists and other natural health care practitioners; publishes a newsletter and resource materials.

Services for the public: Provides information and referrals (send self-addressed and stamped envelope).

Publications: The Herbalist, quarterly newsletter, free with membership, $35.00 (subscription); *Directory of Herbal Education,* $14.00, includes residency and apprenticeship programs, correspondence courses, videotapes and audiotapes, herb journals; recommended reading list, $2.00.

138. Flower Essence Society (FES)

Post Office Box 459, Nevada City, CA 95959
Telephone: 916-265-9163; Fax: 916-265-6467
Contact: Richard Katz, Patricia Kaminski, co-directors

A nonprofit educational and research organization that promotes plant and clinical research on the therapeutic effects of flower essences. Conducts professional and public education, and provides a communication and referral network for teachers, researchers and practitioners of flower essence therapy.

Services for the professional: Maintains practitioner referral network; conducts an annual ten-day intensive training and certification program; offers educational scholarships and small research grants.

Services for the public: Offers classes and seminars internationally; provides referrals to local practitioners; publishes a newsletter.

Publications: Flower Essence Society Newsletter, annual, free with membership (reviewed under Herbal Medicine—Journals and Newsletters).

139. Herb Research Foundation (HRF)

1007 Pearl Street, #200, Boulder, CO 80302
Telephone: 303-449-2265; Fax: 303-449-7849
Contact: Rob McCaleb, president

This nonprofit member-supported research and educational organization is dedicated to providing reliable and scientific botanical data for its members, the public and the media. It supports, encourages and conducts research on all aspects of herbs including safety, benefits, production and conservation, and provides educational information to members, the media, the herbal products industry, government regulatory agencies, legislators and health professionals.

Services: Offers custom search services on hundreds of botanicals; sells information packets on over 150 common herbs and herb-related topics; maintains an extensive on-site library; publishes journal and newsletter.

Publications: *HerbalGram*, quarterly journal, free to members, $25.00 (subscription) (reviewed under Herbal Medicine—Journals and Newsletters); *Herb Research News*, quarterly, free to members; botanical reference items on herb safety, herb dealers and related topics.

140. Northeast Herbal Association (NEHA)

Post Office Box 146, Marshfield, VT 05658-0146
Telephone: 802-456-1402
Contact: Janice Dinsdale, secretary

A nonprofit membership organization serving herbalists in the northeastern United States. Provides information, networking, educational opportunities and legal and political monitoring.

Services for the professional: Holds an annual professional meeting; lists members in resource directory; provides information on educational offerings by members; publishes a newsletter.

Services for the public: Makes referrals to practitioners.

Publications: *NEHA*, tri-annual newsletter, free to members.

Schools

For information about programs in Chinese herbal medicine, see Chinese Medicine—Schools.

141. Avena Botanicals (AB)

20 Mill Street, Rockland, ME 04841
Telephone: 207-594-0694

This small business, owned and run by women, offers an eight-month herbal intensive program, which meets one Saturday per month and is appropriate for health care providers and intermediate herb students. Included are in-depth classes on herbal formulations, topical application of herbs, case-taking with clients, visualization and more. Also offers a full range of classes and workshops on various health-related topics. Visa and MasterCard accepted for payment of fees.

142. The Australasian College of Herbal Studies (ACHS)

Post Office Box 57, Lake Oswego, OR 97034

Telephone: 503-635-6652; Voice Mail: 1-800-48-STUDY; Fax: 503-697-0615

Founded in New Zealand in 1978, the college opened an office in the United States in 1991. Offers numerous correspondence courses including an 800-hour diploma course in herbal studies and certificate courses in herbal studies, natural therapies, flower essences, iridology, homeopathy and aromatherapy. Major credit cards are accepted for payment of fees.

143. Blazing Star Herbal School (BSHS)
Post Office Box 6, Shelburne Falls, MA 01370
Telephone: 413-625-6875
Contact: Gail Ulrich, herbalist/director

Offers a seven-month course in therapeutic herbalism, a clinically oriented program encompassing study of the organ systems, herbal therapies and the use of case studies. For the lay public, the school offers comprehensive apprenticeship programs which give students the skills necessary to become accomplished herbalists. Programs include wild plant identification, herbal therapeutics, the art of herbal preparation, and more. The school also sponsors a variety of workshops and an annual Women's Herbal Conference each August.

144. California Institute of Integral Studies (CIIS)
765 Ashbury Street, San Francisco, CA 94117
Telephone: 415-753-6100, x270; Fax: 415-753-1169
See chapter 1: General—Schools.

145. California School of Herbal Studies (CSHS)
Post Office Box 39, Forestville, CA 95436
Telephone: 707-887-7457
Contact: James Green, director; Evelyn Leigh, admissions and communications

Offers a 480-hour intensive training program in foundations and therapeutic herbalism, a two-semester program which covers all aspects of herbalism and includes hands-on experience working with medicinal herbs. The school awards a certificate to those who successfully complete the course of study. The program is accredited for continuing education credits for nurses. A limited number of work/study positions are available to qualified students. A second year apprenticeship program affords interested students the opportunity to pursue further study by assisting in running the Student Wellness Center and participating in related activities. These courses are most appropriate for those with a strong interest and some previous experience in herbalism. In addition the school offers a six-evening introductory course on herbalism, a nine-month weekend course on body systems and herbal wellness, a six-month weekend course on medicinal plants of the Bay area, and a four-weekend intensive on practical applications of herbs and essential oils.

146. East West School of Herbalism (EWSH)
Post Office Box 712, Santa Cruz, CA 95061
Telephone: 408-336-5010; Fax: 408-336-3227
Contact: Manager

Offers two correspondence courses, each designed by the well-known herbalist Michael Tierra. The home study course in herbal medicine is a twelve-lesson program, appropriate for beginning students, those pursuing a theoretical basis in the principles of oriental medicine and food therapy, and sellers, growers and manufacturers of herbal and health products. The professional herbalist course, a thirty-six lesson program, covers western, Chinese and Ayurvedic herbalism and is appropriate for herbal professionals and those seeking more in-depth knowledge. The school also sells several Chinese herbal healing tools and a few books on herbology.

147. Herbal Healer Academy International (HHAI)
HC 32 97-B, Mountain View, AR 72560
Telephone: 501-269-4177; Fax: 501-269-5424
Contact: Marijah McCain, N.D., M.H.

Offers a twenty-two lesson home-study course in herbal medicine, in which students learn to make herbal salves, liniments and tinctures and to apply principles of natural medicine. Upon completion of the program, a certificate for herbology is awarded. For those with previous training in alternative healing, the academy also offers an advanced healing course. In addition, a one-year, home-study certificate course in reflexology is also offered (see also chapter 4: Reflexology—Schools). All courses are appropriate for both professionals and the lay public. Visa and MasterCard accepted for payment of fees.

148. Herbally Yours (HY)
Post Office Box 26, 209 Changewater Road, Changewater, NJ 07831
Telephone: 908-689-6140 (Mondays only); 908-735-4469 (Tuesday - Saturday)

Offers a variety of classes on herb-related topics including herbal preparations, the kitchen medicine cabinet, herbs for women, and external herbal preparations.

149. International School of Herbal Cultures (ISHC) (Herbal Essence, Inc.)

8524 Whispering Creek Trail, Fort Worth, TX 76134
Telephone: 817-293-5410
Contact: Judy Griffin, president and master herbalist

Offers a sixteen-hour course with demonstrations entitled "Around the World with Herbs" which covers medicinal herbs from Chinese, East Indian, American Indian, western, Mediterranean, South, Central, and Mexican American cultures. Also offers "Healing From the Heart: the Texas Flower Essences and Aromatherapy Texas Essential Oils," a practitioners' course on subtle body healing. Both programs are also available as correspondence courses. In addition, the school sponsors workshops and lecture demonstrations on female tonic herbs, aromatherapy for health and beauty, American Indian herbalism, western herbalism, and medicinal teas and compresses from the garden.

150. Oriental Medical Institute of Hawaii (OMIH)

181 South Kukui Street, Suite 206, Honolulu, HI 96813
Telephone: 808-536-3611; 808-537-3873; Fax: 808-537-5821
Contact: Kathy Low, office manager
See Chinese Medicine/Acupuncture—Schools.

151. Rocky Mountain Center for Botanical Studies (RMCBS)

Post Office Box 19254, Boulder, CO 80308-2254
Telephone: 303-442-6861
Contact: Feather Jones, director; Marian Barone, faculty coordinator

Offers a seven-month, evening certification program, "The Essence of Herbalism," and a one-year certification program, "Western Herbalism," both emphasizing the study of North American bioregional plant medicines and including hands-on experience and training in natural herbal therapies. Noncertificate courses, which can be taken individually or as an eight-week series, are offered for those who want to learn the basics of herbalism or increase their knowledge about herbs. Workshops by noted herbalists from around the country are given periodically.

152. Rocky Mountain Herbal Institute (RMHI)

Post Office Box 579, Hot Springs, MT 59845

Telephone: 406-741-3811
Contact: Roger W. Wicke, Ph.D., director

Offers training in traditional Chinese herbal sciences to health professionals. The basic course is a one-year program with three one-week intensives in Hot Springs, Montana, covering traditional Chinese health assessment, pulse palpation and tongue inspection, materia medica, herbal formulation, and environmental health issues. Textbooks and a series of homework assignments are mailed prior to attendance at each intensive. Second year courses include advanced topics such as integrating western medical ideas with traditional Chinese methods. In addition, RMHI occasionally offers short seminars for the general public on local herb identification, a comparison of herbal traditions of the world, the use of traditional Chinese health principles to design a healthy diet, and traditional Chinese medicine and environmental issues. The courses were designed by Dr. Wicke, a graduate of the American College of Traditional Chinese Medicine and a practicing herbalist since 1983.

153. SAGE
Post Office Box 420, East Barre, VT 05649
Telephone: 802-479-9825
Contact: Rosemary Gladstar

A ten-lesson correspondence course on the science and art of herbology which features in-depth study of medicinal herbology and hands-on herbal preparation. Also offers an apprenticeship program consisting of two one-week sessions at Sage Mountain. The program includes hands-on demonstrations, field trips, discussions and other herb-related activities.

154. School of Natural Medicine (SNM)
Post Office Box 7369, Boulder, CO 80305-7369
Telephone: 303-443-4882; Fax: 303-443-4882
Contact: Farida Sharan, director

Offers several home-study programs: a twelve-lesson master herbalist course which provides the foundation for naturopathic and herbal treatment in correlation with iridology and integrates other forms of treatment such as acupuncture, osteopathy and allopathic medicine; a fourteen-lesson master iridology course; and a twelve-lesson naturopathy course. The school also offers a summer program on herbology which consists of workshops, lectures, field trips and more. A natural physician course is also offered. (See also Naturopathy—Schools.)

Treatment Centers/Referrals

See Herbal Medicine—Organizations for referrals to individual practitioners.

Product Suppliers

For additional information on Chinese medicinal herbs, see Chinese Medicine/Acupuncture—Product Suppliers.

155. American Botanical Council Bookstore
Post Office Box 201660, Austin, TX 78720-1660
Telephone: 800-373-7105; Fax: 512-331-1924
Credit Cards: Visa, MasterCard

Publishes and sells the Botanical Booklet Series, eight-page booklets providing a wealth of information on different medicinal plants. Also sells books on general herbology, medicinal plants and Chinese herbs as well as back issues of the journal *HerbalGram* and *Classical Botanical Reprints,* articles containing information on the uses of medicinal plants reprinted from technical and academic journals.

156. Avena Botanicals
20 Mill Street, Rockland, ME 04841
Telephone: 207-594-0694
Credit Cards: Visa, MasterCard

This small business, owned and run by women, grows, harvests and prepares a variety of herbal remedies and sells them to retail stores, health care practitioners and individuals. More than half of the herbs used in their products are certified organically grown or wildcrafted.

157. Blessed Herbs
109 Barre Plains Road, Oakham, MA 01068
Telephone: 800-489-HERB (4372); Fax: 508-882-3755
Credit Cards: Visa, MasterCard

Offers a full line of herbal products including medicinal herbs, herbal oils and salves, liquid herbal extracts and aromatherapy oils, herbal equipment and books. All herbs are certified organically grown or wildcrafted.

158. East West School of Herbalism
Post Office Box 712, Santa Cruz, CA 95061

Telephone: 408-336-5010; Fax: 408-336-3227
Credit Cards: Visa, MasterCard

Sells several Chinese herbal healing tools and a few herbology books.

159. Ellon USA
644 Merrick Road, Lynbrook, NY 11563
Telephone: 516-593-2206; 800-423-2256 (800-4-BE-CALM); Fax: 516-593-9668
Credit Cards: Visa, MasterCard, Discover, American Express

Manufactures and sells thirty-eight flower remedies. Remedies can be ordered directly from the company or purchased over-the-counter at retail outlets. Also manufactures animal remedies under the name HomeoPet.

160. Frontier Cooperative Herbs
3021 78th Street, Post Office Box 118, Norway, IA 52318-0118
Telephone: 800-786-1388
Credit Cards: Visa, MasterCard

Sells their own product lines of organic and Chinese herbs in bulk, herbal extracts, essential oils, and combination homeopathic remedies. Also sells other manufacturers' essential oils, homeopathic remedies, herbal and Ayurvedic products.

161. Gaia Herbs, Inc.
12 Lancaster County Road, Harvard, MA 01451
Telephone: 508-772-5400; 800-831-7780; Fax: 508-772-5764
Credit Cards: Visa, MasterCard, American Express

Manufactures herbal products made from plants grown by certified organic growers or gathered by wildcrafters. Inventory includes fresh and freshly dried single plant extracts, Chinese and Ayurvedic plant extracts, compounds, elixirs, oils and salves. Products are sold to retail outlets and to individuals.

162. Green Terrestrial
Post Office Box 266, Milton, NY 12547
Telephone: 914-795-5238
Credit Cards: Visa, MasterCard

This family-owned business sells healing products primarily made from plants they grow or wildcraft themselves, or from plants grown by other herbalists. Items available through their catalog include flower essences, alcohol extracts, oils and salves, tea blends, dried herbs, books, tapes and related products. Green Terrestrial also sponsors an annual gathering which includes workshops and intensives on various aspects of herbal healing.

163. Herb Pharm

Post Office Box 116, Williams, OR 97544
Telephone: 503-846-6262 (Customer Service); 800-348-4372 (Orders); Fax: 503-846-6112 (Orders)
Credit Cards: Visa, MasterCard

This family-owned business produces herbal extracts and compounds from certified organically grown herbs grown on their farm or purchased from other organic growers and wildcrafters. Also sells selected books and pamphlets on the health-related use of herbs.

164. Herbal Healer Academy International

HC 32 97-B, Mountain View, AR 72560
Telephone: 501-269-4177; Fax: 501-269-5424
Credit Cards: Visa, MasterCard

Sells a wide variety of products including homeopathic remedies, Bach Flower Essence remedies, Chinese medicinal herbs, bulk herbs, herb seeds, essential oils, books, videotapes and audiotapes. The academy will also prepare customized herbal formulas upon request. Some volume discounts are available.

165. Herbally Yours

Post Office Box 26, 209 Changewater Road, Changewater, NJ 07831
Telephone: 908-689-6140 (Mondays only); 908-735-4469 (Tuesday - Saturday)
Credit Cards: None

Sells a variety of herbal products including extracts from Herbalist & Alchemist, an herbal supplier, herbal health teas, compound herbal extracts, books, herbal animal products and more. Wholesale and retail.

166. Herbs and Spices

1944 Eastern Avenue S.E., Grand Rapids, MI 49507
Telephone: 616-245-6268
Credit Cards: Visa, MasterCard

Sells herbs and spices for medicinal and culinary uses in whole, cut and powder forms, in sizes ranging from one ounce to one pound. Also sells essential oils, gelatin capsules and a small selection of books about herbs and their uses.

167. Horizon Herbs
Post Office Box 69, Williams OR 97544-0069
Telephone: 503-846-6704
Credit Cards: None

This small, family-owned company cultivates organically grown medicinal plants and sells organically grown or wild-harvested seeds, live roots and medicinal herbs. Catalog includes almost 200 medicinal species including commonly used healing and native plants as well as some more unusual plants from other countries.

168. Indiana Botanic Gardens
Post Office Box 5, Hammond, IN 46325
Telephone: 219-947-4040; Fax: 219-947-4148
Credit Cards: Visa, MasterCard, Discover

Sells a variety of herbal formulas, homeopathic remedies, Chinese medicinal herbs, books and essential oils.

169. Intra American Specialties
3014 North 400 West, West Lafayette, IN 47906-5231
Telephone: 317-497-9785; Fax: 317-497-9381
Credit Cards: None

Compiles and sells *Directory of Herbal Education,* a guide to herbal resident and correspondence courses available in the United States and Canada, as well as selective herbology-related books and videotapes.

170. Jean's Greens
Herbal Tea Works
R.R. 1, Box 55J Hale Road, Rensselaerville, NY 12147
Telephone: 518-239-TEAS (8327); Fax: 518-239-8327
Credit Cards: None

Offers a complete selection of herbal teas and herbal tea combinations made from fresh dried organic and wildcrafted herbs. Herbal extracts, oils, capsules, creams and lotions are also available, as well as a full range of accessories and information products for humans and animals.

171. Mayway Corp.
1338 Cypress Street, Oakland, CA 94607
Telephone: 510-208-3113; Fax: 510-208-3069; 800-909-2828 (Orders only)
Credit cards: Visa, MasterCard

Sells a wide variety of Chinese herbal extracts, concentrated powders and formulas made under Mayway's own label, Plum Flower, and through an exclusive arrangement with Lanzhou Pharmaceutical Works, a prestigious manufacturer of herbal patents in China.

172. Motherlove herbal company
280 Stratton Park, Bellevue, CO 80512
Telephone: 303-493-2892; Fax: 303-493-2892
Credit Cards: None

Sells only those salves, oils and tinctures which are made from fresh herbs, have been used by the proprietors and which they know to be safe, effective and cruelty-free.

173. Mountain Rose Herbs
Post Office Box 2000, Redway, CA 95560
Telephone: 800-879-3337; Fax: 707-923-7867
Credit Cards: Visa, MasterCard

Offers a full line of herbal healing oils, teas, extracts, seeds, remedies, books, videotapes and related products. Many of these items are made from certified organically grown or wildcrafted herbs. Some of the formulas were developed by herbalist and author Rosemary Gladstar. All items are produced in small quantities in order to ensure freshness and quality.

174. Nature's Herb Company
1010-46th Street, Emeryville, CA 94608
Telephone: 510-601-0700; Fax: 510-547-4234
Credit Cards: Visa, MasterCard

Sells a wide range of herbs in sizes ranging from one ounce to one pound. Also sells health-related herbal teas, essential oils and Mother Tinctures.

175. Nature's Way Products, Inc.
Post Office Box 4000, 10 Mountain Springs Parkway, Springville, UT 84663
Telephone: 801-489-1520
Credit Cards: None

Manufactures and distributes a wide variety of natural health care products made from certified organically grown or wildcrafted herbs, for sale in health and nutrition stores throughout the country. Offerings include homeopathic medicines, single herbs and combination herbal formulas, herbal extracts, and other natural over-the-counter medicines.

176. Penn Herb Company, Ltd.
603 North 2nd Street, Philadelphia, PA 19123-3098
Telephone: 215-925-3336; 800-523-9971; Fax: 215-925-7946
Credit Cards: Visa, MasterCard, Discover

Mills, encapsulates, processes and sells medicinal dried herbs and herbal products, most in whole, cut, powder and capsule form. Single herbs and herbal formulas blended for specific common ailments are also available.

177. Perelandra
Post Office Box 3603, Warrentown, VA 22186
Telephone: 703-937-2153; Fax: 703-937-3360
Credit Cards: Visa, MasterCard, Discover

Sells a variety of items including flower essences prepared from plants grown in the Perelandra garden and related flower essence products.

178. Pro Natura
5341 Derry Avenue, Agoura Hills, CA 91301
Telephone: 818-760-0147; Fax: 818-889-4041
Credit Cards: Visa, MasterCard

Produces and sells herbal remedies which are available to health professionals only. Also sells selected publications on natural healing.

179. SAGE Mountain Herb Products
Post Office Box 420, East Barre, VT 05649
Telephone: 802-479-9825
Credit Cards: No

Affiliated with SAGE (see Herbal Medicine—Schools), this is a small, family-run herb business. All products are made of organically grown or wildcrafted herbs. Sells a limited number of tinctures, salves and natural skin care products.

180. Simplers Botanical Co.
Post Office Box 39, Emeryville, CA 95436

Telephone: 707-887-2012; 800-652-7646
Credit Cards: None

Owned and operated by herbalist and author James Green, this company manufactures and sells herbal compounds, extracts, glycerites, oils, aromatic hydrosols, aromatherapy skin care and health products, herbal products for animals, and other botanical health specialties. Only organically cultivated or ethically wild-harvested plants are used to make these products. Also offers herbal publications and educational resources.

181. Starwest Botanicals, Inc.
11253 Trade Center Drive, Rancho Cordova, CA 95742
Telephone: 916-638-8100; 800-800-HERB (4372); Fax: 916-638-8293
Credit Cards: Visa, MasterCard

Distributes Chinese herbs, homeopathic remedies, aromatherapy essential oils and accessories, as well as Boericke and Tafel homeopathic products. This certified organic processor also offers custom milling, formulation and blending, and private label/packaging. Wholesale only.

182. Terra Firma Botanicals, Inc.
28653 Sutherlin Lane, Eugene, OR 97405
Telephone: 503-485-7726
Credit Cards: Visa, MasterCard

A small family-run business which prepares and sells flower oils and single and combination herb extracts for use as healing aids. Wholesale orders are accepted from professional health care practitioners and retail concerns. All others retail.

183. Trout Lake Farm
149 Little Mountain Road, Trout Lake, WA 98650
Telephone: 509-395-2025; Fax: 509-395-2645
Credit Cards: None

Grows certified organically grown herbs and markets them to manufacturers of herbal teas, homeopathic medicines, nutritional supplements, pet products and phytopharmaceuticals. Through their sister company, Flora Laboratories, they manufacture liquid over-the-counter Class C liquid drugs of botanical substances and also custom-manufacture liquid extracts according to buyer specifications.

184. Turtle Island Herbs

4949 North Broadway, #101A, Boulder, CO 80304
Telephone: 303-442-2215; Fax: 303-786-9667
Credit Cards: None

Manufactures and sells single and combination herb extracts, herbal preparations and related products. Bulk discounts and custom formulas are available. Products are sold to retail outlets, distributors and professional herbalists.

185. Wild Weeds

302 Camp Weott Road, Post Office Box 88, Ferndale, CA 95536
Telephone: 707-786-4906; 800-553-WILD (9453) (Orders); Fax: 800-836-WILD (9453) (Orders)
Credit Cards: Visa, MasterCard

Offers a wide variety of medicinal herbal products, including fresh dried herbs, herbal teas, seeds and oils. Also sells herbalist supplies, essential oils, and books on herbalism, aromatherapy and women's care. Some items may be purchased wholesale. Bulk discounts are available.

Homeopathy

Homeopathy is a natural system of medicine which was developed by Samuel Hahnemann, M.D., in Germany almost 200 years ago. It is based on the "law of similars" —like cures like. This means that natural substances that in large amounts will make a healthy person sick, when administered in very minute doses, will heal the condition in a sick person. These very small doses, also called remedies, act to stimulate an individual's immune and defense system so that the body can heal itself. There are currently more than 2,000 homeopathic remedies, with more being added to the homeopathic repertoire every day. There are two major approaches to homeopathic treatment: classical homeopathy uses only one remedy at a time, determined by detailed information provided by the patient; non-classical or modern homeopathy combines the use of several remedies to treat a given condition. In most states, only individuals licensed to practice medicine may prescribe homeopathic remedies; however, many such remedies are also available for purchase by the general public in pharmacies, health food stores and supermarkets. Homeopathy can be used to treat a variety of medical conditions, including allergies, colds, digestive ailments, headaches, and some injuries, among many others.

Organizations

186. American Institute of Homeopathy (AIH)
925 East 17th Avenue, Denver, CO 80218-1407
Telephone: unavailable
Contact: Karen Kaiser Nossaman, executive secretary

The oldest national medical organization in the United States. This professional membership organization for homeopathic medical physicians, dentists and osteopaths represents the political and professional interests of homeopathic medicine to the federal government and organized medicine through legislatures, courts, medical licensing boards, health agencies, the media, community groups and the health care community. Promotes original clinical research and homeopathic teaching programs in private clinics and academic medical centers.

Services for the professional: Holds an annual scientific conference; plays an active role in conveying information to medical students; co-ordinates efforts with the various state homeopathic societies; engages in political activism; publishes a journal.

Publications: *Journal of the American Institute of Homeopathy,* quarterly, $45.00 (subscription) (reviewed under Homeopathy—Journals and Newsletters); *Introduction to Homeotherapeutics,* monograph, intermediate text on homeopathy including Material Medica and Repertory, $20.00; *AIH President's Newsletter,* monthly, free to members.

187. The Boiron Research Foundation (BRF)
6 Campus Boulevard, Building A, Newtown Square, PA 19073
Telephone: 610-325-0918

A nonprofit foundation established to conduct and promote basic and clinical research in homeopathy in the United States.

Services: Conducts medical and pharmacological research; maintains international information centers, a databank and library; encourages exchange of information among physicians, scientists and pharmacists; sponsors educational and training programs; publishes reports, books and research data in scientific and medical journals.

Publications: Copies of published reports on research are available through the foundation.

188. The Council for Homeopathic Certification (CHC)
1709 Seabright Avenue, Santa Cruz, CA 95062
Telephone: 408-421-0565
Contact: Richard Pitt, vice president/secretary

This nonprofit organization works to promote excellence in classical homeopathic practice and promote the inclusion of homeopathy within the recognized scope of practice of all health care professions.

Services for the professional: Offers certification in classical homeopathy (CCH) based on educational training, case submissions, written examination in both homeopathy and human sciences, and oral examination.

Services for the public: Provides a directory of certified classical homeopaths.

189. Homeopathic Academy of Naturopathic Physicians (HANP)

Post Office Box 69565, Portland, OR 97201
Telephone: 503-795-0579; Fax: 503-829-8541
Contact: Christa Louise, executive director

A specialty membership organization of licensed naturopathic physicians and the interested public, affiliated with the American Association of Naturopathic Physicians. The society promotes the practice of homeopathy through the education of naturopathic physicians and other homeopaths.

Services for the professional: Provides board certification of naturopathic physicians in classical homeopathy, granting the title of Diplomate of the Homeopathic Academy of Naturopathic Physicians; holds an annual case conference; encourages the development and improvement of homeopathic curriculum at naturopathic colleges; publishes a journal and directory of diplomates.

Services for the public: Sponsors an annual conference; provides referrals to diplomates of the HANP; publishes a journal.

Publications: Simillimum, quarterly journal, free with membership, $40.00 (subscription) (reviewed under Homeopathy—Journals and Newsletters).

190. International Foundation for Homeopathy (IFH)

Post Office Box 7, Edmonds, WA 98020
Telephone: 206-776-4147; Fax: 206-776-1499
Contact: Fred Bishop, executive director

A nonprofit membership educational organization promoting the highest standards of homeopathic practice and education, public awareness of classical homeopathy through education and research, and the establishment of homeopathic medical schools.

Services for the professional: Offers extensive postgraduate courses for professionals; sponsors IFH professional case conference; publishes magazine and conference proceedings, directory of IFH-trained homeopaths, and yearly book of cases cured with homeopathy.

Services for the public: Offers courses for lay people; provides general information on homeopathy and referrals to homeopaths (send self-addressed stamped envelope).

Publications: Resonance, bimonthly magazine, $40.00 (member subscription) (reviewed under Homeopathy—Journals and Newsletters); *IFH Directory of Professional Course Postgraduates,* free with membership, $5.00 nonmembers; *Information Booklet,* 16 pages, $4.00; *Proceedings of the IFH Professional Case Conferences,* free to supporting members, $32.50 nonmembers; First Aid Chart, free to members.

191. National Center for Homeopathy (NCH)

801 North Fairfax Street, Suite 306, Alexandria, VA 22314
Telephone: 703-548-7790; Fax: 703-548-7792
Contact: Sharon Stevenson, executive director

This nonprofit membership organization of professionals and lay persons is dedicated to promoting homeopathy through education, publication, research and membership services.

Services for the professional: Conducts educational seminars and training programs; holds an annual conference; interfaces with the media, government and the health insurance industry; coordinates a network of 220 local homeopathic study groups; offers an affiliated study group program; maintains a library of texts, journals and monographs; distributes literature and sells homeopathic books and products; publishes a newsletter.

Services for the public: Conducts educational seminars and training programs; sells books and products.

Publications: Homeopathy Today, newsletter, 11 times a year, $40.00 (subscription) (reviewed under Homeopathy—Journals and Newsletters).

192. The North American Society of Homeopaths (NASH)

10700 Old Country Road, #15, Plymouth, MN 55441
Telephone: 612-593-9458; Fax: 612-593-0097
Contact: Val Ohanian

A professional membership organization of homeopathic doctors and students, as well as the interested public, dedicated to developing and maintaining high standards of homeopathic practice in the United States. NASH works toward developing a qualified, certified and distinct homeopathic profession and supports the public in receiving high quality homeopathic care.

Services for the professional: Certifies homeopaths and provides a registry of these individuals; works toward the development of standardized high quality education in classical homeopathy; offers regular and continuing education; works toward legal recognition of the profession and increased public awareness; supports research and networking with homeopathic organizations internationally; supports the public's freedom to choose homeopathic treatment and remedies; publishes newsletter and journal.

Services for the public: Provides referrals to certified homeopaths; provides information on homeopathy, professional training, first aid and acute care.

Publications: The American Homeopath, annual journal, $20 (subscription) (reviewed under Homeopathy—Journals and Newsletters).

Schools

193. Acupressure-Acupuncture Institute (AAI)
9835 Sunset Drive, Suite 206, Miami, FL 33176
Telephone: 305-595-9500; Fax: 305-274-0675
See Chinese Medicine/Acupuncture—Schools.

194. Animal Natural Health Center (ANHC)
1283 Lincoln Street, Eugene, OR 97401
Telephone: 503-342-7665; Fax: 503-344-5356
Contact: Richard Pitcairn, D.V.M., Ph.D.

Offers an in-depth professional training program in veterinary homeopathy for licensed veterinarians.

195. Atlantic Academy of Classical Homeopathy (AACH)
c/o Lawrence Galante, 209 First Avenue, #2, New York, NY 10003
Telephone: 718-518-4593
Contact: Lawrence Galante

Offers a 500-hour certificate program in classical homeopathy, comprised of a one-year basic course which presents an introduction to this modality, followed by a two-year advanced studies course. In addition, students are required to attend advanced seminars which they may take at their own pace. For those unable to attend the classes, the academy offers an off-site option, which allows students to study with AACH-approved instructors throughout the world. Advanced seminars are offered throughout the year and are open to all who are interested.

196. The Australasian College of Herbal Studies (ACHS)
Post Office Box 57, Lake Oswego, OR 97034
Telephone: 503-635-6652; Voice Mail: 1-800-48-STUDY; Fax: 503-697-0615
See Herbal Medicine—Schools.

197. Boiron Institute (BI)
1208 Amosland Road, Norwood, PA 19074
Telephone: 800-258-8823
Contact: Warren Bell, R. Ph.

Administered by Boiron USA, the American subsidiary of a French homeopathic pharmaceutical company, the institute offers "An Introduction to Homeopathy for the Practicing Pharmacist," a home-study continuing education program approved by the American Council on Pharmaceutical Education. The course provides pharmacists with an overview of homeopathy and its role in contemporary health care practice.

198. The British Institute of Homeopathy (BIH)
520 Washington Boulevard, Suite 423, Marina Del Rey, CA 90292
Telephone: 310-306-5408; Fax: 310-827-5766
Contact: Terry S. Jacobs, USA registrar

Founded in London in 1986, BIH programs teach both classical and modern homeopathy. In the United States, two home-study programs are offered. The 300-hour diploma course consists of 29 written lessons, supplemented by audiotapes and videotapes. Students who successfully complete the course are awarded a diploma of the British Institute of Homeopathy. The 350-hour post-graduate course consists of 26 written lessons, audiotapes, videotapes and practical work, and leads to a doctorate of homeopathic medicine. In the U.S., these courses are recognized by the Federation of Homeopaths, The College of Homeopathy, and the Alternative Medicine Foundation.

199. Five Elements Center (FEC)
115 Route 46, Building D, Suite 29, Mountain Lakes, NJ 07046
Telephone: 201-402-8510, ext. 908; Fax: 201-402-9753
Contact: Jane Cicchetti, director

Offers a two-year program in essentials of constitutional homeopathy, each year consisting of 110 credit hours which may be used toward certification in classical homeopathy. Also offers several levels of individual courses in homeopathy: a one and one-half hour overview of the subject; a four-hour course on homeopathic remedies for home use; in-depth courses on case analysis; a homeopathy workshop in which students learn to use homeopathy for self-treatment and which provides a basis for further study; and a beginning course in veterinary homeopathy, appropriate for both pet owners and veterinary professionals. Visa, MasterCard and Discover accepted for payment of tuition for all courses.

200. Hahnemann College of Homeopathy (HCH)
828 San Pablo Avenue, Albany, CA 94706
Telephone: 510-524-3117; Fax: 510-524-2447
Contact: Neda Tomasevich, administrator

Designed for students who plan to practice homeopathy on a full-time basis, this is a part-time training program in classical homeopathy for licensed medical professionals. The 864-hour program meets in four-day sessions, nine times a year for four years, and consists of academic course work and clinical training. No previous background in homeopathy is required. This is the only course in the United States accredited at the advanced level by the Council on Homeopathic Education.

201. Homeopathy Works (HW)
124 Fairfax Street, Berkeley Springs, WV 25411
Telephone: 304-258-2541; Fax: 304-258-6335

Offers free introductory classes in classical homeopathy every Saturday and hosts a large local study group which meets there regularly. Also manufactures homeopathic remedies for Washington Homeopathic Products (see Homeopathy—Product Suppliers) and functions as a museum, displaying and interpreting the history of homeopathy.

202. New England School of Homeopathy (NESH)
115 Elm Street, Suite 210, Enfield, CT 06082
Telephone: 800-NESH-440; Fax: 203-253-5041
Contact: Mary Anne Dietschler, coordinator

Offers three levels of homeopathic study: introductory, intermediate and advanced. A clinic course meeting over five weekends provides students the opportunity to take the cases of many patients, integrating all aspects of homeopathic study and practice. Level I, an introductory course, lays the groundwork for those interested in a career in homeopathy and is also appropriate for individuals who want to learn homeopathy for their own purposes; Level II, a one-year intermediate course, teaches students to analyze cases and manage a homeopathic practice; Level III, an eighteen-month advanced course, includes guest lectures by internationally known, highly experienced homeopathic practitioners.

203. The Northwestern Academy of Homeopathy (NAH)
10700 Old Country Road #15, Suite 350, Plymouth, MN 55441
Telephone: 612-593-9458; Fax: 612-593-0097
Contact: Eric Sommermann, dean

Offers a three-year, 1,152-hour professional training program in classical homeopathy, consisting of classroom instruction and clinical training, leading to a certificate of completion. Appropriate for licensed health care practitioners; students with no previous medical training must complete designated basic medical science courses at an accredited college.

204. Oregon College of Oriental Medicine
10525 S.E. Cherry Blossom Drive, Portland, OR 97216
Telephone: 503-253-3443; Fax: 503-253-2701
See Chinese Medicine/Acupuncture—Schools.

205. Pacific Academy of Homeopathic Medicine (PAHM)
1678 Shattuck Avenue, #2, Berkeley, CA 94709
Telephone: 510-420-8839; Fax: 510-655-4982
Contact: Cindy Muller, administrative coordinator

Offers two programs of study in foundations of classical homeopathy. The one-year program covers basic homeopathic principles, first aid and acute self-limiting conditions, and is designed for students who want to understand the basics of home treatment as well as for those preparing for in-depth study in the field. A certificate in acute homeotherapeutics is awarded upon completion. The three-year professional program explores in-depth the nature and cure of acute and chronic disease and is appropriate for those pursuing a career as a professional homeopath. A certificate in homeopathy is awarded upon completion. Both programs meet one weekend per month for lectures; students are required to complete twenty-five to forty hours of home study per month in between weekend lectures. The academy is a member of the North American Council for Classical Homeopathy, a council of homeopathic schools working cooperatively to develop and standardize homeopathic curricula.

Treatment Centers/Referrals

See Homeopathy—Organizations for referrals to individual practitioners.

206. The Natural Health Clinic
Bastyr University (BU), 144 N.E. 54th Street, Seattle, WA 98105-9916
Telephone: 206-523-9585; Fax: 206-527-4763
See Naturopathy—Treatment Centers/Referrals.

207. Shealy Institute for Comprehensive Health Care
1328 East Evergreen, Springfield, MO 65803

Telephone: 417-865-5940; Fax: 417-865-6111
See chapter 1: General—Treatment Centers/Referrals.

Product Suppliers

208. Biological Homeopathic Industries
11600 Cochiti S.E., Albuquerque, NM 87123
Telephone: 505-293-3843; 800-621-7644 (Orders only); Fax: 505-275-1672
Credit Cards: Visa, MasterCard

Produces and distributes combination homeopathic preparations created by Dr. H-H Reckeweg, a well-known German homeopath. Also distributes the product line of BHI's parent company, HEEL, a leading German homeopathic manufacturer, and the books of Menaco, the publishing division of BHI. Markets these products primarily to health care practitioners but also to health food stores.

209. Boericke & Tafel
2381 Circadian Way, Santa Rosa, CA 95407
Telephone: 800-876-9505, x100; Fax: 707-571-8237
Credit Cards: Visa, MasterCard

Offers a full line of homeopathic remedies including tonics and syrups, sports medicines and children's remedies. Products may be purchased directly from the company or through local health food stores.

210. Boiron USA
6 Campus Boulevard, Building A, Post Office Box 449, Newtown Square, PA 19073
Telephone: 800-BLU-TUBE (258-8823)
Credit Cards: Visa, MasterCard, American Express

This United States office of an international company manufactures and distributes homeopathic products made of substances from the botanical, mineral and animal kingdoms including remedies, storage equipment, homeopathic kits, topical and personal care products, as well as books on homeopathy. No longer serving as a retail outlet, orders for Boiron products are processed through: C.O. Bigelow Chemists, 414 Sixth Avenue, New York, NY 10011; Telephone: 800-793-LIFE, Fax: 212-228-8107; and by Hickey Chemists, 888 Second Avenue, New York, NY; Telephone: 800-698-4425 (New York City only), 800-724-5566 (all others), Fax: 212-980-1533.

211. Dolisos America, Inc.
3014 Rigel Avenue, Las Vegas, NV 89102
Telephone: 702-871-7153; 800-DOLISOS (365-4767); Fax: 702-871-9670
Credit Cards: None

This full-service homeopathic company, in business since 1936, offers practitioners classical homeopathic remedies, allergens, organotherapy, gemmotherapy, lithotherapy, oligotherapy and a variety of combination remedies, custom combinations, kits and books. Remedies are available in pellet, liquid or tablet form in a range of potencies.

212. Homeopathic Educational Services
2036 Blake Street (Retail and Shipping Address); 2124 Kittredge Street (Mailing and Billing Address), Berkeley, CA 94704
Telephone: 510-649-0294 (Information/catalogs); 800-359-9051 (Orders only); Fax: 510-649-1955
Credit Cards: Visa, MasterCard

Directed by Dana Ullman, well-known writer of several books on homeopathy, this company is the largest distributor in the United States of homeopathic books, family medicine kits, children's products, a variety of homeopathic formulas and veterinary products, as well as audiotapes, videotapes, software and related products.

213. Longevity Pure Medicine
9595 Wilshire, Suite 202, Beverly Hills, CA 90212
Telephone: 310-273-7423; 800-628-0202; Fax: 310-859-9930
Credit Cards: None

Produces and distributes to retail outlets different combination homeopathic formulas for treatment of common ailments. Medicines are sold over-the-counter and, for ease of use, are named by the symptoms they treat. Wholesale only.

214. Merz Apothecary
4716 North Lincoln Avenue, Chicago, IL 60625
Telephone: 312-989-0900; 800-252-0275 (Orders Only); Fax: 312-989-8108
Credit Cards: Visa, MasterCard, American Express

Sells bulk herbs, homeopathic remedies and publications.

215. Newton Laboratories Homeopathic Medicine
612 Upland Trail, Conyers, GA 30207

Telephone: 404-922-2644; Fax: 404-388-7768
Credit Cards: Visa, MasterCard

Sells single and combination homeopathic remedies for adults and children as well as remedy kits for first aid, common ailments, childbirth labor and chronic fatigue. Also sells homeopathic medicines, lotions and ointments for treating dogs, cats and horses. Informational flyers on various aspects of homeopathy are available upon request.

216. Standard Homeopathic Company
210 West 131st Street, Box 61067, Los Angeles, CA 90061
Telephone: 213-321-4284; 800-624-9659; Fax: 310-516-8579
Credit Cards: Visa, MasterCard

Manufactures and sells a large stock of homeopathic medicines including rare and hard-to-find remedies. Product line includes single remedies in tincture, tablet and pellet form, combination remedies in tablet form, cell salts, and homeopathic medicines for children. The catalog contains an index arranged by symptom and the appropriate remedies for each. Free literature on a variety of homeopathy-related topics is available upon request.

217. Washington Homeopathic Products, Inc.
4914 Del Ray Avenue, Bethesda, MD 20814
Telephone: 301-656-1695 (Orders, business and information); 800-336-1695 (Orders only); Fax: 301-656-1847
Credit Cards: Visa, MasterCard

Manufactures and sells single and combination remedies, tinctures, ointments and oils. Also has another retail outlet, Homeopathy Works, in Berkeley Springs, West Virginia. (See Homeopathy—Schools.)

Naturopathy

Naturopathy is based on a philosophical approach incorporating the following principles of healing: 1) the prescription of treatments which do no harm, are noninvasive, and have minimal risk of side effects; 2) the use of treatments which support the restoration of the body's ability to heal itself; 3) identification of the cause of an ailment rather than the simple treatment of the symptoms; 4) evaluation of the whole person, including physical, emotional, spiritual, environmental and other factors; 5) prevention of disease through encouragement of healthy lifestyle choices; 6) education of the patient and support for the patient's taking personal responsibility for good health. Naturopaths have bachelor's degrees and are trained in four-year programs which lead to the degree of doctor of naturopathic medicine (N.D.). Although currently licensed only in Alaska, Arizona, Connecticut, Hawaii, Montana, New Hampshire, Oregon and Washington, with several additional states pursuing licensure, naturopaths may practice in all fifty states. Naturopathy employs a variety of therapies including herbal medicine, physical medicine, homeopathy, nutrition, exercise and hydrotherapy, and may be used to treat a wide range of acute and chronic ailments.

Organizations

218. American Association of Naturopathic Physicians (AANP)
2366 Eastlake Avenue East, Suite 322, Seattle, WA 98102
Telephone: 206-323-7610; Fax: 206-323-7612
Contact: Leah Maslow, administrative assistant

A nonprofit national membership organization of naturopathic physicians involved in promoting naturopathy and the public health through work on licensing and accreditation, standards of practice, public information and education, scientific research, and participation on the state and federal level to represent and further the profession.

Services for the professional: Sponsors an annual convention; offers a malpractice insurance program; maintains referral and practice mentor programs; publishes a journal, newsletter, *AANP Directory, AANP Action* and educational and promotional brochures.

Services for the public: Provides a referral service to AANP member physicians and accredited schools; offers a Patient Assistance Support System (PASS) which helps patients select the health insurance policy most suited to their needs.

Publications: *Journal of Naturopathic Medicine,* quarterly, free to members, $65.00 (subscription) (reviewed under Journals and Newsletters); *The Naturopathic Physician,* quarterly newsletter, free to members; *AANP Directory,* providing a complete listing of members, state associations, state boards, specialty societies, schools and corporate sponsors; *AANP Action,* quarterly publication on planning and initiatives on national issues, free to members.

219. American Naturopathic Medical Association (ANMA)
Post Office Box 96273, Las Vegas, NV 89193
Telephone: 702-897-7053
Contact: Stephen Nugent, N.M.D., Ph.D., president

A professional membership organization of doctors from many different disciplines with sufficient training in natural health care as well as doctors of naturopathy. ANMA supports research leading to higher standards of naturopathic practice and monitors legislation nationally relating to natural health care, especially as it relates to naturopathy.

Services for the professional: Sponsors an annual convention offering approved continuing medical education credits; offers scholarships and educational guidance; sends letters to members providing information regarding legislation, educational, licensing and registration opportunities.

Publications: ANMA Update, quarterly newsletter, free to members.

Schools

220. Bastyr University (BU)

144 N.E. 54th Street, Seattle, WA 98105-9916
Telephone: 206-523-9585; Fax: 206-527-4763
Contact: Stephen E. Bangs, director, marketing and admissions

Offers a 323-credit program leading to a doctorate in naturopathic medicine, a 226-credit program leading to a master of science in acupuncture and oriental medicine, a 171.5-credit program leading to a master of science in acupuncture, and a 91-credit program leading to a bachelor of science in oriental medicine (see also Chinese Medicine/Acupuncture—Schools). Graduates of the naturopathic medicine program are eligible to take the Naturopathic Physicians licensing examination. (The results of this exam are used by all states which license individuals to practice naturopathic medicine.)

221. National College of Naturopathic Medicine (NCNM)

11231 S.E. Market Street, Portland, OR 97216
Telephone: 503-255-4860
Contact: Admissions Office

The oldest naturopathic medical school in North America, the college offers a four-year graduate program consisting of classroom studies and clinical practice, leading to the degree of doctor of naturopathic medicine. Graduates who successfully complete the program are eligible to take the licensing board examinations in those states with licensing laws: Alaska, Arizona, Connecticut, Hawaii, Montana, New Hampshire, Oregon and Washington. The school is currently developing postdoctoral programs in naturopathic obstetrics, homeopathy, and classical Chinese medicine, each of which will consist of one year of intensive academic and clinical training. The college is accredited by the Council on Naturopathic Medical Education, a specialized accreditor recognized by the U.S. Secretary of Education. Financial aid is available through several federal programs.

222. School of Natural Medicine (SNM)
Post Office Box 7369, Boulder, CO 80305-7369
Telephone: 303-443-4882; Fax: 303-443-4882
Contact: Farida Sharan, director

Offers several home-study programs: a twelve-lesson naturopathy course covering the theory, practice and philosophy of naturopathy; a twelve-lesson master herbalist course (see Herbal Medicine—Schools); and a fourteen-lesson master iridology course. The school also offers a natural physician course which includes all three home-study courses, as well as attendance at the foundation summer school and clinical training. Also offered is a summer program on herbology (see Herbal Medicine—Schools).

223. Southwest College of Naturopathic Medicine (SCNM)
6535 East Osborn Road, Suite 703, Scottsdale, AZ 85251
Telephone: 602-990-7424; Fax: 602-990-0337
Contact: Dr. Michael J. Cronin, president

Southwest College, which was established in 1992, offers a four-year graduate medical program covering a wide variety of natural therapies including botanical and homeopathic medicine, manipulation, nutrition, and acupuncture. Also offers a three-year accelerated program. Both program options lead to the degree of doctorate in naturopathic medicine. The college offers public education programs on a wide variety of natural health care topics. In addition, Southwest Naturopathic Medical Center opened in 1995 and provides naturopathic medical care to the Scottsdale community. The college has been approved as a candidate for accreditation by the Council of Naturopathic Medicine. A limited number of jobs are available through the school's work/study program.

Treatment Centers/Referrals

See Naturopathy—Organizations for referrals to individual practitioners.

224. The Natural Health Clinic
Bastyr University
144 N.E. 54th Street, Seattle, WA 98105-9916
Telephone: 206-523-9585; Fax: 206-527-4763

The teaching clinic for the health science programs at Bastyr University, the clinic provides natural health care for the community. Facilities include a natural medicine dispensary, physiotherapy modalities, laboratory, library, a hydrotherapy department for colonics, steam and sitz baths, whirlpool and constitutional hydrotherapy. Clinic services include naturopathic medicine, nutritional counseling, women's health care, homeopathy, physical medicine, counseling, pediatrics, massage and sports medicine. The newest addition to the program is the Acupuncture and Oriental Medicine Clinic with a Chinese herbal medicine dispensary.

225. Southwest College of Naturopathic Medicine
6535 East Osborn Road, Suite 703, Scottsdale, AZ 85251
Telephone: 602-990-7424; Fax: 602-990-0337

Southwest College of Naturopathic Medical Center provides naturopathic medical care to the community. In addition, naturopathic physicians and students conduct public education programs on a wide variety of health care topics such as self-care and first aid, stress management, and women's health issues.

Product Suppliers

See Herbal Medicine—Product Suppliers, and Homeopathic Medicine—Product Suppliers for additional listings.

226. Morrills' New Directions
Post Office Box 30, Orient, ME 04471
Telephone: 800-368-5057; Fax: 207-532-0895
Credit Cards: Visa, MasterCard

The catalog's subtitle is *Your Natural Pet Care Catalog* and, as the name indicates, they sell natural products for pets including nutritional supplements, natural remedies and herbal solutions as well as books on this topic.

CHAPTER 3: MANIPULATIVE THERAPIES

Chiropractic

By far the most widely accepted of the alternative therapies included in this book, chiropractic focuses primarily on the relationship between the spinal column and the central nervous system. Chiropractors seek to adjust "subluxations," misalignments of the spinal vertebrae, which interfere with the healthy functioning of the nervous system. Elimination of subluxations allows the nervous system to freely transmit impulses throughout the body which, in turn, assists the body in healing itself. This therapy is used extensively to treat back, neck and shoulder pain, as well as other disorders of the muscular, skeletal and nervous systems. Doctors of Chiropractic (D.C.) have an Associate's degree, at minimum, followed by four years of study at a school of chiropractic. Chiropractors are licensed in all fifty states. Chiropractic treatment is covered under many medical insurance programs.

Organizations

227. American Chiropractic Association (ACA)
1701 Clarendon Boulevard, Arlington, VA 22209
Telephone: 703-276-8800; 800-368-3083; Fax: 703-243-2593
Contact: J. Ray Morgan, executive vice president

A nonprofit membership organization dedicated to the advancement of chiropractic and service to the chiropractic profession.

Services for the professional: Sponsors regional seminars and an annual convention; provides yearly listing in the *ACA Membership Directory*; maintains media relations and public relations programs; airs public service announcements; ensures representation on a federal level to help shape national policy; supports research; maintains an information clearinghouse and information resource center; sells products; monitors state and federal legal actions; offers insurance programs; publishes journals, newsletter and specialty publications.

Services for the public: Provides referrals to practitioners and information on chiropractic.

Publications: Journal of the American Chiropractic Association, monthly, free to members, $80 (subscription) (reviewed under Manipulative Therapies—Journals and Newsletters); *ACA Today,* monthly newsletter, free to members; *ACA Membership Directory,* annual, one copy free to members, $100 nonmembers.

228. Association for Network Chiropractic (ANC)

444 North Main Street
Longmont, CO 80501
Telephone: 303-678-8101; Fax: 303-678-8089
Contact: Dr. Donald Epstein, president

A membership organization devoted to the promotion of network spinal analysis, a model of chiropractic treatment, and to the creation of a forum for communication on the healing arts.

Services for the professional: Conducts seminars and workshops for health care practitioners on network spinal analysis; sponsors an annual convention; conducts ongoing research; publishes a newsletter, journal in development.

Services for the public: Acts as a referral and information resource for network spinal analysis and doctors worldwide who utilize this model in their practice.

Publications: *The Network Release,* quarterly newsletter, free to members.

229. The Council on Chiropractic Education (CCE)

7975 N. Hayden Road, Suite A-210, Scottsdale, AZ 85258
Telephone: 602-443-8877; Fax: 602-483-7333

CCE is authorized by the U.S. Department of Education to provide accreditation for chiropractic programs and institutions. These programs are reviewed against a set of rigorous professional standards in order to assure the public of the quality and integrity of chiropractic education. Benefits of accreditation also include participation in various federal and state government programs, ability to sit for state licensure examinations in all fifty states, facilitation of the transfer of credits among educational institutions, encouragement of donor grants, and assurance for students of the quality of chiropractic education at an institution.

Services: Provides a listing of accredited chiropractic institutions; publishes a variety of materials.

Publications: *Official Directory of the Federation of Chiropractic Licensing Boards,* annual, $20, $15/students (available through the Federation of Chiropractic Licensing Boards, 901 54th Avenue, Suite 101, Greeley, CO 80634, Telephone: 303-356-3500); *Standards for Chiropractic Programs and Institutions.*

230. Federation of Chiropractic Licensing Boards (FCLB)
901 54th Avenue, Suite 101, Greeley, CO 80364
Telephone: 970-356-3500; Fax: 970-356-3599
Contact: Gail Royster, administrative assistant

A nonprofit organization established in 1933 as the professional association for government regulatory boards responsible for chiropractic licensure. Promotes excellence in standards for chiropractic licensure, accurate information, networking, resources and education.

Services for the professional: Sponsors an annual educational conference; holds regional meetings; provides an online computerized disciplinary databank; publishes a directory of licensing requirements and newsletter.

Publications: *Official Directory of the Federation of Chiropractic Licensing Boards,* annual, $20 (individual subscription), $15 (student subscription); *FCLB News,* periodic newsletter, free to members.

231. Foundation for Chiropractic Education and Research (FCER)
1701 Clarendon Boulevard, Arlington, VA 22209
Telephone: 703-276-7445; Fax: 703-276-8178
Contact: Mary E. Johnson, director of communications

An independent research foundation promoting education and research on chiropractic. Areas of research include back pain, carpal tunnel syndrome, migraine and tension headaches, infantile colic, otitis media, primary hypertension, asthma and scoliosis. Also sponsors cost-effectiveness studies, randomized clinical trails and patient satisfaction studies.

Services for the professional: Sponsors an annual research-oriented conference; offers a literature search service: offers discounts on products and services; provides free financial planning; publishes a variety of materials including a journal, newsletter, and doctor and patient education materials

Services for the public: FCER's Staying Well Division publishes educational materials designed for chiropractic patients.

Publications: *Spinal Manipulation,* quarterly research reviews, $45.00 (member subscription), $50.00 (nonmember subscription); *JNMS: Journal of the Neuromusculoskeletal System,* quarterly, free to members, $58.00 (individual subscription), $118.00 (institutional subscription), $35.00 (student subscription); *Advance,* bimonthly newsletter, free to members; *FCER News*

Alert, monthly newsletter, $79 (member subscription), $87 (nonmember subscription); *The Weekend Chiropractic*, a fax service summarizing weekly developments affecting the chiropractic profession, $99 (member subscription), $125 (nonmember subscription); doctor and patient education materials including pamphlets, newsletters, books and booklets, videotapes, audiotapes and special programs.

232. International Chiropractors Association (ICA)

1110 N. Glebe Road, Suite 1000, Arlington, VA 22201
Telephone: 203-528-5000; 800-423-4690; Fax: 203-528-0523
Contact: Dr. Dana Rose, director of professional affairs

The oldest national chiropractic organization representing practitioners, educators, students and lay persons. Promotes the interests of chiropractic as a separate and distinct drugless profession through advocacy, research and education.

Services for the professional: Sponsors seminars and conferences; offers insurance programs and limited legal counsel; provides media/political updates; airs radio public service announcements; works toward staff privileges for doctors of chiropractic in hospitals and assists their application for privileges; publishes a journal, newsletter, promotional materials for doctors and patients, and conference proceedings.

Services for the public: Provides referrals to member doctors; answers requests for information on the profession.

Publications: *ICA Review*, quarterly journal, free to members, $50 (subscription); *ICA Today;* quarterly newsletter, free to members; patient brochures, books and manuals, practice marketing material, research and information on chiropractic, conference proceedings, videotapes, children's materials.

233. Sacro Occipital Research Society International, Inc. (SORSI)

Post Office Box 8245, Prairie Village, KS 66208
Telephone: 913-649-3475; Fax: 913-649-2676
Contact: Candice Binyon, director

A nonprofit association dedicated to advancing the practice of Sacro Occipital Technique (SOT) and SOT cranial as a method of chiropractic through education, research and legislative activity. Membership is open to doctors, chiropractic assistants and students.

Services for the professional: Provides instructional courses, materials, videotapes and books on Sacro Occipital Technique of chiropractic and SOT-Craniopathy. SOT Board Certification available.

Publications: *Technical Report*, quarterly newsletter, free to members; a variety of books on Sacro Occipital Technique.

234. World Chiropractic Alliance (WCA)
2950 North Dobson Road, Suite 1, Chandler, AZ 85224
Telephone: 800-347-1011; Fax: 602-732-9313
Contact: Terry A. Rondberg, D.C., president

A nonprofit association serving to promote the aims, essence and growth of chiropractic. The alliance works toward defining the arena of chiropractic, gaining public and professional acceptance, opposing universal immunization, and promoting public relations efforts, research and standards of care.

Services for the professional: Maintains a referral list; provides lobbying representation; produces public relations tools; offers a malpractice insurance program; provides financial and professional services, offering advice and information; publishes a journal and newsletter.

Services for the public: Provides a referral service; publishes informational brochures.

Publications: *The Chiropractic Journal*, monthly, free to doctors of chiropractic; *True Health*, newspaper, ten times a year, written for the public and distributed through chiropractic offices only.

Schools

235. Cleveland Chiropractic College (CCC)
590 North Vermont Avenue, Los Angeles, CA 90004
Telephone: 213-660-6166; 800-466-CCLA; Fax: 213-660-5387
Contact: Paul Forgetta, director of admissions

Offers a ten-trimester, 4,845-hour program, including more than 700 hours of clinical training and internship, leading to the degree of doctor of chiropractic. The college also offers preceptorship programs to qualified students, as well as a variety of continuing education courses. The program is accredited by the Council on Chiropractic Education. Federal grants, loans and work/study programs, and some private grants and scholarships are available.

236. Life College (LC)
School of Chiropractic, 1269 Barclay Circle, Marietta, GA 30060
Telephone: 404-424-0554; 800-394-5433; Fax: 404-429-4819
Contact: Deborah Michel

Offers a fourteen-quarter program leading to the degree of doctor of chiropractic, and a four-quarter chiropractic technician program leading to a diploma. The school is accredited by the Commission on Accreditation of the Council on Chiropractic Education. Financial aid from federal, state and local sources, including grants, loans and work study, are available. Life College publishes *Today's Chiropractic,* a bimonthly publication, $6.00/issue, $24.00 (subscription).

237. Life Chiropractic College West (LCCW)
2005 Via Barrett, San Lorenzo, CA 94580-1368
Telephone: 510-276-9013; 800-788-4476; Fax: 510-276-0984
Contact: Suzanne C. Smith, admissions director

Offers a 4,856-hour program including 554 hours of clinical experience leading to the degree of doctor of chiropractic. The program is accredited by the Commission on Accreditation of the Council on Chiropractic Education. A department of continuing and postgraduate education offers postgraduate programs and continuing education seminars including a one-year, 100-hour certification program and a three-year, 360-hour diplomate program of the Council on Applied Chiropractic Sciences of the International Chiropractors Association. Financial aid is available through a variety of grant, loan, work/study and scholarship programs.

238. Los Angeles College of Chiropractic (LACC)
16200 East Amber Valley Drive, Whittier, CA 90604
Telephone: 310-947-8755; Fax: 310-947-5724
Contact: Charlene Frontiera, director of admissions

Offers the ADVANTAGE program of chiropractic education, which encourages students to develop competencies rather than learn subjects. Lab and hands-on experiences are emphasized and lecture time is reduced. A preceptor program is available to students once they have completed the program's clinical requirements; a postceptor program is available to graduates awaiting licensure. The college is accredited for the doctor of chiropractic degree by the Commission on Accreditation of the Council on Chiropractic Education. Financial aid in the form of grants, scholarships and loans are available.

239. The National College of Chiropractic (NCC)
200 East Roosevelt Road, Lombard, IL 60148-4583
Telephone: 708-629-2000; 800-826-NATL; Fax: 708-268-6554
Contact: Jo Beth Castleberry, director of admissions.

Offers a four-year, 239-credit, 4,849-hour program consisting of classroom study and clinical training, leading to the degree of doctor of chiropractic. The college is accredited by the Commission on Accreditation of the Council on Chiropractic Education, the State Education Department of New York, and the Commission of Higher Education of the North Central Association of Colleges and Schools. Federal and state loans, grants and scholarships, as well as some work/study positions and fellowships, are available.

240. New York Chiropractic College (NYCC)
2360 State Route 89, Seneca Falls, NY 13148-0800
Telephone: 315-568-3039; Fax: 315-568-3015
Contact: Fred P. Zuccala, director of admissions

Offers a three and one-half year, 5,005-hour program of study, including two trimesters of internship at one of the college's three outpatient clinics, leading to the degree of doctor of chiropractic. The program is accredited by the Commission of Accreditation of the Council on Chiropractic Education and regionally accredited by the Commission on Higher Education, Middle States Association of Colleges and Schools. Financial aid from federal, state and private sources is available.

241. Northwestern College of Chiropractic (NWCC)
2501 West 84th Street, Bloomington, MN 55431
Telephone: 612-888-4777; 800-888-4777; Fax: 612-888-6713
Contact: Henry P. Kaynes, director of admissions

Awards the doctor of chiropractic degree to those students who complete the five-year, ten-semester program. The curriculum consists of course work in basic, chiropractic and clinical sciences and a twelve-month internship and preceptorship. The college is accredited by the Commission on Accreditation of the Council on Chiropractic Education and by the Commission on Institutes of Higher Education of the North Central Association of Colleges and Schools. A wide variety of federal, state, institutional and private financial aid programs are available.

242. Parker College of Chiropractic (PCC)
2500 Walnut Hill Lane, Dallas, TX 75229-5668
Telephone: 214-438-6043; 800-438-6932, Admissions

Offers a nine-trimester program of course work and practical training leading to the doctor of chiropractic degree. The program is accredited by the Council on Chiropractic Education and the Southern Association of Schools and Colleges.

243. Sherman College of Straight Chiropractic (SCSC)
2020 Springfield Road, Post Office Box 1452, Spartanburg, SC 29304
Telephone: 803-578-8770; 800-849-8771; Fax: 803-599-7145
Contact: Susan S. Newlin, director of admissions

Offers a thirteen-quarter program leading to the degree of doctor of chiropractic. A continuing education program offers workshops for license renewal, noncredit courses for chiropractors and seminars for spouses. Financial aid is available through a variety of federal grant, loan and work/study programs, as well as through college-based scholarship and loan programs. The college is accredited by the Commission on Accreditation of the Council on Chiropractic Education. It is currently accredited by the Commission on Accreditation of the Southern Association of Colleges and Schools (a federally recognized agency) and the Commission on Accreditation of the Straight Chiropractic Academic Standards Association (not a federally recognized agency).

244. Texas Chiropractic College (TCC)
5912 Spencer Highway, Pasadena, TX 77505
Telephone: 713-487-1170; Fax: 713-487-2009
Contact: Robert Cooper, director of admissions

Offers a 4,970-hour, 245-credit program, consisting of academic course work and clinical training, leading to the doctor of chiropractic degree. Also offers postgraduate diplomate programs and continuing education courses. The college is accredited by the Commission on Accreditation of the Council on Chiropractic Education and by the Southern Association of Colleges and Schools. Various programs of grants, loans, scholarships and work/study are available.

Treatment Centers/Referrals

See also Chiropractic—Organizations for referrals to individual chiropractic practitioners.

245. Life Chiropractic College West
22336 Main Street, Hayward, CA 94541
Telephone: 510-889-1700; Fax: 510-889-7975

The college maintains a clinic offering chiropractic care by qualified interns supervised by doctors of chiropractic. This consists of a complete consultation and history, physical examination, spinal examination including range of motion studies, postural analysis, palpation and instrumentation, and a program of care formulated with the guidance of clinical faculty. A sliding fee scale is available for those in financial need. In addition, the clinic offers weekly free orientations called Life Talks and teaches patients about ongoing health care maintenance through nutrition, exercise and other natural approaches.

246. Life College

School of Chiropractic, 1269 Marclay Circle, Marietta, GA 30060
Telephone: 404-424-0554; Fax: 404-429-4819

The college operates three chiropractic health care centers, one on campus, one in Atlanta and one in Marietta. Treatments are performed by student chiropractors under the supervision of experienced professional chiropractors.

247. Los Angeles College of Chiropractic

16200 East Amber Valley Drive, Whittier, CA 90604
Telephone: 310-947-8755; Fax: 310-947-5724

The college operates an on-campus chiropractic health center and two out-patient clinics, one in Glendale and one in Pasadena, California.

248. The National College of Chiropractic

200 East Roosevelt Road, Lombard, IL 60148-4583
Telephone: 708-629-2000; 800-826-NATL; Fax: 708-268-6554

NCC has six teaching clinics serving the community: one in Chicago, one in Aurora, two on campus, and two in association with the Salvation Army in Chicago. On-campus facilities include the National College Chiropractic Center and the Student Clinic. All clinics perform a full range of chiropractic patient services with treatments performed by senior interns under the supervision of licensed chiropractic physicians.

249. New York Chiropractic College

2360 State Route 89, Seneca Falls, NY 13148-0800
Telephone: 315-568-3039; 315-568-3015

Maintains three off-campus public health care centers in Syracuse, Levittown, and Buffalo, New York, and one on-campus clinical facility. Students provide chiropractic care for members of the community under licensed, practicing doctors of chiropractic.

250. Parker College of Chiropractic
2500 Walnut Hill Lane, Dallas, TX 75229-5668
Telephone: 214-438-6043; 800-438-6932, Admissions

The college runs two clinics, the ALPHA Clinic in Irving, Texas, and the BETA Clinic in Dallas, Texas. They offer lower cost treatment consisting of patient consultation, comprehensive examination, x-rays as indicated, and chiropractic adjustments of the spine with physical therapy modalities if appropriate. Services are performed by interns in conjunction with licensed doctors of chiropractic.

251. Sherman College of Straight Chiropractic
2020 Springfield Road, P.O. Box 1452, Spartanburg, SC 29304
Telephone: 803-578-8770, 800-849-8771; Fax: 803-599-7145

At the Sherman College Chiropractic Health Center, students, under supervision of clinic staff, offer chiropractic care to the community. Located in the E. C. Taylor Building, there are twenty-one treatment rooms with modern chiropractic analytical and adjusting equipment.

252. Texas Chiropractic College
5912 Spencer Highway, Pasadena, TX 77505
Telephone: 713-487-1170; Fax: 713-487-2009

The Texas Chiropractic Clinic is open to the general public, faculty, and staff and their families Monday through Saturday. Student interns offer chiropractic health services under the supervision of licensed doctors of chiropractic. The clinic sees more than 450 patients per day and is equipped with modern adjusting tables, an x-ray department, clinical laboratory, departments of physical therapeutics and rehabilitation as well as a computerized tomography (CT scan) unit.

Craniosacral Therapy

Dr. John Upledger, an osteopathic physician and doctor of science, is credited with expanding upon the work of osteopathic physician Dr. William G. Sutherland in the 1900s in the development of Cranial Osteopathy. Upledger further developed, investigated and substantiated a new bodily system based on manipulation of the cranial bones of the skull, called the craniosacral system. This system is composed of the layered membranes of the brain and spinal cord, the cerebral spinal fluid within this membrane, and the structures within the membrane system that control the flow of the fluid. Like the cardiovascular and respiratory systems, the craniosacral system has its own rhythm and is thought to influence a wide variety of total body functions through its effect on the nervous and endocrine systems. Craniosacral therapists locate areas of restricted movement in the bones of the skull and the vertebrae and reestablish motion in these areas. This is done through very light hands-on manipulation of the bones of the skull, realigning them and freeing the membranes to allow freer circulation of cerebral spinal fluid from the cranium to the sacrum. Craniosacral therapy has been used to treat migraine headaches, temporomandibular joint problems, chronic fatigue, back pain, arthritis, gastrointestinal problems, acute systemic infections, depression, infant distress problems such as colic and asthma, and for immune system enhancement. It is practiced by osteopathic physicians, medical doctors, psychologists, dentists, nurses, chiropractors, physical and occupational therapists, and licensed body workers.

Organizations

253. The Cranial Academy (CA)
3500 DePauw Boulevard, Suite 1080, Indianapolis, IN 46268-1136
Telephone: 317-879-0713; Fax: 317-879-0718
Contact: Patricia Crampton, executive director

A component society of the American Academy of Osteopathy, The Cranial Academy is a membership organization established to ensure the continuation of the teaching of William G. Sutherland, D.O.

Services for the professional: Sponsors an annual conference; maintains member information directory and acts as a referral service; offers Category 1-A continuing medical education; conducts competency testing; offers scholarships; publishes a newsletter, books and brochures.

Services for the public: Provides referral service; distributes publications (brochures).

Publications: *The Cranial Letter,* quarterly newsletter, free to members; various books and brochures on cranial osteopathy (order list available).

254. New Mexico School of Natural Therapeutics (NMSNT)
117 Richmond N.E., Albuquerque, NM 87106
Telephone: 505-268-6870; Fax: 505-268-0818
See chapter 4: Massage—Schools.

255. The Upledger Institute (UI)
11211 Prosperity Farms Road, Palm Beach Gardens, FL 33410
Telephone: 407-622-4333; Fax: 407-622-4771

An educational and clinical resource center integrating holistic techniques with conventional health care approaches.

Services for the professional: Offers courses in craniosacral and other therapies; acts as an international networking system of Upledger-trained professionals; sponsors a research conference through the Upledger Foundation; publishes an alumni directory of advanced practitioners for patient referrals.

Services for the public: Conducts workshops; provides referrals to licensed health care practitioners.

Schools

256. Colorado Cranial Institute (CCI)
1080 Hawthorn Avenue, Boulder, CO 80304
Telephone: 303-449-0322
Contact: Peggy Daugherty, Telephone: 303-329-0413

Offers a variety of training programs which combine lectures and slides on the functional anatomy of the membrane system, cerebrospinal fluid and related information. Hands-on methods and sequences are demonstrated and followed by closely supervised practice. Programs are appropriate for those with a strong interest in developing hands-on skills and those who are already practicing bodywork or counseling.

257. National Institute of Craniosacral Studies (NICS)
7827 North Armenia Avenue, Tampa, FL 33604-3806
Telephone: 813-933-6335; Fax: 813-935-0583
Contact: Dallas Hancock, founder and president

Craniostructural Technique℠ uses gentle hands-on procedures which enable the therapist to adjust the alignment and function of the craniosacral system. The institute offers weekend workshops in Craniosacral Techniques℠ and Craniosacral Integration℠ at locations throughout the United States. Craniostructural Techniques℠ workshops cover craniosacral concepts, anatomy, physiology, muscle testing, and more. Craniostructural Integration℠ workshops cover advanced techniques and build upon information presented in the Techniques workshops. Programs are appropriate for health care professionals. Visa and MasterCard are accepted for payment of workshop fees.

258. New Mexico School of Natural Therapeutics
117 Richmond N.E., Albuquerque, NM 87106
Telephone: 505-268-6870; Fax: 505-268-0818
See chapter 4: Massage—Schools.

259. The Upledger Institute, Inc. (UI)
11211 Prosperity Farms Road, Palm Beach Gardens, FL 33410
Telephone: 407-622-4333; Fax: 407-622-4771

Founded in 1985 by the well-known osteopath John E. Upledger, the institute offers workshops and other programs in the field of craniosacral therapy. Courses are offered throughout the United States and are appropriate for doctors and therapists in all disciplines. Depending on the regulations of an individual's professional state board, attendance at workshops may be eligible for continuing education credits.

Treatment Centers/Referrals

See Craniosacral Therapy—Organizations for referrals to individual practitioners.

Osteopathy

This therapeutic system of medicine, founded by Dr. Andrew T. Still in the late 19th century, is based on a preventive and holistic approach to patient care. Doctors of osteopathy are physicians who have attended a four-year osteopathic medical school, completed a one-year internship, taken a possible two- to six-year additional residency in a specialty area such as internal medicine, and have passed a state medical board examination licensing them to practice in a particular state. Osteopathic treatment focuses on the musculoskeletal system, nutrition, environmental factors, and the patient as a whole in order to understand and effect the underlying causes of disease and support the body's natural process of healing. Osteopathic medicine may utilize hands-on manipulation and palpation in the diagnosis and treatment of disease, emphasizing the interdependence of all bodily systems on both structural and organic levels.

Organizations

260. American Academy of Osteopathy (AAO)
3500 DePauw Boulevard, Suite 1080, Indianapolis, IN 46268-1136
Telephone: 317-879-1881; Fax: 317-879-0563
Contact: Stephen J. Noone, CAE, director

A professional society for doctors of osteopathy, the academy's mission is to teach, explore, advocate and advance the study and application of the science and art of total health care management, emphasizing palpatory diagnosis and osteopathic manipulative treatment.

Services for the professional: Provides listing in annual directory; maintains an advocacy program for osteopathic manipulative medicine; promotes research; offers a fellowship program; acts as a referral service; promotes the development of osteopathic skills; provides access to the American Osteopathic Board of Special Proficiency in Osteopathic Manipulative Medicine (certifying board); offers discounts on registration at nine continuing medical education programs in OMM; publishes a journal, newsletter and yearbook.

Services for the public: Provides referrals to physicians who utilize osteopathic manipulative treatment as part of their practice of osteopathic medicine.

Publications: The AAO Journal, quarterly $25.00 (subscription) (reviewed under Manipulative Therapies—Journals and Newsletters); *The AAO Yearbook,* annual, price varies; *The AAO Newsletter,* 8 issues, $25.00 (subscription); *AAO Directory,* annual, $35.00.

261. The American Association of Colleges of Osteopathic Medicine (AACOM)

6110 Executive Boulevard, Suite 405, Rockville, MD 20852-3991
Telephone: 301-468-0990
Contact: Bonnie A. Saylor, director of member services

An association of the sixteen member osteopathic medical colleges in the United States dedicated to the advancement of osteopathic medical education.

Services: Keeps the osteopathic medical community up-to-date on key areas of osteopathic medical education through an extensive network of published data and analysis; monitors and interacts with the U.S. Congress and federal agencies; sponsors recruitment and retention programs; maintains a centralized application service to assist students interested in enrolling in a college of osteopathic medicine.

Publications: *Osteopathic Medical Education Brochure,* yearly, free in small quantities; *College Information Booklet,* yearly, $2.00; *Debts and Career Plans of Osteopathic Medical Students,* yearly, $13.00; *Annual Statistical Report,* yearly, $14.00; various brochures and booklets.

262. American Osteopathic Association (AOA)

142 East Ontario Street, Chicago, IL 60611-2864

Telephone: 312-280-5800; 800-621-1773; Fax: 312-280-5893
Contact: Robert E. Draba, Ph. D.

A membership organization for osteopathic physicians dedicated to the advancement of osteopathic medicine by supporting educational excellence, research and the delivery of quality and cost-effective health care; participates in the development of health care policy and the expansion of osteopathic medical care nationwide.

Services for the professional: Sponsors annual meeting and seminars; conducts a specialty certification program; maintains mandatory program of continuing medical education for members; sponsors research activities; maintains a physicians' placement service; inspects and accredits colleges and hospitals; maintains library and biographical archives on osteopathic medicine and history; awards grants and scholarships.

Services for the public: Publishes brochures on osteopathic referral sources, osteopathic medicine, and osteopathic medical education and licensing of doctors of osteopathy (including a listing of osteopathic medical colleges).

Publications: *American Osteopathic Association Yearbook and Directory,* annual, $76.00; *Journal of the American Osteopathic Association,* monthly, $20 (subscription) (reviewed under Manipulative Therapies—Journals and Newsletters).

Schools

There are sixteen osteopathic colleges, all of which offer four-year programs leading to the degree of doctor of osteopathy (D.O.). All of the schools require applicants to have completed a minimum of ninety credits toward a baccalaureate degree, with preference being given to those students who have already received their degrees. Application to any of the schools is made through the American Association of Colleges of Osteopathic Medicine Application Service (AACOMAS), 6110 Executive Boulevard, Suite 405, Rockville, MD 20852. Telephone: 301-468-2037.

263. Chicago College of Osteopathic Medicine (CCOM)
Midwestern University
555 31st Street, Downers Grove, IL 60515-8213
Telephone: 708-515-6472; 800-458-6253
Contact: Office of Admissions

Founded in 1900, CCOM is a college of Midwestern University. The four-year program begins with two years of a basic science curriculum and "hands-on" course work in osteopathic manipulative medicine, emergency medicine and early introduction to clinical medicine. The last two years include student rotations through urban, suburban and rural clinical clerkships. The college has its own clinical facilities, including the Chicago Osteopathic Hospital and Medical Center and the Olympia Fields Osteopathic Hospital and Medical Center. Financial aid is available through local, state, federal and private assistance programs.

264. College of Osteopathic Medicine of the Pacific (COMP)
309 East Second Street, College Plaza, Pomona, CA 91766-1889
Telephone: 909-623-6116; Fax: 909-629-7255
Contact: Office of Admissions

Founded in 1977, the college serves the primary health care needs of the western United States. The curriculum is a four-year, full-time academic and clinical program divided into three phases: introduction to basic science, correlated system teaching incorporating basic and clinical sciences in the study of organ systems, and clinical experience beginning in the third year. Students are required to complete twenty-two clinical rotations of four weeks each. Financial aid is available.

265. Kirksville College of Osteopathic Medicine (KCOM)
800 West Jefferson, Kirksville, MO 63501
Telephone: 816-626-2237; 800-626-KCOM, Ext. 2237
Contact: Office of Admissions

Dr. Andrew Taylor Still, the father of osteopathy, founded the first school of osteopathy in 1892, the American School of Osteopathy, now the Kirksville College of Osteopathic Medicine. The college prepares physicians for primary care or specialty training, although emphasizing primary care with a focus on practice in rural and underserved areas. In addition, the college has a strong biomedical and scientific research program and offers pre- and postdoctoral fellowship programs in academic and scientific medicine. The first two years of training consist of basic science courses and some clinical courses and experiences. In the third and fourth years, students conduct clinical rotations for approximately ninety weeks in all aspects of medicine at regional site training hospitals. Financial aid is available through scholarships, loans and other sources.

266. Lake Erie College of Osteopathic Medicine (LECOM)
1858 West Grandview Boulevard, Erie, PA 16509
Telephone: 814-866-6641
Contact: Office of Admissions

Founded in 1993, the LECOM program is comprised of three phases: phase one emphasizes introductory science course work; phase two focuses on pathology, pharmacology, neuroanatomy and the clinical aspects of the organ systems; phase three consists primarily of clinical training. Financial aid through federal loan programs is available.

267. Michigan State University College of Osteopathic Medicine (MSU-COM)

C110 East Fee Hall, Michigan State University, East Lansing, MI 48824-1316
Telephone: 517-353-7740; Fax: 517-353-9862
Contact: Office of Admissions

MSUCOM was the first state-assisted and university-based school of its kind, established by act of the Michigan legislature in 1969. It provides a four-year program leading to the doctor of osteopathy degree. In addition, it operates a joint D.O./Ph.D. degree in a medical scientist training program as well as masters and doctoral degrees in a graduate study program. The curriculum focuses on training family physicians, medical scientists and educators. It includes an eleven-semester program in extensive basic science, behavioral science and clinical education in an organ-systems approach. Clinical training is conducted in community hospitals, ambulatory care centers and physicians' offices. Approximately 85 percent of each entering class is from Michigan. Financial aid, primarily in the form of loans, is available.

268. New York College of Osteopathic Medicine (NYCOM) of New York Institute of Technology

Post Office Box 8000, Old Westbury, NY 11568-8000
Telephone: 516-626-6947
Contact: Office of Admissions

The NYCOM is a four-year program which emphasizes ambulatory primary care and osteopathic manipulative medicine. The program focuses on the health care problems of the inner city and rural communities. The first two years consist of study in the basic sciences and clinical sciences with computer-assisted instruction such as patient simulation software. Third- and fourth-year students rotate preceptorship-clinical clerkships at affiliated hospitals, physicians' offices and NYCOM ambulatory health care centers, with a rural clinical clerkship program for third-year students in upstate New York. Several other programs are available: a combined baccalaureate/osteopathic physician early admission program is offered to selected qualified students, allowing students to earn B.S./D.O. degrees in seven years rather than eight; a three-year accelerated program for newly emigrated physicians in osteopathic medicine; a college-coordinated post-doctoral program at affiliated hospitals including college-sponsored internship and residency programs approved by the American Osteopathic Association; and a fellowship program in osteopathic manipulative medicine established in 1982 based on outstanding interest and academic performance, adding an extra year to the program. Special effort is made to recruit women and members of minority groups, and financial aid is available through grants, scholarships and loans.

269. Nova Southeastern University College of Osteopathic Medicine (NSUCOM)

1750 N.E. 167th Street, North Miami Beach, FL 33162-3017
Telephone: 305-949-4000
Contact: Office of Admissions

Chartered in 1979, the college's four-year curriculum includes two years of basic sciences and didactic studies in the clinical sciences with an emphasis on community medicine, geriatrics, rural medicine and minority medicine. In the third year, hands-on training including clinical rotations in affiliated hopsitals, clinics, health centers and osteopathic medical offices is the focus of study. After twenty-two months of clinical training, students begin a senior internship seminar consisting of basic and clinical science correlations and preparation for internship, residency and practice. Financial aid is available, as are a limited number of part-time work assignments.

270. Ohio University College of Osteopathic Medicine (OUCOM)

102 Grosvenor Hall, Athens, OH 45701
Telephone: 614-593-2500
Contact: Office of Admissions, External Affairs

Focusing on training primary care physicians in the disciplines of family medicine, internal medicine and pediatrics, the college was created by the Ohio legislature in 1975. The curriculum is divided into three phases, each integrating the clinical and basic science aspects of medicine. Traditional classroom and laboratory instruction is complemented by the Continuum Primary Care curriculum, blending basic and clinical sciences with new technologies such as computer-simulated patient cases and interactive telemedicine. The college's centers for osteopathic regional education consist of a network of community and city hospitals, clinics and physicians' offices which offer third- and fourth-year students a wide range of clinical patient care experiences. The school provides professional financial aid counseling, strategy workshops and computerized budget planning;

awards scholarships; and assists students in finding alternative forms of financial assistance. It conducts several programs to encourage the enrollment of minorities, women and the educationally and economically disadvantaged.

271. Oklahoma State University
College of Osteopathic Medicine (OSUCOM)
111 West 17th Street, Tulsa, OK 74107-1898
Telephone: 918-582-1972; 800-677-1972
Contact: Admissions Office

Founded in 1972, OSUCOM's program focuses on educating primary care physicians for general practice. The curriculum emphasizes a student-centered approach and includes simulated clinical experiences, problem-based methods, small-group learning, and opportunities for independent study. Year one of the program covers basic biomedical sciences and clinical knowledge; in year two, students learn about specialized clinical care and procedures related to each body system; in years three and four, the emphasis is on actual clinical experience, including observation of patients in hospitals and clinics and supervised patient contact in small towns and rural areas throughout Oklahoma. For those interested in pursuing a career in medical research and/or academic medicine, a D.O/Ph.D. program is also available. Financial aid is available through loan, scholarship and work/study programs.

272. Philadelphia College of Osteopathic Medicine (PCOM)
4170 City Avenue, Philadelphia, PA 19131-1696
Telephone: 215-871-1000; 800-999-6998
Contact: Office of Admissions

Offers a curriculum which combines classroom instruction and clinical training throughout the four-year program. Courses in the basic and clinical sciences, as well as in subjects relating to current health care issues, are included. The college also offers a postdoctoral program consisting of rotating internships, and residency and fellowship programs in primary care, and medical and surgical subspecialties. In addition, five-year programs leading to the degree of D.O./M.B.A. and D.O/M.P.H are also available. Continuing education courses and weekend seminars are offered for practicing osteopathic physicians. Financial aid is available through a number of scholarship and loan programs.

273. University of Health Sciences, College of Osteopathic Medicine (UHS/COM)

2105 Independence Boulevard, Kansas City, MO 64124-2395
Telephone: 816-283-2000; 800-234-4UHS; Fax: 816-283-2303
Contact: Associate Dean for Student Affairs/Registrar

Course work, clinical and preceptorship training are the major components of this program which emphasizes training for a career in primary care. Federal and private financial aid programs are available.

274. University of Medicine and Dentistry of New Jersey (UMDNJ)

School of Osteopathic Medicine
Admissions Office, Suite 162, 1 Medical Center Drive, Academic Center, Stratford, NJ 08084
Telephone: 609-566-7050
Contact: Admissions Office

Offers a program of professional education consisting of academic instruction and clinical training. Year one focuses on the study of the basic sciences; year two stresses the integration of the basic sciences and clinical medicine; years three and four emphasize the development of clinical competence through hands-on experience. Approximately 87 percent of the student body are New Jersey residents. A variety of scholarship, loan and work/study programs are available.

275. University of New England (UNECOM)

College of Osteopathic Medicine
11 Hills Beach Road, Biddeford, ME 04005
Telephone: 207-283-0171
Contact: Office of Admissions and Enrollment

The curriculum for this program covers basic and clinical sciences, human behavior and community medicine. Course work, preceptorships and clinical training are all components of the program. Preference for admission is given to applicants residing in New England states. A wide variety of financial aid programs is available.

276. University of North Texas (UNT)

Texas College of Osteopathic Medicine
Health Science Center at Fort Worth
3500 Camp Bowie Boulevard, Fort Worth, TX 76107-2699
Telephone: 817-735-2204; 800-535-TCOM; Fax: 817-735-5098
Contact: Jane Hall Absher, associate director, Office of Medical Student Admissions

UNT's program consists of classroom instruction, specialized workshops, preceptorships and clinical rotations. Ninety percent of each entering class is comprised of Texas residents; the other ten percent may include individuals from out-of-state. Some financial aid is available.

277. University of Osteopathic Medicine and Health Sciences
College of Osteopathic Medicine and Surgery (UOMHS/COMS)
3200 Grand Avenue, Des Moines, IA 50312
Telephone: 515-271-1400; 800-240-2767
Contact: Admissions Office

Offers a program which consists of two and one-half years of lecture and laboratory study and one and one-half years of clinical training. The curriculum emphasizes the teaching of sciences and clinical medicine in relation to preventive care and treatment of the whole person. Financial aid programs, including federal and private loans, scholarships and work/study, are available.

278. West Virginia School of Osteopathic Medicine (WVSOM)
400 North Lee Street, Lewisburg, WV 24901
Telephone: 304-645-6270
Contact: Admissions Office

This program consists of two years of preclinical training and two years of clinical rotation, and focuses on training family physicians to work in rural West Virginia and Appalachia. Preference for admission is given to students coming from these areas. A full range of financial aid programs is available.

Treatment Centers/Referrals

To locate a doctor of osteopathy in a specific geographic area, the American Academy of Osteopathy provides a list of state referral sources consisting of state osteopathic medical associations, hospitals that are members of the American Osteopathic Hospital Association, colleges and foundations. In addition, the American Osteopathic Association publishes an annual *Yearbook and Directory of Osteopathic Physicians* (ISSN 0084-358X) which includes an alphabetical and geographical listing of U.S. and foreign osteopathic physicians as well as osteopathic health care facilities. See Osteopathy—Organizations for the address and telephone number of each of these organizations.

CHAPTER 4: BODYWORK

Acupressure/Shiatsu

The ancient healing art of shiatsu or acupressure was developed in China and Japan more than 5,000 years ago. Using the same points on the body into which acupuncture needles are inserted, acupressure stimulates these points with finger pressure, releasing muscle tensions that obstruct the free flow of energy within the body. As these tensions are released, blood and the nutrients carried by the blood are able to flow more freely, and are believed to improve circulation and speed healing of the affected area. Acupressure can be self-administered to relieve pain caused by tension-related problems such as headaches, backaches and neck tension. In addition, when performed regularly, acupressure can be used as a preventive measure to enable the body to maintain good health and vitality.

Organizations

279. International Macrobiotic Shiatsu Society (IMSS)
1122 "M" Street, Eureka, CA 95501-2442
Telephone: 707-445-2290; Fax: 707-445-2391
Contact: Patrick McCarty, director

A membership organization based on the teachings of Shizuko Yamamoto on shiatsu and macrobiotics.

Services for the professional: Courses to train as a macrobiotic shiatsu practitioner are available at different locations throughout the United States.

Services for the public: Offers a series of seminars to introduce the public to shiatsu and macrobiotics.

Publications: *Healthways*, newsletter, three times a year, $20.00 (subscription) (reviewed under Acupressure/Shiatsu—Journals and Newsletters).

280. Jin Shin Do® Foundation for Bodymind Acupressure™ (JSDFBA)
366 California Avenue, Suite 16, Palo Alto, CA 94306
Telephone: 415-328-1811
Contact: Iona Marsaa Teeguarden, M.A., director

A trade organization founded to promote the art of Jin Shin Do® Acupressure (JSD). Serves as a networking vehicle for authorized JSD teachers, facilitates research, and provides the public and professionals with informational materials.

Services for the professional: Offers workshops and training programs (see Acupressure/Shiatsu—Schools); publishes teaching materials; provides a listing in membership directory; publishes newsletter.

Services for the public: Offers introductory classes (see Acupressure/Shiatsu—Schools); sells products (see Acupressure/Shiatsu—Product Suppliers); provides referrals to JSD teachers and acupressurists through the membership directory.

Publications: *Acupressure News,* annual, $2.50; *Jin Shin Do Foundation Directory of Certified Teachers and Practitioners*, $1.00; *Jin Shin Do Acupressure Newsletter,* distributed only to authorized JSD teachers.

Schools

281. Acupressure Institute (AI)
1533 Shattuck Avenue, Berkeley, CA 94709
Telephone: 510-845-1059; Fax: 510-845-1496
Contact: Joella Caskey, administrator; Michael Reed Gach, president

Offers a number of acupressure training programs: a 150-hour basic training program in acupressure massage, leading to certification as an acupressure massage technician; several 200-hour acupressure specialization programs; and an 850-hour acupressure therapy program, which is appropriate for students who want to become recognized acupressure professionals, enabling graduates to work with other health care practitioners. All these programs may be pursued on a part-time basis or through full-time intensives. The institute also offers advanced training to graduates of other massage schools.

282. Acupressure-Acupuncture Institute (AAI)
9835 Sunset Drive, Suite 206, Miami, FL 33176
Telephone: 305-595-9500; Fax: 305-274-0675
Contact: Nancy Browne, administrative director

Offers an eight-month, 500-hour massage therapy program, particularly appropriate for those who want to specialize in shiatsu, leading to a diploma in massage therapy and eligibility for the Florida state licensing examination. See also chapter 2: Chinese Medicine/Acupuncture—Schools for information about the institute's Acupuncture Physician Program.

283. Boulder School of Massage Therapy (BSMT)
3285 30th Street, Boulder, CO 80301-1451
Telephone: 800-442-5131; Fax: 303-541-9068
See Massage—Schools.

284. G-Jo Institute (GJI)
Post Office Box 8060, Hollywood, FL 33084
Telephone: 305-791-1562
Contact: Michael Blate, executive director; Gail Watson, administrative director

Offers certification as a Master of G-Jo acupressure through a correspondence course in G-Jo, the simplest form of acupressure. The course consists of training manuals, a training videotape and audiocassette. Students who complete the Master of G-Jo acupressure certification test receive a certificate of master from the institute.

285. Jin Shin Do® Foundation for Bodymind Acupressure™
366 California Avenue, Suite 16, Palo Alto, CA 94306
Telephone: 415-328-1811
Contact: Iona Marsaa Teeguarden, director

For those interested in becoming registered Jin Shin Do® acupressurists or authorized Jin Shin Do® teachers, as well as other serious students, the foundation offers Jin Shin Do[R] BodyMind acupressure classes including Module I, a 150-hour beginning course of Jin Shin Do® theories and techniques; Module II, a 100-hour intermediate program of modality technique and practice; and Module III, a 70-hour program offered periodically, which is required for teacher authorization and trademark licensure. For the lay public, short introductory classes are also available.

286. Jin Shin Jyutsu®, Inc.
8719 East San Alberto Drive, Scottsdale, AZ 85258
Telephone: 602-998-9331; Fax: 602-998-9335
Contact: David Burmeister, director

Offers seminars in the art of Jin Shin Jyutsu®, a form of bodywork that releases the tensions in one's energy pathways that can cause various symptoms in the body.

287. New Mexico School of Natural Therapeutics (NMSNT)
117 Richmond N.E., Albuquerque, NM 87106
Telephone: 505-268-6870; Fax: 505-268-0818
See Massage—Schools.

288. The Ohashiatsu Institute (OI)
12 West 27th Street, New York, NY 10001
Telephone: 212-684-4190; Fax: 212-447-5819
Contact: Cynthia Lucash, registrar

Offers a program that trains students in Ohashiatsu, a method of bodywork which combines traditional Japanese shiatsu with exercise, meditation and eastern healing philosophy. The curriculum is comprised of three, two-part levels: beginning, intermediate and advanced, plus courses in anatomy and oriental diagnosis, and consists of lectures, demonstrations, practice meditation and exercises. Courses are taught at the institute's headquarters in New York City as well as at branch schools and other locations throughout the United States. A work/study option is available. Upon completion of this program, students may enroll in the postgraduate training program in order to become certified Ohashi instructors or consultants. Also offered is a series of one-day and weekend enrichment courses, some of which are appropriate for professionals who have not previously taken classes at the institute. Yoga for Ohashiatsu and T'ai Chi Ch'uan for Ohashiatsu classes are available, and the institute is also interested in cosponsoring other appropriate programs.

289. The Reilly School of Massotherapy (RSM)
67th Street and Atlantic Avenue, Post Office Box 595, Virginia Beach, VA 23451
Telephone: 804-428-0446; Fax: 804-422-4631
See Massage—Schools.

290. Santa Barbara College of Oriental Medicine (SBCOM)
1919 State Street, Suite 204, Santa Barbara, CA 93101
Telephone: 805-682-9594; Fax: 805-682-1864
See chapter 2: Chinese Medicine/Acupuncture—Schools.

Treatment Centers/Referrals

See Acupressure/Shiatsu—Organizations for referrals to individual practitioners.

291. The American Foundation of Traditional Chinese Medicine
505 Beach Street, San Francisco, CA 94133
Telephone: 415-776-0502; Fax: 415-776-9053
See chapter 2: Chinese Medicine/Acupuncture—Treatment Centers/Referrals.

292. East West Academy of Healing Arts
450 Sutter Street, Suite 210, San Francisco, CA 94108
Telephone: 415-788-2227
See chapter 2: Chinese Medicine/Acupuncture—Treatment Centers/Referrals.

293. Emperor's College of Traditional Oriental Medicine
1807-B Wilshire Boulevard, Santa Monica, CA 90403
Telephone: 310-453-8300; Fax: 310-829-3838
See chapter 2: Chinese Medicine/Acupuncture—Treatment Centers/Referrals.

Product Suppliers

294. Acupressure Institute
1533 Shattuck Avenue, Berkeley, CA 94709
Telephone: 510-845-1059 (In California); 800-442-2232 (All Others); Fax: 510-845-1496
Credit Cards: Visa, MasterCard, Discover, Others

Through its *Hands-On Health Care Catalog*, the institute sells instructional videotapes, visualization audiotapes, books, charts, equipment and other products for personal healing.

295. Jin Shin Do® Foundation for Bodymind Acupressure™
366 California Avenue, Suite 16, Palo Alto, CA 94306
Telephone: 415-328-1811
Credit Cards: None

Offers books, booklets, charts, audiotapes and videotapes on Jin Shin Do® acupressure and Taoist meditation and exercise techniques, along with other products such as the "acu-releaser," adjustable wooden balls for self-acupressure of the back.

296. The Ohashiatsu Institute
12 West 27th Street, New York, NY 10001
Telephone: 212-684-4190; Fax: 212-447-5819
Credit Cards: Visa, MasterCard

The institute runs a bookstore which sells Ohashiatsu books, videotapes, charts, clothing and related products. Items may also be purchased by mail.

Applied Kinesiology (AK)

Developed in the 1960s by chiropractor Dr. George Goodhart, applied kinesiology (AK) is a diagnostic system using muscle testing, posture and gait analysis, range of motion, palpation, and motion analysis to evaluate an individual's structural, biochemical, emotional and mental condition. AK is used with other diagnostic methods by health professionals trained in clinical diagnosis, such as chiropractors, osteopaths, dentists and medical doctors. Because specific muscle functions are seen to be related to different body systems, AK can be used to identify problems that involve muscle, nerve, nutritional, energetic, vascular, and lymphatic imbalances.

Organizations

297. International College of Applied Kinesiology (ICAK)
Post Office Box 905, Lawrence, KS 66044-0905
Telephone: 913-542-1801; Fax: 913-542-1746
Contact: Terry Kay Underwood, executive director

A nonprofit membership organization for health care professionals with a license to diagnose, including chiropractors, dentists, medical doctors, naturopaths, osteopaths, podiatrists and Ph.D.s in psychology. ICAK's goal is to further the knowledge of professionals in the practice of AK through professional development and advance education in health care.

Services for the professional: Offers educational programs on basic, intermediate and advanced levels; provides a listing of comprehensive educational programs qualifying for continuing education credits; awards diplomate status in AK; sponsors an annual meeting and regional meetings; conducts clinical research and public relations activities; provides a listing in annual membership directory for referrals; publishes a newsletter, proceedings and other materials.

Services for the public: Provides referrals to practitioners and information on AK; sells various publications.

Publications: *ICAK-USA News Update,* quarterly newsletter, free to members; *A.K. Sports,* semiannual newsletter, free to members; *A.K. Review,* collection of selected papers, free to members, $30.00 nonmembers; *Proceedings,* annual, free to member doctors, $25.00 to other members; *Index of Collected Papers,* free to members; *Membership Directory,* annual, one copy free to members, $14.00 additional copy for members, $16.00 nonmembers; *A.K. Review,* annual journal, free to members, $15.00 nonmembers.

298. Touch for Health Foundation (THF)

Post Office Box 5547, Sherman Oaks, CA 91413

Telephone: 818-509-9945; 800-826-0364; 213-340-4154 (international); Fax: 818-509-9946

Contact: Arthur Smukler, director of marketing

A not-for-profit foundation promoting research, funding education and gathering and reporting information on health promotion and touch healing, particularly in the Touch for Health methods.

Services for the professional: Offers educational programs in Touch for Health for chiropractors, massage therapists and physical therapists; the International College of Kinesiology based in Zurich, Switzerland, certifies instructors through faculty members in twenty-five countries and serves as a forum for research and presentation of papers at its annual meeting; publishes and distributes a training manual, charts, and a videotape used in training and educating the public.

Services for the public: Provides information on available courses for lay people.

Publications: TFH Foundation Newsletter, quarterly, $15-$50 (subscriptions). Twenty-five associations worldwide also publish newsletters or magazines, various books, charts, videotapes and reference packets (see Applied Kinesiology—Product Suppliers).

Schools

299. International College of Applied Kinesiology (ICAK)

Post Office Box 905, Lawrence, KS 66044-0905

Telephone: 913-542-1801; Fax: 913-542-1746

See Applied Kinesiology—Organizations.

300. The Reilly School of Massotherapy (RSM)

67th Street and Atlantic Avenue, Post Office Box 595, Virginia Beach, VA 23451

Telephone: 804-428-0446; Fax: 804-422-4631
See Massage—Schools.

301. The Siskiyou Essence Company (SEC)
Post Office Box 353, 485 East Main Street, Suite 3, Ashland, OR 97520
Telephone: 503-482-5311
Contact: Debra Hurt

Offers a training program in specialized kinesiology, also known as muscle testing, which is used to discover emotional, psychological or energy imbalances. Also offered are introductory classes in vibrational healing and the Chakras. See also chapter 5: Energy Medicine—Schools.

302. Touch for Health Foundation (THF)
Post Office Box 5547, Sherman Oaks, CA 91413
Telephone: 818-509-9945; 800-826-0364; 213-340-4154 (international); Fax: 818-509-9946
See Applied Kinesiology—Organizations.

Treatment Centers/Referrals

See Applied Kinesiology—Organizations for referrals to individual practitioners.

Product Suppliers

303. Touch for Health Foundation
Post Office Box 5547, Sherman Oaks, CA 91413
Telephone: 818-509-9945; 800-826-0364; 213-340-4154 (international); Fax: 818-509-9946
Credit Cards: Visa, MasterCard

Sells Touch for Health-related educational materials including books, charts, reference packets, videotapes and related products.

Hellerwork

Joseph Heller, first president of the Rolf Institute, developed Hellerwork in the mid-1970s. It consists of three aspects: deep connective tissue massage focusing on the fascia (the tissue that surrounds all muscles), movement re-education, and emotional/mental work with the client. Hellerwork consists of a series of eleven sessions, approximately ninety minutes long, each focusing on a different area of the body in a prearranged sequence. It seeks to realign the body, allow freer and more effective movement, release vitality, increase sense of self, and enhance openness and awareness.

Schools

304. California Hellerwork Training
2211 Corinth Avenue, Suite 204, Los Angeles, CA 90064
Telephone: 310-477-8151; 800-484-9988

Offers workshops and intensives in Hellerwork which may be taken individually or as part of the Hellerwork practitioner training program.

305. Hellerwork, Inc.
406 Berry Street, Mount Shasta, CA 96067
Telephone: 916-926-2500; 800-392-3900; Fax: 916-926-6839

Offers a 1,250-hour certification program in Hellerwork practitioner Training. The program consists of six fourteen-day intensives and an eighteen-month independent study. Intensives are offered throughout the year at various locations across the United States. A four-phase special training for health care professionals is also offered. A geographic directory to Hellerwork practitioners is available.

Massage

Massage therapy uses hands-on techniques to manipulate the body's soft tissue through touch, movement and pressure. It is used to treat a wide range of conditions from specific physical problems and injuries to generalized management of stress and tension. Massage is appropriate for all ages with specific techniques for infants, pregnant women, and other groups. It is thought to influence various bodily systems, including blood supply to the tissues, energy levels, elimination of toxic waste stored in muscles, functioning of the immune system, posture and flexibility, and blood pressure. In addition, it may be used to address local problems such as carpal tunnel syndrome, backache, sprained ligaments and pulled muscles.

Organizations

306. American Massage Therapy Association (AMTA)
820 Davis Street, Suite 100, Evanston, IL 60201-4444

Telephone: 708-864-0123; Fax: 708-864-1178
Contact: Keith A. Miller, director of communications

A national professional membership association which promotes the practice of massage therapy through public awareness, professional development, maintenance of high ethical and educational standards, and involvement with legislation and regulation.

Services for the professional: Conducts an accreditation/approval process for massage schools; provides continuing education and advanced certification programs; provides funding and assistance in research, education and voluntary outreach programs; maintains national public relations and legislation programs; acts as a central networking resource; sponsors spring national education conference and fall national convention; publishes a newsletter, journal, annual membership registry, promotional and educational brochures, books, pamphlets, and audiotapes and videotapes.

Services for the public: Provides information on training, national referrals to qualified practitioners and general information on massage therapy (national consumer referral service telephone number 708-864-0123).

Publications: *Massage Therapy Journal*, quarterly, free to members, $20 (subscription) (reviewed under Massage—Journals and Newsletters); *Hands On*, quarterly newsletter ($15 of annual dues allocated to subscription to newsletter); products and publication guide, free to members.

307. Associated Bodywork and Massage Professionals (ABMP)
28677 Buffalo Park Road, Evergreen, CO 80439-7347
Telephone: 303-674-8478; 800-458-2267; Fax: 303-674-0859
Contact: Sherri Williamson, president; Valerie Cass, publications manager

An international professional membership organization affiliated with over twenty-five massage and bodywork organizations worldwide. ABMP promotes ethical practices, protects the rights of practitioners, educates the public on the benefits of massage and bodywork and provides a variety of services and benefits to its members.

Services for the professional: Provides liability insurance policy; acts as an international referral service; offers discounts on massage and bodywork supplies, education and services; promotes international networking; actively works with legislative, municipal and regulatory committees; publishes various handbooks, directories and a journal.

Services for the public: Provides referrals to practitioners by geographic area; offers career information (directory of schools, organizations and state boards); provides information on various techniques.

Publications: Successful Business Handbook (free with membership); *Massage and Bodywork Yellow Pages*, a resource guide for products and services (free to members); *Touch Training Directory,* information on approximately 500 schools and seminars, state massage boards and alternative health organizations internationally, free to members, $12.95 to public; *Massage and Bodywork Quarterly,* quarterly magazine, free to members, $15 (subscription) (reviewed under Massage—Journals and Newsletters).

308. International Association of Infant Massage (IAIM)

U.S. Chapter
2350 Bowen Road, Post Office Box 438, Elma, NY 14059-0438
Telephone: 716-652-9789; 800-248-5432; Fax: 716-652-1990
Contact: Christine M. Weber, office manager; Mindy Zlotnick, outreach coordinator

A nonprofit membership association dedicated to promoting nurturing touch and communication between parents, caregivers and infants through support of training, education and research.

Services for the professional: Conducts a four-day certification course for nurses, massage therapists, social workers, parent advocates, childbirth educators, doctors and midwives working with healthy babies as well as special needs populations; offers inservices and demonstrations for professional groups and conferences; supplies material and audiovisual presentations; provides consultation services.

Services for the public: Offers parent/baby classes ages three weeks to crawling, as well as classes for older infants, children and teenagers; private instruction available; provides referrals to practitioners and instructors through membership directory.

Publications: *Gentle Touch Warehouse* catalog, quarterly, free with membership; *Tender Loving Care Newsletter,* quarterly, free with membership; membership roster.

309. International Myomassethics Federation, Inc. (IMF)

17172 Bolsa Chica, #60, Huntington Beach, CA 92649
Telephone: 800-433-4463
Contact: Sherry L. Lynch, president

A professional membership association of individuals practicing various forms of therapeutic touch. IMF's purpose is to improve the image and quality of massage services, educate the public on the variety, means and benefits of therapeutic touch, and establish and foster high personal and professional standards of practice.

Services for the professional: Sponsors an annual conference; offers professional insurance programs through affiliation with Associated Bodywork and Massage Professionals; offers certification programs in myomassology and related fields for individuals and schools; provides continuing education programs and resource information; promotes professional networking opportunities; maintains affiliations with state organizations; publishes a quarterly magazine.

Services for the public: Provides professional referrals for massage and bodywork.

Publications: *Intra-Myomassethics Forum* or *The Forum*, quarterly, free with membership.

310. National Association of Nurse Massage Therapists (NANMT)

147 Windward Avenue, Osprey, FL 34229
Telephone: 813-966-6288; Fax: 407-625-5995
Contact: Barbara Harris, B.A., R.N., L.M.T., president

A national, not-for-profit professional membership organization for nurses and health care professionals who practice massage and other therapeutic forms of bodywork. The association is committed to promoting and integrating these modalities as a complementary therapy to technological procedures in nursing and medicine, promoting nurse massage therapists as specialists within the nursing profession, and promoting massage and bodywork as an adjunct to the existing health care system.

Services for the professional: Maintains a referral system and provides information; offers continuing education opportunities; sponsors national conventions and conferences; actively participates in advocacy efforts and monitoring of legislation; provides listing in membership directory; promotes networking with other nurse massage therapists; supports education of the medical community and the general public about bodywork therapies; publishes newsletter.

Services for the public: Provides referrals and information.

Publications: *Nurse's Touch*, quarterly newsletter, free to members; *Membership Directory*, annual, free to members, $75/nonmembers.

311. United States Sports Massage Federation (USSMF)

Sports Massage Training Institute
2156 Newport Boulevard, Costa Mesa, CA 92657
Telephone: 714-642-0735; Fax: 714-642-1729
Contact: M. K. Hungerford, Ph.D.; Kate Montgomery, secretary

A professional membership organization dedicated to promoting peace through sports, continuing education, and community service, increasing public awareness of sports massage, exchanging ideas with other countries, networking, and meeting the needs of the sporting community through the development of sports massage programs.

Services for the professional: Maintains affiliations with professional sports massage therapy organizations; offers continuing education; maintains a national registry of sports massage therapists; offers community services and volunteer programs; promotes networking with other massage and health professionals; publishes federation newsletter and journal.

Services for the public: Provides referrals to sports massage therapists for coaches and athletes.

Publications: *Sports Massage Journal,* quarterly, free with membership; *Beyond Sports Medicine,* monograph, $59.95; *USCMF/ISMF Newsletter,* periodic, free with membership.

Schools

Associated Bodywork and Massage Professionals publishes the *Touch Training Directory,* which provides information on approximately 500 schools and seminars for massage training. The American Massage Therapy Association (AMTA) provides a list of AMTA-affiliated schools, state boards and chapters. (See Massage—Organizations for both.) The Commission on Massage Training Accreditation/Approval, an independent affiliate of the AMTA, sets standards for professional massage therapy education in the United States and Canada.

312. Boulder School of Massage Therapy (BSMT)
3285 30th Street, Boulder, Co 80301-1451
Telephone: 800-442-5131; Fax: 303-541-9068
Contact: Paula Glaser, marketing and recruitment director; Ginger Leeper, registrar

Offers a certification program in massage therapy consisting of 1,000 hours of classroom training, clinical and field experience for persons interested in becoming massage therapists. The school teaches four major approaches to touch therapy: shiatsu, Swedish massage, integrative massage and myofascial therapy. Also offers continuing education courses for practicing massage therapists and other health care practitioners; a hospital-based 360-hour massage therapy advanced course; and beginning courses in basic massage, shiatsu and reflexology. The school has received program approval by the Commission on Massage Training Accreditation/Approval. Financial aid through federal grants and loans is available to qualified students enrolled in the certification program.

313. International Professional School of Bodywork (IPSB)

1366 Hornblend Street, San Diego, CA 92126
Telephone: 619-272-4142; Fax: 619-272-4772
Contact: Barbara Clark; Lana David

Offers several programs in massage therapy: 1) a 120-hour, twelve-week certificate program in massage technician training, completion of which enables an individual to apply for entry-level jobs in licensed massage establishments and health spas or work for holistic health practitioners, chiropractors and physicians. May also be taken as a three-week intensive course; 2) a 150-hour professional massage training program, completion of which qualifies the individual to apply for the massage technician permit in San Diego and many other areas. Requires prior completion of the 120-hour program; 3) a nine-month, 600-hour massage therapy training, which consists of two diploma programs in massage therapy training, one each in western methods and eastern methods. This program meets national organizational standards; 4) a one-year to eighteen-month, 1,000-hour holistic health practitioners' training, which consists of four diploma programs specializing in holistic health. This program also meets national organizational standards, and completion qualifies graduates to practice massage therapy in most states. In addition, the school offers certificate programs in oriental massage, sports massage, Thailand massage, somato-emotional integration, structural integration and neuromuscular therapy. Courses for the general public are offered in such areas as Alexander technique, Feldenkrais Awareness Through Movement, foot reflexology and others. The school's curriculum is approved by the American Massage Therapy Association Commission on Massage Training Accreditation/Approval and as a private postsecondary educational institution by the state of California.

314. The New Center for Wholistic Health Education & Research (NCWHER)

6801 Jericho Turnpike, Syosset, NY 11791
Telephone: 516-364-0808; Fax: 516-364-0989
Contact: Barbara Lawrence

Offers an eighteen-month, 1,072-hour diploma program in massage therapy, consisting of academic course work and practical training. The program is accredited by the American Massage Therapy Association Commission on Massage Training Accreditation/Approval and by the Accrediting Council for Continuing Education and Training. The program is a candidate for approval by the New York State Education Department to grant an associate's degree in this area. Financial aid is available through a variety of grant and loan programs. The center also offers diploma programs in acupuncture and in oriental herbal medicine (see also chapter 2: Chinese Medicine/Acupuncture—Schools) and a program in wholistic nursing (see also chapter 1: General—Schools).

315. New Mexico Academy of Healing Arts
Post Office Box 932, Santa Fe, NM 87504
Telephone: 505-982-6271; Fax: 505-988-2621
Contact: Registrar

Offers 650-hour, 1,000-hour and 1,200-hour programs in massage certification, all of which are approved by the American Massage Therapy Association's Commission on Massage Training Accreditation/Approval. Also offers polarity certification programs accredited by the American Polarity Therapy Association. Students of all programs are required to work a substantial number of hours in the student-staffed clinic which provides low-cost bodywork services to the Santa Fe community. Continuing education courses and introductory courses for the general public are also offered. (See also chapter 5: Polarity Therapy—Schools.)

316. New Mexico School of Natural Therapeutics
117 Richmond N.E., Albuquerque, NM 87106
Telephone: 505-268-6870; Fax: 505-268-0818
Contact: Alison Owens, administrator

Offers a 750-hour course in natural therapeutics which focuses on therapeutic massage and polarity therapy and also includes shiatsu, reflexology, sports massage, herbology and more. Six-month courses begin in February and August; a part-time evening program begins each May. The program is approved by the American Massage Therapy Association Commission on Massage Training Accreditation/Approval. Continuing education programs are offered throughout the year in such areas as craniosacral therapy, advanced polarity, and traditional Chinese medical diagnosis. A 30-hour sports massage course, which fulfills American Massage Therapy Association sports massage certification requirements, is offered annually. (See also chapter 5: Polarity Therapy—Schools.)

317. Pacific College of Oriental Medicine (PCOM)
7445 Mission Valley Road, Suite 105, San Diego, CA 92108
Telephone: 619-574-6909; 800-729-0941; Fax: 619-574-6641
Contact: David Orman, admissions counselor

Offers a number of certificate programs: a 112-hour massage technician program leading to eligibility for a massage license in San Diego; a 555-hour massage therapist program, which includes the 112 hours required for the massage technician program, and consists of classroom instruction and supervised clinical work; a 1,115-hour holistic health practitioner program, which includes all course work forming the massage technician and massage therapist programs, as well as additional courses and supervised clinical work; a tui na (Chinese physical therapy massage) program; a Chinese health and exercise program; and an oriental body therapist program. (See also chapter 2: Chinese Medicine/Acupuncture—Schools.)

318. The Reilly School of Massotherapy (RSM)

67th Street and Atlantic Avenue, Post Office Box 595, Virginia Beach, VA 23451
Telephone: 804-428-0446; Fax: 804-422-4631
Contact: Gary Blavert, director

A department of the Association for Research and Enlightenment (ARE), the school teaches Swedish-style massage techniques, based on the work of Dr. Harold Reilly and the Edgar Cayce readings. Two courses of study are offered: a 225-hour program which is completed over an eight-month period, and a 600-hour program consisting of two three-month semesters. Part-time enrollment in the 600-hour program is also available. Completion of these programs leads to either a certificate in massage therapy for the 225-hour program or a diploma in massage therapy for the 600-hour course. The school also offers a 105-hour course in basic and intermediate Jin Shin Do. In addition, beginner's massage workshops and special workshops in areas such as Reiki, Jin Shin Do, applied kinesiology and biofeedback are offered throughout the year. Limited financial assistance for the two massage programs is available.

319. Sarasota School of Natural Healing Arts (SSNHA)

8216 South Tamiami Trail, Sarasota, FL 34238
Telephone: 800-966-7117; Fax: 813-966-4414
Contact: Isabelle Dunkeson, director

Offers a 600-hour program in massage therapy and a 2,700-hour program in acupuncture and traditional Chinese medicine, both of which are intended to prepare students to take the Florida state board examination to work as professionals in these fields. The school's employment placement service provides job referral and placement assistance for its graduates. Educational classes in yoga, T'ai Chi Chuan, finger pressure treatment for stress, and reflexology are offered to the lay public periodically throughout the year.

320. Somatic Learning Associates (SLA)
8950 Villa La Jolla Drive, #2162, La Jolla, CA 92037
Telephone: 619-436-0418; Fax: 619-457-3615
Contact: Kate Jordan

Offers an advanced certification program in massage therapy, posture and movement education for pregnancy, the post-partum period, and infancy, appropriate for massage and physical therapists, midwives, nurses and childbirth educators. Has also compiled an annotated bibliography, *Bodywork for the Childbearing Year,* and sells books on the same subject.

321. Swedish Institute, Inc. (SI)
School of Massage Therapy and Allied Health Sciences
226 West 26th Street, New York, NY 10001
Telephone: 212-924-5900; Fax: 212-924-7600
Contact: Jean M. Eckhardt, co-director

Offers a three-trimester, 657-hour program of Swedish massage training, leading to a diploma and eligibility for licensing examinations in New York and several other states. The curriculum is accredited by the Career College Association, a national accrediting agency, by the American Massage Therapy Association and the Alliance of Massage Therapists. Federal grants and loans are available.

322. Touch Research Institute (TRI)
University of Miami Medical School, Department of Pediatrics (D-820)
Post Office Box 016820, Miami, FL 33101
Telephone: 305-547-6781; Fax: 305-547-6488
Contact: Tiffany Field, director

The first center in the world for basic and applied research on the sense of touch, the institute also develops training and education programs for scientists, health care professionals and the general public. Their work/study program provides university undergraduates and high school students with training in a variety of career opportunities related to the study of touch.

Treatment Centers/Referrals

See Massage—Organizations for referrals to individual practitioners.

Product Suppliers

323. Best of Nature
Post Office Box 3164, Long Branch, NJ 07740
Telephone: 908-747-2874 (in New Jersey); 800-228-6457 (all others)
Credit Cards: Major credit cards

Nationally distributes bodywork products, including massage oils, blends and lotions, massage tables, yoga mats and accessories, books, audiotapes, compact discs, and charts, etc.

324. Blue Ridge Tables, Inc.
South Industrial Park, Route 6, Box 490, Corinth, MS 38834
Telephone: 800-447-2723
Credit Cards: Visa, MasterCard, Discover

Sells portable and stationary bodywork tables, a massage chair, face rest, travel bags, bolsters, and arm and foot extensions.

325. Body Support Systems
Post Office Box 337, Ashland, OR 97520
Telephone: 503-488-1172; 800-448-2400; Fax: 503-488-5959
Credit Cards: Visa, MasterCard, American Express

Manufactures and sells the bodyCushion, a support system used to alleviate pressure on the neck, shoulders, lower back, etc. Also sells related products such as portable tables, bodyCushion covers and instructional videotapes. Appropriate for use by massage therapists, acupuncturists, chiropractors and other health care professionals.

326. Custom Craftworks
1030 Tyinn Street, #5, Eugene, OR 97402
Telephone: 503-345-2712; 800-627-2387; Fax: 503-345-4377
Credit Cards: Visa, MasterCard, Discover

Makes and sells portable, stationary and electric lift tables and related accessories for use by bodywork professionals.

327. Colorado Healing Arts Products
4635 Broadway (Street Address), Boulder, CO 80303; Post Office Box 2247 (Mailing Address), Boulder, CO 80306
Telephone: 800-728-2426
Credit Cards: Visa, MasterCard, Discover

Manufactures massage and therapy equipment, as well as a variety of other massage and bodywork products such as oils, massage table sheets and travel covers. These items are also sold locally through their retail operation, The Massage Store. Products are primarily appropriate for massage therapists, chiropractors, physical therapists and nurse massage therapists. Information on how to select a massage table is available upon request.

328. Gentle Touch

See International Association of Infant Massage, below.

329. Golden Ratio Bodyworks

Post Office Box 440, Emigrant, MT 59027
Telephone: 406-333-4578 (Customer Service); 800-796-0612 (Orders only); Fax: 406-333-4769
Credit Cards: Visa, MasterCard, American Express, Discover

Sells bodywork tools for use by healing professionals, including massage tools and equipment, pads, packs, oils, creams and lotions, as well as anatomical charts, books, videotapes, audiotapes and compact discs.

330. Golden Ratio Woodworks

Highway 89, Seven Point Ranch, Emigrant, MT 59027
Telephone: 406-333-4578; 406-333-4346; 800-345-1129; Fax: 406-333-4769
Credit Cards: Visa, MasterCard, American Express, Discover

Makes and sells portable, stationary and electric bodywork tables and massage chairs, using replenishable woods and other environmentally responsible materials. Also sells cushions, linens, oils, lotions and other bodywork accessories.

331. Innerpeace

"The Sheet People"
Post Office Box 648, Easthampton, MA 01027
Telephone: 800-949-7650
Credit Cards: Visa, MasterCard

Sells 100 percent cotton flannel linens for massage tables. Fabric samples included with brochure. Wholesale orders to schools and stores; retail orders to individuals.

332. International Association of Infant Massage/Gentle Touch Warehouse Catalog
2350 Bowen Road, Post Office Box 438, Elma, NY 14059-0438
Telephone: 716-652-6949; Fax: 716-652-1990
Credit Cards: None

Sells books, audiotapes, videotapes, and related infant massage products.

333. Living Earth Crafts®
600 East Todd Road, Santa Rosa, CA 95407
Telephone: 707-584-4443; 800-358-8292; Fax: 707-585-6167
Credit Cards: Visa, MasterCard, American Express

Manufactures and sells portable, stationary, electric and specialty bodywork tables and supplies using environmentally safe materials. Also sells massage lotions, oils, linens and related accessories.

334. Montgomery Woods
See New Generation Products, below.

335. Mountain Laurel Massage Tables
Post Office Box 407, Windsor, VT 05089
Telephone: 802-674-9337
Credit Cards: Visa, MasterCard

Sells massage tables and related accessories including futon mats and covers, face cradles and carrying cases. Also sells yoga meditation cushions.

336. New Generation Products
Montgomery Woods
6721 East Akron Street, Mesa, AZ 85205-9005
Telephone: 800-850-5552
Credit Cards: None

Builds and sells bodywork tables and related accessories.

337. Oakworks
Post Office Box 99, Glen Rock, PA 17327-0099
Telephone: 717-235-6807; 800-558-8850 (Customer Service); Fax: 717-235-6798
Credit Cards: Visa, MasterCard

Manufactures and sells the Portal Pro (patent pending) and the Desktop Portal, bodywork equipment which allows patients to be treated in a seated supported position. Also sells traditional portable and stationary tables and bodywork accessories (oils, carrying cases, music, tools, etc.).

338. Pure Pro Massage Oils, Inc.
955 Massachusetts Avenue, #232, Cambridge, MA 02139
Telephone: 800-900-PURE
Credit Cards: Visa, MasterCard

Begun by massage therapists who wanted to create affordable, quality massage oils, this company offers scented and unscented oils in a variety of sizes. Bulk discounts are available on oils purchased by the case or in five-gallon cubes. Also sells massage music, books and related products, all of which are appropriate for use by bodywork professionals.

339. Ultra-Light
3140 Roy Messer Highway, White Pine, TN 37890
Telephone: 615-674-8111; 800-999-1971
Credit Cards: Visa, MasterCard

Manufactures and sells ultra-light portable bodywork tables. Tables come in three sizes, the lightest of which weighs under nineteen pounds, the heaviest just over twenty-one pounds. Customization available.

Reflexology

Reflexology is based upon the theory that every part of the body, every organ and every gland has a corresponding reference point on the foot, hand and ear. Usually working with the reference points on the feet, reflexology can be used to treat a wide range of health problems, such as acne, back pain, high blood pressure, intestinal problems, migraine headaches, and urinary difficulties, as well as to relieve stress and promote relaxation. Reflexology offers a means of treating pain in a specific area of the body without actually working on the area directly and, with limited instruction, can be self-administered. The healing capabilities of this therapy are believed to lie in the manipulation of the reference points which correspond to the injured or ailing part of the body, resulting in assistance to the body's own healing ability to resolve the problem through improved blood circulation, elimination of bodily poisons, and a reduction in stress.

Organizations

340. American Reflexology Certification Board (ARCB)
Post Office Box 620607, Littleton, CO 80162
Telephone: 303-933-6921
Contact: Barbara J. Mosier, administrative secretary

A nonprofit corporation acting as an independent testing agency for the field of reflexology.

Services for the professional: Certifies the competency of professional reflexologists to meet basic standards; acts as a national registration board for certified practitioners; sponsors a national conference; publishes a newsletter.

Services for the public: Represents the interests of the public through certifying competency and upgrading the standards of practice. Provides referrals to certified practitioners.

Publications: Reflexology Today, semiannual newsletter, free to members; conference transcripts, $20.00; a variety of brochures on testing, public relations, and various reflexology associations (free to certificants).

341. International Council of Reflexologists (ICR)
4311 Stockton Boulevard, Sacramento, CA 95820
Telephone: 916-455-5381
Contact: Christine Issel, director

A professional membership organization providing a communication network for reflexologists internationally and supporting the development of local and regional associations and sponsored conferences.

Services for the professional: Sponsors a biennial international conference; publishes a newsletter.

Publications: ICR Newsletter, quarterly, free to members.

Schools

342. Herbal Healer Academy International (HHAI)
HC 32 97-B, Mountain View, AR 72560
Telephone: 501-269-4177; Fax: 501-269-5424
Contact: Dr. Marijah McCain, N.D., M.H

Offers a home-study certificate course in reflexology, consisting of written work and case studies. Although there is no time limit for completion, students are encouraged to complete the program within one year. Visa and MasterCard accepted.

343. International Academy of Advanced Reflexology (IAAR)
145 Northampton Street, Easton, PA 18042
Telephone: 610-258-1525; Fax: 610-258-1525
Contact: Lorraina J. Telepo, C.R.R., director

Offers a thirty-hour, four-day course which provides basic reflexology practitioner training. Also offers a certification program in reflexology practitioner training which consists of three 30-hour courses, one full year of practice, and documented case histories.

344. International Academy of Reflexology Studies (IARS)
4759 Cornell Road, Suite D, Cincinnati, OH 45242
Telephone: 513-489-9328; Fax: 513-489-9354
Contact: Marcia L. Aschendorf, director of studies

For the professional, the academy offers a fourteen-month, 600-hour program of training for reflexologists consisting of 450 hours of classroom instruction and 150 hours of clinical lab. For the lay public, they offer self-help classes on the hands, ears, couples (this is a class on feet), and mother and child. Each class teaches the student how to maintain a feeling of wellness through the application of reflexology techniques.

345. International Institute of Reflexology (IIR)
5650 First Avenue North (Street Address), St. Petersburg, FL 33710; Post Office Box 12642 (Mailing Address), St. Petersburg, FL 33733-2642
Telephone: 813-343-4811; Fax: 813-381-2807
Contact: Dwight C. Byers, president

Offers two-day seminars consisting of theory and hands-on practice in the method of foot reflexology originally developed by Eunice Ingham. Seminars are held year-round in various locations throughout the eastern United States. Instructors are all long-term professional certified reflexologists.

346. Laura Norman & Associates Reflexology Center (LNARC)
41 Park Avenue, Suite 8A, New York, NY 10016
Telephone: 212-532-4404

Offers reflexology training through workshops and through a 72-hour, three-level certification program, all of which are appropriate for health professionals and the lay public. Laura Norman is a New York State licensed massage practitioner and a well-known authority on reflexology. A work/study program is available.

347. New Mexico School of Natural Therapeutics (NMSNT)
117 Richmond N.E., Albuquerque, NM 87106
Telephone: 505-268-6870; Fax: 505-268-0818
See Massage—Schools.

348. New York Open Center (NYOC)
83 Spring Street, New York, NY 10012
Telephone: 212-219-2527; Fax: 212-219-1347
See chapter 1: General—Schools.

Treatment Centers/Referrals

See Reflexology—Organizations for referrals to certified practitioners.

Product Suppliers

349. Ingham Publishing, Inc.
Post Office Box 12642, Saint Petersburg, FL 33733-2642
Telephone: 813-343-4811
Credit Cards: Visa, MasterCard, Discover

Sells books and wall charts on reflexology.

350. International Academy of Advanced Reflexology
145 Northampton Street, Easton, PA 18042
Telephone: 610-258-1525; Fax: 610-258-1525
Credit Cards: None

Sells a reflexology documentary videotape and a reflexology foot chart.

Rolfing

Founded by Dr. Ida P. Rolf and originally called Structural Integration, Rolfing focuses on the connective tissue that surrounds the muscles (the fascia) using deep tissue manipulation to bring the body into a state of alignment with gravity. Misalignments and postural compensations occur as a reaction to life events, accidents, injuries, poor movement habits and emotional traumas. The body tends to remember these changes and become fixed in unbalanced positions, with the shortened fascia holding it in place. Through ten sessions, each focusing on a different predetermined area of the body, realignment of the head, chest, pelvis and legs is sought. Rolfing may be used for relief from pain and stress, increased flexibility and energy, performance enhancement, improvement in the spinal curvature, and deeper psychological awareness.

Schools

351. Rolf Institute of Structural Integration (RISI)
Post Office Box 1868 (Mailing Address), Boulder, CO 80306-1868; 205 Canyon Road (Street Address), Boulder, CO 80302
Telephone: 303-449-5903; 800-530-8875; Fax: 303-449-5978
Contact: Liesel Orend, education director

Provides pretraining in foundations of bodywork and Rolfing training, completion of which allows graduates to become certified Rolfers. Also provides advanced Rolfing training, movement integration training, workshops and seminars for continuing education. In addition, a variety of books and other printed materials are available, a list of which is available from the institute.

CHAPTER 5: ENERGY MEDICINE

This approach to health and healing influences the electromagnetic human energy system through various therapeutic interventions. Based on ancient concepts from Indian and Chinese traditions, energy is seen as underlying all matter. Its pattern of flow thus has direct effects on the physical, mental, emotional and spiritual aspects of the individual. Energy flow that is impeded, blocked or disrupted can produce symptomology from the earliest stages of pain or discomfort to the later development of disease. It is felt that treating the human energy system directly reaches the underlying source of the problem and helps the body move toward self-healing and health.

General

Organizations

352. International Society for the Study of Subtle Energies and Energy Medicine (ISSEEM)

356 Goldco Circle, Golden, CO 80401
Telephone: 303-278-2228; Fax: 303-279-3539
Contact: C. Penny Hiernu, executive director

An interdisciplinary nonprofit membership organization for the study of consciousness, energy medicine and mind/body self-regulation supporting research, scholarship and clinical application of these principles to foster health and promote healing.

Services: Sponsors an annual conference, seminars and workshops; publishes a journal, newsletter, and membership directory.

Publications: *Subtle Energies*, journal, 3 issues annually, $50.00 (subscription) (reviewed under Energy Medicine—Journals and Newsletters); *Bridges*, quarterly newsletter, free to members.

Schools

353. Barbara Brennan School of Healing
Post Office Box 2005, East Hampton, NY 11937
Telephone: 516-329-0951; Fax: 516-324-9745

Offers a four-year professional Healing Science training program, a comprehensive, all-encompassing vocational training in which students learn to perceive and heal illness on all levels of the human energy field, while developing themselves spiritually as healers. Five-day classes are held five times annually at the school. Also offers an Introduction to Healing Science, three and one-half day intensive workshops in which participants learn the basic techniques of perceiving the aura and balancing/strengthening the field, as well as the fundamental principles of Healing Science. This program is a prerequisite for the four-year program. Workshops are held six to eight times annually at locations throughout the United States, and are eligible for continuing education credits for nurses and acupuncturists.

354. The Siskiyou Essence Company
Post Office Box 353, 485 East Main Street, Suite 3, Ashland, OR 97520
Telephone: 503-482-5311
Contact: Debra Hurt

Offers a training program in specialized kinesiology, also known as muscle testing, which is used to discover emotional, psychological or energy imbalances. Also offers introductory classes in vibrational healing and the Chakras. (See also chapter 4: Applied Kinesiology—Schools.)

Product Suppliers

355. Pegasus Products, Inc.
Post Office Box 228, Boulder, CO 80306
Telephone: 303-667-3019; 800-527-6104 (Orders only); Fax: 303-667-3624
Credit Cards: Visa, MasterCard, American Express, Discover

Offers flower remedies, gem elixirs, elemental elixirs, aromatherapy essential oils, books, audiotapes and related products for sale at the wholesale and retail levels.

356. The Siskiyou Essence Company
Post Office Box 353, 485 East Main Street, Suite 3, Ashland, OR 97520

Telephone: 503-482-5311
Credit Cards: None

Sells vibrational essences intended to restore equilibrium to the body, heart, mind and spirit.

357. Tools for Exploration
4460 Redwood Highway, Suite 2, San Rafael, CA 94903
Telephone: 415-499-9050; 800-456-9887 (Orders Only); Fax: 415-499-9047
Credit Cards: Visa, MasterCard

Distributes products, books and audiotapes for enhancing energy, consciousness and health. Many products are unusual and hard to find; some are widely known. Biofeedback instruments, light and color products, energy health products, acupuncture products, and tools for professionals are some of the items sold.

Polarity Therapy

This form of energetic healing was developed by Dr. Randolph Stone (1890-1982) and is based on ancient health systems such as Ayurveda and oriental medicine. The therapy addresses the flow and balance of energy in the body. Through the placement of the practitioner's hands on the client's body, areas of energy that were blocked may be opened up, balanced, and returned to their natural pattern of flow, relieving symptomotology and supporting optimum health and well being. Polarity therapy consists of four therapeutic methods: bodywork, diet, simple exercises that relax and balance the flow of energy, and self-awareness.

Organizations

358. American Polarity Therapy Association (APTA)
2888 Bluff Street, Suite 149, Boulder, CO 80301
Telephone: 303-545-2080; Fax: 303-545-2161
Contact: Gary Peterson, executive director

A nonprofit membership organization dedicated to the advancement of polarity therapy in America through supporting the expansion of knowledge in the field, establishing professional standards, increasing public awareness, and cooperating with other professional organizations and public agencies in the oversight of practitioners.

Services for the professional: Certifies practitioners at two levels; accredits polarity training courses; provides promotional materials and advertising;

offers listing in the annual membership directory for referrals; holds networking forums; offers low cost professional liability insurance.

Services for the public: Hosts three educational conferences per year; provides referrals to polarity practitioners and trainings; publishes a newsletter.

Publications: *Energy*, quarterly newsletter, free to members; *Annual Membership Directory*, $3.00; *Membership List* (by alphabetical or zip code order), $15.00 members, $20.00 nonmembers; *APTA Polarity Therapy, Energy Healing and Related Topics Bibliography*, $5.00.

Schools

359. New Mexico Academy of Healing Arts (NMAHA)
Post Office Box 932, Santa Fe, NM 87504
Telephone: 505-982-6271; Fax: 505-988-2621
Contact: Registrar

Offers polarity certification programs accredited by the American Polarity Therapy Association. Students are required to work a substantial number of hours in the student-staffed clinic which provides low-cost bodywork services to the Santa Fe community. Continuing education courses and introductory courses for the general public are also offered. (See also chapter 4: Massage—Schools.)

360. New Mexico School of Natural Therapeutics (NMSNT)
117 Richmond N.E., Albuquerque, NM 87106
Telephone: 505-268-6870; Fax: 505-268-0818
Contact: Alison Owens, administrator

Offers a 750-hour course in Natural Therapeutics which focuses on therapeutic massage and polarity therapy and also includes shiatsu, reflexology, sports massage, herbology and more. Six-month courses begin in February and August; a part-time evening program begins each May. Continuing education programs are offered throughout the year in such areas as craniosacral therapy, advanced polarity, and traditional Chinese medical diagnosis. (See also chapter 4: Massage—Schools.)

361. New York Open Center (NYOC)
83 Spring Street, New York, NY 10012
Telephone: 212-219-2527; Fax: 212-219-1347
See chapter 1: General—Schools.

Treatment Centers/Referrals

See Polarity Therapy—Organizations for referrals to individual practitioners.

Product Suppliers

362. American Polarity Therapy Association Bookstore
2888 Bluff Street, Suite 149, Boulder, CO 80301
Telephone: 303-545-2080; Fax: 303-545-2161
Credit Cards: Visa, MasterCard

Sells books written by Randolph Stone, D.C., founder of polarity therapy, as well as books on polarity therapy written by other authors. Also sells audiotapes of annual American Polarity Therapy Association conferences, and videotapes and charts. Volume discounts available.

Reiki

This Japanese word describes any type of healing work based on life force energy. There are various schools of Reiki, including the Usui method and the Radiance technique, all based on the channeling of higher frequency energies by the practitioner for physical, emotional and spiritual healing. Practitioners undergo a special attunement process thought to open their crown, heart and palm chakras, or energy centers, and link them to the source of energy. It is believed that, through placement of the practitioner's hands on the client's body, Reiki energy is automatically directed to areas in need of healing. Reiki can be used for self-treatment and in conjunction with conventional medical treatments, supporting and speeding recovery and reducing side effects, pain and stress.

Organizations

363. The Radiance Technique Association International, Inc. (RTAI)
Post Office Box 40570, St. Petersburg, FL 33743-0570
Telephone: 813-347-3421
Contact: Maralyn Rose, executive director

A not-for-profit membership organization supporting the practice of the Radiance technique, a stress-reduction and energy balancing technique taught in seminars worldwide.

Services for the professional: Provides information and services for students.

Services for the public: Provides general information on the technique and referrals to authorized instructors by geographic area.

Publications: *The Radiance Technique Newsletter*, three to four times a year, included in membership donation of $10.00 annually.

364. The Reiki Alliance

Post Office Box 41, Cataldo, ID 83810
Telephone: 208-682-3535; Fax: 208-682-4848
Contact: Susan Mitchell, executive director

A worldwide membership organization of Reiki masters who teach the Usui system of healing in thirty-one countries. Supporting clinical research and Reiki certification are new areas being considered by the alliance.

Services for the professional: Promotes exchange between teachers and students; provides a member newsletter and materials for teachers; presents an annual seven-day conference; supports workshops for additional teacher training.

Services for the public: Provides referrals and information on Reiki; newsletter subscriptions and books are also available.

Publications: *The Reiki Alliance*, newsletter, three times a year, free with membership; *Student Book*, available in nine languages, $3.50.

Schools

365. Center for Reiki Training (CRT)

29209 Northwestern Highway, #592, Southfield, MI 48034
Telephone: 810-948-8112; Fax: 810-948-9534
Contact: William L. Rand

Founded by Reiki master/teacher William Rand, this nonprofit organization is dedicated to the promotion of healing through the training and certification of Reiki teachers and students, maintenance of standards for teaching Reiki, research, and support of all Reiki practitioners. Training includes Reiki I and II, advanced Reiki training, and Reiki III/master. Classes are taught throughout the United States and other countries on an ongoing basis. All classes are taught by certified Reiki teachers. Visa and MasterCard accepted for payment of fees. The center also publishes a quarterly newsletter, $5.00 a year, which lists all currently scheduled Reiki classes and includes a form for class enrollment.

366. The Reilly School of Massotherapy (RSM)

67th Street and Atlantic Avenue, Post Office Box 595, Virginia Beach, VA 23451

Telephone: 804-428-0446; Fax: 804-422-4631
See chapter 4: Massage—Schools.

Treatment Centers/Referrals

See Reiki—Organizations for referrals to individual practitioners.

Product Suppliers

367. Center for Reiki Training
29209 Northwestern Highway, #592, Southfield, MI 48034
Telephone: 810-948-8112; Fax: 810-948-9534
Credit Cards: Visa, MasterCard

Sells a variety of Reiki products including instructional audiotapes, books, Reiki tables and related items.

Therapeutic Touch

Therapeutic Touch is based on the concept of the body as an energy system, or fields, that connect and interact with life energy in the surrounding universe. The human energy system thus extends beyond the body and is affected by the energy forces that surround it. Disease is seen as a disruption in the balanced flow of the body's energy fields. Therapeutic Touch practitioners affect these disruptions by moving their hands over the client's body without touching it and directing energy to rebalance the fields, thus aiding its ability to heal. The process consists of several steps: centering, during which the practitioner opens to the source of healing energy; assessment of the client's energy fields, where the practitioner picks up subtle sensory indications of disturbances in the fields; and treatment, where congestions are cleared, energy is added where there is a deficit and the whole system is balanced, or unruffled. Therapeutic Touch, though based on ancient healing practices of laying on of hands, was developed, studied and organized in the 1970s into a method that could be taught by Dora Kunz, a natural healer, and Dolores Krieger, Ph.D., Professor Emeritus of Nursing at New York University. It is currently taught in leading university nursing/medical schools and by private organizations, schools and associations throughout the country.

Organizations

368. Nurse Healers-Professional Associates, Inc. (NH-PA)
Post Office Box 444, Allison Park, PA 15104-0444

Telephone: 412-355-8476

A not-for-profit cooperative of health care professionals organized for the exploration and expansion of healing on theoretical and clinical levels. Works to promote the use of healing modalities among health professionals and excellence in their practice, to support educational and professional standards, and to develop and disseminate knowledge of these healing practices. Focuses on the Krieger/Kunz method of Therapeutic Touch but includes other healing modalities as well.

Services for the professional: Offers classes on various subjects and all levels of Therapeutic Touch; sponsors national conference; promotes networking; provides referrals to qualified Therapeutic Touch teachers; provides seed money for planning and organizing conferences; awards grants for study and research; publishes a bibliography on healing, membership directory of practitioners and teachers of Therapeutic Touch and other modalities, and a quarterly newsletter.

Services for the public: Provides referrals to Therapeutic Touch practitioners and teachers; sells copies of membership directory.

Publications: *Cooperative Connection*, quarterly newsletter, $3.00 donation; *NH-PA Directory*, $75.00 nonmembers; bibliography, complete $5.00, Therapeutic Touch only $3.00.

Schools

369. American Holistic Nurses Association (AHNA)
4101 Lake Boone Trail, Suite 201, Raleigh, NC 27607
Telephone: 919-787-5181; 800-278-2462; Fax: 919-787-4916

Provides telephone referrals to organizations that offer instructional programs in Therapeutic Touch. (See also chapter 1: General—Organizations.)

370. Infinity Institute (II)
4110 Edgeland, Department 800, Royal Oak, MI 48073-2251
Telephone: 810-549-5594

Offers ongoing training in Therapeutic Touch and two full-day workshops. Also teaches courses in basic/self hypnosis, advanced hypnotherapy, and hypnoanalysis. Courses are approved for International Medical and Dental Hypnotherapy Association, National Association of Alcohol and Drug Abuse Counselors, Certified Addiction Councelors, and Michigan nurses continuing education credits. (See also chapter 7: Hypnotherapy—Schools.)

371. Pumpkin Hollow Farm (PHF)
N.E. Theosophical Federation
R.R. 1, Box 135, Craryville, NY 12521
Telephone: 518-325-3583
Contact: Charles Elkind/Loren Wheeler, program managers

Offers workshops and intensives in Therapeutic Touch, some of which are eligible for continuing education credits. Some scholarship assistance is available.

372. University of Colorado Health Sciences Center (UCHSC)
School of Nursing/Center for Human Caring
4200 East 9th Avenue, Campus Box C288-08, Denver, CO 80262
Telephone: 303-270-4331; Fax: 303-270-8660
See chapter 1: General—Schools.

Treatment Centers/Referrals

See Therapeutic Touch—Organizations for referrals to individual practitioners.

CHAPTER 6: MOVEMENT THERAPIES

Alexander Technique

This system of movement re-education addresses postural alignment and what is considered good use of the body. Based on F. M. Alexander's work in the late 1800s to correct his chronic voice problems, the focus is on how the body is aligned and moves and its effect on the entire functioning of the body. It looks at the relationship of the head, neck, and spine and, through a series of lessons, seeks to alter their relationship to each other in positive ways. Through gentle hands-on work and verbal suggestions of lengthening, relaxing, freeing, widening and dropping, a new postural integration is encouraged. The student practices these new structural relationships in everyday activities such as sitting and walking, guided by the practitioner in each session. The Alexander Technique is widely used by performing artists such as dancers, actors, and musicians, where optimal functioning of the body is critical to performance and injury prevention, but can be used by anyone who seeks to change postural habits causing pain, stress and decreased energy and vitality.

Organizations

373. North American Society of Teachers of the Alexander Technique (NASTAT)

Post Office Box 517, Urbana, IL 61801
Telephone: 217-367-6956; 800-473-0620
Contact: Brian McCullough, administrator

A nonprofit educational organization dedicated to promoting the Alexander Technique through establishing standards for the certification of teachers and teacher training courses, providing services to its members, networking, legislative activity and increasing public awareness.

Services for the professional: Maintains a referral service; supports professional development; sponsors conferences; provides a listing of NASTAT-approved training courses; publishes newsletter.

Services for the public: Makes referrals to certified teachers and provides information; publishes and sells books and pamphlets; publishes newsletter.

Publications: *NASTAT News*, quarterly newsletter, $24.00 (subscription); Teacher listings, twice a year, free.

Schools

For a listing of approved Alexander Technique training courses, contact the North American Society of Teachers of the Alexander Technique (see Alexander Technique—Organizations).

374. The Alexander Training Institute of San Francisco (ATISF)
931 Elizabeth Street, San Francisco, CA 94114
Telephone: 415-550-7340
Contact: Stella Moon, administrator

Offers a twelve-quarter, 1,710-hour training program in the Alexander Technique, consisting of academic instruction, practical training and an internship, leading to certification as a teacher of the Alexander Technique. Also offered are four-week, five-week and nine-week noncertificate intensives, which provide an accelerated learning program within ongoing classes.

375. American Center for the Alexander Technique (ACAT)
129 West 67th Street, New York, NY 10023
Telephone: 212-799-0468

A nonprofit organization founded in 1964 by Judith Leibowitz and Deborah Caplan, this was the first teacher certification program of its kind established in the United States for the training of Alexander teachers. The center is dedicated to continuing and supporting the work of F. M. Alexander. ACAT's teacher certification program is a three-year program consisting of three ten-week terms per year, primarily composed of classroom hours and hands-on work. Lectures, demonstrations, readings and discussion provide grounding in the conceptual foundation of the technique. In addition, an independent study program allows students to explore their particular areas of interest. Students receive individual instruction in weekly private sessions and class lessons with a teacher/student ratio of five to one. During the third year, students begin supervised teaching of volunteers. Graduates receive certification from both ACAT and the NASTAT, the North American Society of Teachers of the Alexander Technique. Financial aid is available to students qualifying under federal student loan programs. A list of certified Alexander teachers in private practice in the United States and abroad is available from the center.

Treatment Centers/Referrals

See Alexander Technique—Organizations for referrals to individual practitioners.

Feldenkrais Method

Founded by Moshe Feldenkrais, D. Sc., in the mid-1900s, this system of movement re-education seeks to expand movement options by bringing old movement habits into conscious awareness, breaking the old patterns and creating new, more beneficial ways of moving. There are two parts to the Feldenkrais system. Feldenkrais Awareness Through Movement® consists of verbally directed movement lessons done at the individual's own pace, though usually in a group setting. There are 1,000 basic movements with 3,000 variations. The second modality is functional integration, one-on-one sessions with a practitioner who uses noninvasive, hands-on contact to re-educate the nervous system and develop new movement patterns and possibilities. The Feldenkrais® Method has been used to treat back pain, temporomandibular joint syndrome, postural changes, and other musculoskeletal and neurological conditions, and for performance enhancement.

Organizations

376. The Feldenkrais Guild® (FG)
706 Ellsworth Street, S.W., Post Office Box 489, Albany, OR 97321-0143
Telephone: 503-926-0981, 800-775-2118; Fax: 503-926-0572

The nonprofit professional membership organization of practitioners and teachers of the Feldenkrais® Method. The guild works toward increasing public awareness of the Feldenkrais Method of Somatic Education, maintains the certification and continuing education process of practitioners, protects the quality of the Feldenkrais work, and promotes research on the method's effectiveness.

Services for the professional: Provides professional training and continuing education; publishes membership directory; offers professional liability insurance.

Services for the public: Provides information on the method and referrals to classes, workshops and individual sessions by geographic location; sells books, articles, audiotapes and videotapes.

Publications: *Guild Certified Feldenkrais Practitioners and Teachers*, $3.00; Catalog of Materials, free.

Treatment Centers/Referrals

See Feldenkrais Method—Organizations for referrals to individual practitioners.

Product Suppliers

377. The Feldenkrais Guild®
Post Office Box 489, Albany, OR 97321-0143
Telephone: 503-926-0981, 800-775-2118; Fax: 503-926-0572
Credit Cards: Visa, MasterCard

Sells audiotapes, videotapes, article reprints, books, posters and related Feldenkrais Method products.

The Rosen Method

Based on her work as a physical therapist, Marion Rosen developed the Rosen Method of bodywork and began to teach it in 1971. It is a gentle approach to letting go of unconscious holding and tension, opening the client on a physical, emotional and spiritual level to freer movement, increased awareness, deeper connection with the self, and fuller vitality and self-expression. There are two parts to the method: hands-on bodywork, during which the practitioner locates areas of muscular tension and restricted breath in the client's body, remains there watching, feeling and listening for a response. This facilitates the client in becoming aware of, connecting with, and releasing underlying feelings and thoughts when appropriate in a natural, easy and supportive way. The second part of the approach involves simple movements and movement sequences done alone or with partners, encouraging full range of motion, expansion, release of holding patterns, relaxation, ease, increased sense of balance and fun.

Organizations

378. Rosen Method Professional Association (RMPA)
2550 Shattuck Avenue, Box 49, Berkeley, CA 94704

Telephone: 510-644-4166

A nonprofit group dedicated to the professional support and development of Rosen Method practitioners and to increasing public awareness of Rosen Method bodywork and movement.

Services for the professional: Conducts ongoing training; offers internship programs; provides certification to practitioners; publishes membership directory and newsletter.

Services for the public: Provides referrals to certified practitioners, classes and training; provides information on the Rosen Method.

Publications: *RMPA Views*, quarterly newsletter, $12.00 (subscription).

Schools

379. Rosen Method—The Berkeley Center
825 Bancroft Way, Berkeley, CA 94710
Telephone: 510-531-5442
Contact: Hanna Weare, administrator

Offers a training program in Rosen Method bodywork. Program includes Rosen Method fundamentals and intensives, which emphasize the connections between the body and the emotions and seek to expand understanding of personal relationships and the healing arts.

Treatment Centers/Referrals

See The Rosen Method—Organizations for referrals to individual practitioners.

T'ai Chi Chuan

This moving meditation and martial art is thought to have been developed by a Taoist monk in A.D. 960. Widely practiced in China by people of all ages as a daily health maintenance regimen, T'ai Chi is a system of simple and natural movements which is used to promote health and longevity. Its benefits are believed to reach all levels: mental, spiritual, emotional and physical. T'ai Chi may promote blood circulation, loosen muscles and free joints for greater flexibility, invigorate the body, and enhance the flow of vital energy. Relaxing both the body and the mind, it is thought to facilitate the development of mental clarity and calmness, a sense of grounding and centering, an integration of body and mind, and a deeper connection to and harmony with the universal energy that surrounds us.

Schools

There are schools of T'ai Chi in many local communities throughout the United States. For information on these schools, check the local telephone directory.

380. East West Academy of Healing Arts (EWAHA)
450 Sutter Street, Suite 210, San Francisco, CA 94108
Telephone: 415-788-2227
See chapter 2: Chinese Medicine/Acupuncture—Treatment Centers/Referrals.

381. Living Tao Foundation (LTF)
Post Office Box 846, Urbana, IL 61801
Telephone: 217-337-6113

Offers residential training programs and seminars in all aspects of T'ai Chi, both at the headquarters of the foundation and at various locations throughout the United States. Courses cover Taoist philosophy, Chi exercises, movement and meditation, and much more. Visa, MasterCard and American Express accepted for payment of fees.

382. The New Center for Wholistic Health Education & Research (NCWHER)
6801 Jericho Turnpike, Syosset, NY 11791
Telephone: 516-364-0808; Fax: 516-364-0989
See chapter 1: General—Schools.

383. The Ohashiatsu Institute (OI)
12 West 27th Street, New York, NY 10001
Telephone: 212-684-4190; Fax: 212-447-5819
See chapter 4: Acupressure/Shiatsu—Schools.

384. Sarasota School of Natural Healing Arts (SSNHA)
8216 South Tamiami Trail, Sarasota, FL 34238
Telephone: 800-966-7117; Fax: 813-966-4414
See chapter 4: Massage—Schools.

385. Studio Yoga
Post Office Box 99, Chatham, NJ 07928
Telephone: 201-966-5311; Fax: 201-966-1477
See Yoga—Schools.

Trager[R] Psychophysical Integration

Developed by Dr. Milton Trager over the last sixty years, the Trager[R] approach is a gentle form of movement reeducation that encourages a sense of effortless movement and relaxed awareness as a way of being in the world. The approach consists of two aspects. The first is a hands-on tablework session with the practitioner working in a relaxed state called "hook up." Through rhythmic movements of each part of the client's body, the practitioner seeks to reach the unconscious mind of the client, where holding patterns, tensions and restrictions are thought to originate. The movements influence these patterns and suggest new possibilities of free movement, ease, lengthening, opening, softness and flow. These new sensations are supported by movement work called "Mentastics" done with the client at the end of each session. Through these natural easy movements, clients learn to incorporate the sense of freedom and flow experienced during the tablework into their everyday lives. Clients are encouraged to use these simple movements on a daily basis in order to recall the feeling of Trager[R] work and thus deepen and reinforce the neuromuscular changes that have been experienced in a session.

Organizations

386. The Trager[R] Institute (TI)
21 Locust Avenue, Mill Valley, CA 94941-2806
Telephone: 415-388-2688; Fax: 415-388-2710
Contact: Don Schwartz, administrative director

The nonprofit professional membership organization of practitioners and teachers of the Trager[R] Approach. The institute is responsible for the certification and continuing education of its members, ensuring the quality of the work, increasing public awareness of the Trager[R] Approach, communicating with and encouraging networking of practitioners worldwide, and promoting research on its effectiveness.

Services for the professional: Offers professional training and continuing education for certification in the Trager[R] Approach; sponsors international conferences; offers professional liability insurance; publishes membership directory for referrals and networking; publishes quarterly newsletter.

Services for the public: Provides referrals to classes, workshops and individual practitioners internationally; provides information on the Trager[R] Approach.

Publications: *The Trager[R] Newsletter,* quarterly, free with membership.

Treatment Centers/Referrals

See Trager[R] Psychophysical Integration—Organizations for referrals to individual practitioners.

Yoga

Yoga evolved from an ancient Indian tradition, and focuses on self-realization and the development of spiritual discipline. It encompasses several schools, including hatha yoga, raja yoga, bhakti yoga, karma yoga, tantra yoga and jnana yoga, all of which are based at least in part on the practice of meditation. Hatha yoga, the form most commonly practiced in the United States, also emphasizes poses (called "asanas") and stretches designed to strengthen the body, reduce stress, improve circulation, promote relaxation, and achieve and maintain overall good health. The approach of raja yoga is more inward, focusing on meditation and self-realization. Karma yoga stresses service to others. Bhakti yoga has the strongest religious component, teaching a love for the Divine. Jnana yoga has a strong intellectual component, and tantra yoga emphasizes ceremonies and rituals.

Organizations

387. American Yoga Association (AYA)
513 South Orange Avenue, Sarasota, FL 34236
Telephone: 941-953-5859, 800-226-5859; Fax: 941-364-9153

Post Office Box 18105, Cleveland Heights, OH 44118
Telephone: 216-371-0078; Fax: 941-364-9153
Contact: Linda Gajevski, director of marketing

A nonprofit educational organization dedicated to providing high quality instruction in yoga. Participates in research and direct service programs at federal, state, local and private levels.

Services for the professional: Offers professional training in "Easy Does It Yoga" trainer's course; publishes books, audiotapes and videotapes on yoga; provides stress management training in the business and health care environment.

Services for the public: Maintains teaching centers in Cleveland and Sarasota, offering classes and instructional materials on a primarily introductory level geared toward the general public; publishes instructional books, audiotapes and videotapes, and independent study courses.

Publications: *The American Yoga Association Beginner's Manual* (Simon and Schuster, 1987); *Easy Does It Yoga for Older People* (Harper and Row, 1981); *Basic Yoga* (Parade, 1993), videotape; *Complete Relaxation and Meditation: The 30-minute Workout that Reduces Your Heart Rate Instead of Raising It*, audiotape; free informational sheets on hypertension, menopause and PMS, asthma, heart disease, chronic fatigue, diabetes, arthritis, insomnia, incontinence, AIDS, neck and back pain, weight management, anxiety and headaches.

389. Himalayan International Institute of Yoga Science and Philosophy (Himalayan Institute) (HIIYSP)

RR1 Box 400, Honesdale, PA 18431
Telephone: 717-253-5551; Fax: 717-253-9078
Contact: Suzanne Grady, corporate secretary; Sheela Portersmith, therapy department

A not-for-profit membership organization dedicated to educational, therapeutic, spiritual and charitable work, the institute has worked toward bringing the technique of yoga and meditation to the attention of physicians, psychologists and researchers worldwide.

Services for the professional: Offers training programs for health professionals; sells books, audiotapes and videotapes; sponsors annual congress; publishes journal and newsletter.

Services for the public: Offers educational and therapeutic programs; conducts weekend seminars and residential programs on various health-related topics such as meditation, homeopathy, and hatha yoga; provides holistic medical services and health retreat programs.

Publications: *Yoga International*, bimonthly magazine, free to members, $18.00 (nonmember subscription) (reviewed under Yoga—Journals and Newsletters); *Himalayan Institute Quarterly*, newsletter, free; *The Resource Catalog for Holistic Living*, listing books, audiotapes and videotapes published by Himalayan Publishers.

389. B.K.S. Iyengar Yoga National Association of the United States, Inc. (IYNAUS)

Post Office Box 941, Lemont, PA 16851
Telephone: 814-234-9776; 800-889-YOGA; Fax: 814-234-9776
Contact: F. Dean Lerner, president

This organization is committed to studying, teaching, disseminating and promoting the art, science and philosophy of yoga according to the teachings and philosophy of B. K. S. Iyengar. It serves as a central organization for thirteen regional associations across the U.S. and as a link between the association and Shri B. K. S. Iyengar in Pune, India.

Services for the professional: Maintains a national system of professional standards for certification and teacher training; sells resources such as Iyengar Yoga videotapes, audiotapes, books and articles; publishes a newsletter.

Services for the public: Provides general information as well as a teacher referral service throughout the U.S.

Publications: *IYNAUS Newsletter*, biannual, free with membership; *IYNAUS Bulletin*, periodic, free with membership.

390. International Association of Yoga Therapists (IAYT)
109 Hillside Avenue, Mill Valley, CA 94941
Telephone: 415-383-4587; Fax: 415-381-0876
Contact: Susan Peek, executive administrator

A nonprofit membership organization for the advancement of yoga involved in defining its place in the modern health care system, providing educational programs, formulating certification requirements and standards of practice, and integrating yoga into new areas such as athletics and the creative therapies.

Services for the professional: Sponsors annual conferences; conducts classes and seminars; provides listings in IAYT member directory; sells books on yoga; publishes a newsletter and journal.

Services for the public: Provides referrals to IAYT member practitioners.

Publications: *Journal of the International Association of Yoga Therapists*, annual, free to members, $12.50 (nonmember subscription) (reviewed under Yoga—Journals and Newsletters); *I.A.Y.T. Newsletter*, free to members.

Schools

Yoga International (see Yoga—Journals and Newsletters) published its first annual resource guide, *1995 Guide to Yoga Teachers and Classes* and issues annual updates. This guide provides a listing of schools and individuals who teach yoga, arranged alphabetically by state and city, as well as information on yoga teacher certification programs. A section on international schools is also included.

391. American Yoga Association (AYA)
513 South Orange Avenue
Sarasota, FL 34236
Telephone: For Info: 800-226-5859; Fax: 941-364-9153

Post Office Box 18105, Cleveland Heights, OH
Telephone: 216-371-0078; Fax: 941-364-9153
Contact: Linda Gajerski, director, marketing communications (Ohio telephone)

Offers introductory and advanced classes which include Hatha Yoga exercises, breathing techniques and meditation. Also offers an "Easy Does It Yoga" program for older adults, and an inservice training program at which health care professionals learn to use "Easy Does It Yoga" with their clients. Provides free information on how yoga may be used to treat some common health problems and on how to find a qualified yoga teacher.

392. Bateman Institute for Health Education (BIHE)
43 West 24th Street, New York, NY 10010
Telephone: 212-243-2311; Fax: 212-873-1817
Contact: Allan Bateman; Colleen Blanchette

Offers a certificate program in yoga therapy, a 120-hour program attended over six weekends plus a twenty-hour internship which teaches students to become yoga therapists and teachers. The program is recommended by the International Association of Yoga Therapists. The institute also conducts ongoing classes in yoga and QiGong.

393. The Expanding Light at Ananda (ELA)
14618 Tyler Foote Road, Nevada City, CA 95959
Telephone: 916-292-3496
Contact: Richard McCord, manager

Among many programs, Expanding Light offers workshops and training programs in meditation, self-healing and yoga. Beginning programs are appropriate for the lay public; intermediate and more advanced workshops and training programs are also appropriate for health care paraprofessionals and professionals. Continuing education credits may be awarded to nurses attending some of these programs. Visa and MasterCard accepted for payment of fees.

394. Himalayan International Institute of Yoga Science and Philosophy (Himalayan Institute) (HIIYSP)
RR1 Box 400, Honesdale, PA 18431
Telephone: 717-253-5551; Fax: 717-253-9078
Contact: Suzanne Grady, corporate secretary

Offers seminars, workshops, training programs and residential internships on such topics as hatha yoga, meditation, homeopathy for home use and biofeedback. Audiences for the different programs range from beginning students to health care professionals. Visa and MasterCard accepted for payment of fees.

395. Integrative Yoga Therapy for Body, Mind and Spirit (IYTBMS)
305 Vista de Valle, Mill Valley, CA 94941
Telephone: 800-750-9642; 415-388-6569
Contact: Joseph LePage, director

Offers Integrative Yoga Therapy professional training programs, which combine the theory and practice of yoga with the latest advances in mind/body health, at retreat centers throughout the United States. The program consists of a two-week intensive followed by a three-month program of study and internship in the student's home community; students learn to teach yoga with a focus on health and healing. Through the external degree master's program of Sonoma State University, an extended training program leading to a master's degree in psychology with a focus in yoga and mind-body health is also available.

396. International Sivananda Yoga Vedanta Center (ISYVC)
243 West 24th Street
New York, NY 10011
Telephone: 212-255-4560; Fax: 212-727-7392

14651 Ballantree Lane, Comp. 8, Grass Valley, CA 95949
Telephone: 916-272-9322; Fax: 916-477-6054

Ashram: Post Office Box 195, Woodbourne, NY 12788
Telephone: 914-434-9242; Fax: 914-434-1032

Offers a four-week Yoga teacher training program which covers asanas, pranayama, meditation, yoga theory and more. For those who complete the program, a four-week advanced teacher training course is also available. In addition, the centers offer yoga classes for all levels, meditation and yoga philosophy. The ashram offers weekend retreats throughout the year.

397. The B.K.S Iyengar Yoga Institute of Los Angeles (IYILA)
8233 West Third Street, Los Angeles, CA 90048
Telephone: 213-653-0357
Contact: Leslie Peters, director

The institute offers a three-year training program in Iyengar yoga for teachers and serious students, and includes basic poses, yoga philosophy, anatomy and physiology of yoga poses, asanas and pranayama, and more. Also offered are introductory, continuing, and advanced classes for the general public, and classes specifically designed for children.

398. Iyengar Yoga Institute of San Francisco (IYISF)
2404 27th Avenue, San Francisco, CA 94116
Telephone: 415-753-0909
Contact: Natasha Sevilla, director

Offers a two-year, 48-credit advanced studies/teacher training program, leading to a yoga instructor certificate of completion. This program is appropriate for those training to be teachers, teachers continuing their education and for interested students of yoga. For the lay public, the institute offers continuous public classes, workshops, retreats and intensives which are appropriate for students of all levels. Visa and MasterCard accepted for payment of fees.

399. Kundalini Yoga Center (KYC)
401 Lafayette, 3rd Floor, New York, NY 10003
Telephone: 212-475-0212
Contact: Ravi Singh, director

Offers ongoing yoga classes and special intensives in Kundalini yoga, a blend of breathing, movement, meditation, relaxation and more.

400. Mt. Madonna Center (MMC)
445 Summit Road, Watsonville, CA 95076
Telephone: 408-847-0406; Fax: 408-847-2683
Contact: Jaya Maxon, advertising coordinator

Offers retreats and weekend programs on a variety of topics including yoga, healing and spiritual growth. Programs include Ayurveda workshops, yoga workshops and yoga teacher training intensives.

401. Satchidananda Ashram - Yogaville (SA-Y)
Route 1, Box 1720, Buckingham, VA 23921
Telephone: 804-969-3121; Fax: 804-969-1303

Offers classes in hatha yoga, raja yoga, meditation and related topics, all based on the Integral Yoga teachings of Sri Swami Satchidananda, the founder of the Integral Yoga Institutes. Also offered are several levels of yoga teacher certification programs: teacher training, which provides students with the skills needed to instruct Integral Yoga hatha beginners; advanced teacher training, where students learn to teach beginning and intermediate students; and prenatal yoga teacher training, which teaches the standard asanas that pregnant women can use as well as asanas used specifically for pregnancy.

402. Studio Yoga (SY)

Post Office Box 99, Chatham, NJ 07928
Telephone: 201-966-5311; Fax: 201-966-1477
Contact: Theresa Rowland, director

For the professional, a one-year first degree certificate course is offered, which covers principles of yoga, anatomy and physiology, teaching of beginners, and more. One-year advanced degree certificate programs are also offered, which include training in teaching more advanced students and therapeutic work. Those who complete the third degree certificate program may apply for certification testing through the National Iyengar Yoga Association. For the lay public, offers classes in Iyengar yoga for beginners, mid-level and advanced students. Classes are given for men, women and children; private and corporate classes are also available. Classes are taught by certified instructors at locations throughout New Jersey and Pennsylvania. Also offered are classes in meditation, Pranayama, T'ai Chi and QiGong. Visa, MasterCard and Discover accepted for payment of fees.

Treatment Centers/Referrals

See also Yoga—Organizations for referrals to individual practitioners. In addition, the journal *Yoga International* publishes an annual resource guide listing schools and individual yoga teachers.

403. Himalayan International Institute of Yoga Science and Philosophy (Himalayan Institute)

RR1 Box 400, Honesdale, PA 18431
Telephone: 717-253-5551; Fax: 717-253-9078

Offers holistic health services including stress management skills, biofeedback, relaxation training, yoga instruction and shiatsu.

Product Suppliers

404. American Yoga Association (AYA)
513 South Orange Avenue, Sarasota, FL 34236
Telephone: 941-953-5859; For Info: 800-226-5859; Fax: 941-364-9153

Post Office Box 18105, Cleveland Heights, OH 44118
Telephone: 216-371-0078; Fax: 941-364-9153
Credit Cards: Visa, MasterCard

Sells instructional books, audiotapes and videotapes by Alice Christensen, founder of the American Yoga Association. Also offers free information on the use of yoga to treat some common health problems and how to find a qualified yoga teacher.

405. Himalayan International Institute of Yoga Science and Philosophy (Himalayan Institute)
RR1 Box 400, Honesdale, PA 18431
Telephone: 717-253-5551; Fax: 717-253-9078
Credit Cards: Visa, MasterCard

Sells books, audiotapes and videotapes on meditation, yoga, holistic health and related topics.

406. Iyengar Yoga Institute of San Francisco
2404 27th Avenue, San Francisco, CA 94116
Telephone: 415-753-0909
Credit Cards: Visa, MasterCard

Sells books, periodicals, videotapes, audiotapes and yoga clip art.

407. Tools for Yoga
Post Office Box 99, Chatham, NJ 07988
Telephone: 201-966-5311; Fax: 201-966-1477
Credit Cards: Visa, MasterCard, Discover

Sells yoga mats, yoga audiotapes and videotapes, books on yoga, meditation, ayurveda and homeopathy, and related products. Bulk discounts available on most items. Custom orders welcome.

408. Yoga Mats

Post Office Box 885044, San Francisco, CA 94188
Telephone: 415-626-7378; 800-829-6580; 800-720-YOGA
Credit Cards: Visa, MasterCard

As the name of the company indicates, they make and sell 100 percent cotton yoga mats, as well as shiatsu mats, cushions and pillows for use in yoga practice. Products are sold at the wholesale and retail levels.

409. Yoga Pro Products

Post Office Box 7612, Ann Arbor, MI 48107
Telephone: 313-668-0263; 800-488-8414 (For Orders)
Credit Cards: Visa, MasterCard

Sells yoga equipment that facilitates learning and practicing the full range of yoga postures.

410. Yoga Research Foundation

6111 S.W. 74th Avenue, Miami, FL 33143
Telephone: 305-666-2006
Credit Cards: Visa, MasterCard

Among the products sold by the foundation are books, audiotapes and videotapes on yoga philosophy, hatha yoga exercises and meditation.

CHAPTER 7: SELF-REGULATORY TECHNIQUES

These therapeutic tools are used to influence a person's mind/body state, i.e., their physiological reactions, mental and emotional states, and behavior, through the power of the mind. They are thought to foster health by lessening stress, pain and anxiety, by promoting positive attitudes and a sense of control and participation in one's health, and by enhancing immune system function. They are used in a variety of settings for a wide range of problems including cancer, substance abuse, preoperative preparation, weight loss, cardiovascular disorders, stress management, and in the treatment of many acute and chronic diseases.

Biofeedback

Biofeedback teaches an individual to become aware of processes and sensations in the body that are not normally apparent, and to learn to bring them under conscious control with the use of special equipment. An individual is hooked up to a biofeedback instrument which measures such physiological variables as skin temperature and heart rate and translates those measurements to either visual readouts or auditory tones. The individual then attempts to alter those measurements and thus affect the body function(s) being measured. Since the equipment is designed to detect even minute changes in measurements, the patient's effort to affect body processes is reinforced by every positive change in measurement, no matter how small, and the patient is further encouraged to bring these processes into conscious awareness and control. Over time, the goal is to be able to influence these sensations and processes without the aid of the biofeedback instruments. This therapeutic approach is often used to treat stress-related ailments such as migraine headaches, high blood pressure and gastrointestinal disorders.

Organizations

411. Association for Applied Psychophysiology and Biofeedback (AAPB)
10200 West 44th Avenue, #304, Wheat Ridge, CO 80033-2840
Telephone: 303-422-8436; 800-477-8892; Fax: 303-422-8894
Contact: Francine Butler, Ph. D., executive director

Founded in 1969 as the Biofeedback Research Society and later known as the Biofeedback Society of America, this membership society is dedicated to the study of biofeedback and applied psychophysiology.

Services for the professional: Offers continuing education programs; sponsors an annual conference; offers workshops; serves as an information resource: publishes a journal, newsletter and other publications.

Services for the public: Offers an information fact sheet and an eight-page information brochure on biofeedback (send legal-size self-addressed stamped envelope); provides referrals to state chapter chairmen; provides list of practitioners.

Publications: *Biofeedback and Self-Regulation,* quarterly journal, free to members in certain categories, $55 (individual subscription) (reviewed under Biofeedback—Journals and Newsletters); *Biofeedback,* news magazine, 3 times a year, free to members; *Membership Directory,* annual; *Annual Meeting Proceedings,* $15 members, $30 nonmembers; *AAPB Survey of Instruments and Software for Biofeedback-Applied Physiology,* $8.00 members, $10.00 nonmembers; *Biofeedback: A Client Information Paper,* one copy free, multiple copies available at member and nonmember rates; *Biofeedback: An Information Kit,* $4.00 members, $10.00 nonmembers.

412. Biofeedback Certification Institute of America (BCIA)
10200 West 44th Avenue, #304, Wheat Ridge, CO 80033
Telephone: 303-420-2902; Fax: 303-422-8894
Contact: Francine Butler, Ph. D., executive director

The credentialing organization working in conjunction with the Association for Applied Psychophysiology and Biofeedback.

Services for the professional: Offers credentialing in biofeedback to health care professionals, both general certification and specialty certification; currently developing a listing of training programs that meet the BCIA criteria for didactic training in biofeedback.

Services for the public: Provides a register of certified biofeedback practitioners.

413. The Mankind Research Foundation (MRF)
1315 Apple Avenue, Silver Spring, MD 20910
Telephone: 301-587-8686; Fax: 301-585-8959
See chapter 1: General—Organizations.

Schools

414. Biofeedback Institute of Los Angeles (BILA)
3810 South Robertson Boulevard, #216, Culver City, CA 90232
Telephone: 310-841-4970; 800-246-3526; Fax: 310-841-0923
Contact: Marjorie K. Toomim, director

Offers professional training in clinical biofeedback, focusing on stress and stress-related disorders and their treatment with biofeedback-assisted relaxation, imagery and cognitive behavior modification procedures. Courses are appropriate for health care professionals, teachers, and paraprofessionals interested in biofeedback therapy and related modalities. Also offers professional training in neurofeedback for work with attention deficit disorders, learning disabilities, mild head trauma, addictions and other cognitive disorders, and leads to neurofeedback certification. The training programs are approved by the Biofeedback Certification Institute of America, Biofeedback Society of California, and the American Dental Association. The institute is approved by the American Psychological Association to offer continuing education credit for psychologists.

415. Biofeedback Instrument Company (BIC)
255 West 98th Street, New York, NY 10025
Telephone: 212-222-5665
Contact: Philip Brotman, Ph.D.

Offers a monthly course in biofeedback certification training for professionals, approved for American Psychological Association continuing education credit and nationwide certification.

416. Himalayan International Institute of Yoga Science and Philosophy (Himalayan Institute) (HIIYSP)
RR1 Box 400, Honesdale, PA 18431
Telephone: 717-253-5551; Fax: 717-253-9078
See chapter 6: Yoga—Schools.

417. Institute for Holistic Healing Studies (IHHS)
San Francisco State University
1600 Holloway Avenue, San Francisco, CA 94132

Telephone: 415-338-1200; Fax: 415-338-0573
See chapter 1: General—Schools.

418. The Reilly School of Massotherapy (RSM)
67th Street and Atlantic Avenue, Post Office Box 595, Virginia Beach, VA 23451
Telephone: 804-428-0446; Fax: 804-422-4631
See chapter 4: Massage—Schools.

Treatment Centers/Referrals

See also Biofeedback—Organizations for referrals to individual practitioners. In addition, local hospitals may offer biofeedback services through departments of neurology, psychology or behavioral medicine.

419. Biofeedback Institute of Los Angeles
1450 10th Street, Suite 402, Santa Monica, CA 90491-2831
Telephone: 213-933-9451

The institute offers a full service program of counseling, psychotherapy, biofeedback training, and stress and pain management. Eleven separate programs are available: 1) treatment center for stress-related disorders such as headaches, back pain, insomnia, anxiety, diabetes, hypertension and more. Treatment includes extensive biofeedback training; 2) post-traumatic stress center uses biofeedback-assisted treatment procedures; 3) the EEG training center uses EEG biofeedback to affect brain wave frequency patterns for such conditions as learning disabilities, chronic fatigue, head injury, stroke, hyperactivity, insomnia, and other conditions; 4) substance abuse center offers outpatient treatment based on Peniston's research and the Menninger Clinic model. The program features EEG alpha/theta brain wave training as well as group, individual, marriage and family counseling; 5) incontinence training with EMG biofeedback; 6) diabetic's service center uses biofeedback and relaxation training to gain control of blood sugar levels and temperature training to control neuropathy; 7) hypnosis and hypnotherapy for habit control, eating disorders, fears and phobias, insomnia, pain control and other conditions with the addition of biofeedback instrumentation and training; 8) biodynamic fitness utilizes EMG measurement of muscles in action to prevent work-related pain and injury; 9) psychotherapy and counseling through cognitive behavior modification therapy monitored with biofeedback instruments; 10) workplace pain and injury prevention training; 11) healing center for abused and disabled children and parents uses stress management, sensory development and creativity. In addition, as a community service, treatment is available for selected clients who have no insurance or other ability to pay. Treatment is given by professional training course interns for a $5.00 voluntary donation.

420. Georgetown University Medical Center
Behavioral Medicine Programs
3800 Reservoir Road, N.W., Washington, DC 20007-2197
Telephone: 202-687-8770; Fax: 202-687-6658
Contact: Rebecca E. Chen, coordinator, specialty programs
See chapter 1: General—Treatment Centers/Referrals.

421. The Menninger Clinic
Clinical Resources
Post Office Box 829, Topeka, KS 66601-0829
Telephone: 913-273-7500; 800-351-9058

This innovative mental health center, established in 1925, has been a leader in the use of biofeedback therapy. In addition, it utilizes hypnotherapy, relaxation therapy, art therapy, fitness therapy and patient education as well as traditional forms of medical and psychiatric treatment to support the integration of more constructive forms of behavior. Treatment programs consist of outpatient services, partial hospital services, residential treatment, and acute hospital services. All patients receive an individualized treatment plan formulated by a team of health professionals supervised by a psychiatrist. Conditions treated include chemical dependency, sleep disorders, dyslexia, chronic illness, depression and manic depression, headache treatment, trauma recovery, anxiety disorders and more. The clinic is licensed by the state of Kansas and is accredited by the Joint Commission on Accreditation of Healthcare Organizations. It is an approved hospital for Blue Cross, Medicare and many other insurance carriers.

422. The New Center for Wholistic Health Education & Research
6801 Jericho Turnpike, Syosset, NY 11791-4413
Telephone: 516-496-7766
See chapter 1: General—Treatment Centers/Referrals.

423. Shealy Institute for Comprehensive Health Care
1328 East Evergreen, Springfield, MO 65803
Telephone: 417-865-5940; Fax: 417-865-6111
Contact: Nancy Almirall, R.N., administrator
See chapter 1: General—Treatment Centers/Referrals.

Product Suppliers

424. Biocomp Research Institute
3710 South Robertson Boulevard, #216, Culver City, CA 90232
Telephone: 310-841-4970; 800-246-3526
Credit Cards: None

Designs, manufactures and sells biofeedback equipment.

425. Biofeedback Instrument Company
255 West 98th Street, New York, NY 10025
Telephone: 212-222-5665
Credit Cards: Visa, MasterCard, American Express

Sells biofeedback instrumentation and stress tapes for clinical applications.

426. The Relaxation Company
20 Lumber Road, Roslyn, NY 11576
Telephone: 516-621-2727; 800-788-6670 (Orders); Fax: 516-621-2750
Credit Cards: Visa, MasterCard

Develops and sells products that promote relaxation, including audiotapes, compact discs and massage oils.

427. Tools for Exploration
4460 Redwood Highway, Suite 2, San Rafael, CA 94903
Telephone: 415-499-9050; 800-456-9887 (Orders Only); Fax: 415-499-9047
Credit Cards: Visa, MasterCard
See chapter 5: Energy Medicine—General—Product Suppliers.

Hypnotherapy

Though viewed with suspicion and disdain as recently as the 1950s, hypnotherapy has gradually gained acceptance over the last forty years. Derived from the Greek word *hypnos,* which means sleep, hypnosis is an altered state in which the conscious mind is relaxed and the subconscious mind is alert and receptive to suggestions. When given suggestions which are within the realm of one's value system, an individual is able to accept those suggestions in a way not possible when the conscious mind is in control. Hypnotherapy refers to the use of this relaxed state of mind to explore an individual's long-held attitudes and their origins and to make suggestions which will reprogram certain undesirable behaviors. Hypnotherapy can be used to treat stress, high blood pressure, smoking addiction, poor eating habits, some chronic and acute pain problems, and many other conditions.

Organizations

428. Academy of Scientific Hypnotherapy (ASH)
Post Office Box 12041, San Diego, CA 92112
Telephone: 619-427-6225; Fax: 619-427-5650
Contact: W. E. Kemery, Ph.D., F.A.S.H.

A nonprofit worldwide membership organization serving as a referral service to qualified professionals in the field of hypnotherapy and as an information resource for the public and members of the academy.

Services for the professional: Offers a referral service; provides certification to practitioners; maintains a library and statistics; conducts legal and political activities.

Services for the public: Provides referrals to professionals in the healing arts properly trained in hypnosis; disseminates information on the art and science of hypnosis.

Publications: *Hypnotherapy in Review,* published periodically, free to members and to the public; bulletins to members.

429. American Association of Professional Hypnotherapists (AAPH)
Post Office Box 29, Boones Mill, VA 24065-0029
Telephone: 703-334-3035
Contact: William Brink, executive director

A professional organization with a national and international membership dedicated to strengthening the role of hypnosis as a therapeutic modality, promoting high standards of professional practice, sharing ideas and techniques, and providing information on training and continuing education opportunities.

Services for the professional: Conducts educational activities; encourages high standards of professional conduct; publishes a national and international listing of member hypnotherapists; publishes a newsletter discussing clinical practice issues.

Services for the public: Provides public education on the increasing use of hypnosis in healing and personal growth.

Publications: *Hypnotherapy Today,* quarterly newsletter, free with membership; *National Register of Professional Hypnotherapists,* annual directory, free with membership.

430. American Guild of Hypnotherapists (AGH)

2200 Veterans Boulevard, New Orleans (Kenner), LA 70062
Telephone: 504-468-3223; Fax: 504-468-3213
Contact: Dr. Reg Sheldrick
National Headquarters: 7117 Farnam Street, Omaha, NE 68132

A nonprofit international organization for professional hypnotherapists, hypnotists, chiropractors, medical doctors, psychologists, counselors, attorneys, nurses, law enforcement officials, and others who use hypnosis in their professional practice. The purpose of the guild is to register hypnotherapists, professional hypnotists and others whose professional governing bodies allow the use of hypnosis in their practice, provide training seminars, and establish standards of professionalism and education.

Services for the professional: Conducts training and continuing education programs; offers a scholarship program for bachelors, master and doctoral degree programs at Southwest University, New Orleans, (Kenner), LA; conducts active legislative program opposing anti-hypnosis state laws; publishes a journal, newsletter and membership directory.

Publications: *Journal of Hypnotherapy*, periodic, free to members; periodic newsletters; *AGH Directory of Registrants*, free to members.

431. The American Society of Clinical Hypnosis (ASCH)

2200 East Devon Avenue, Suite 291, Des Plaines, Illinois 60018-4534
Telephone: 708-297-3317; Fax: 708-297-7309

A not-for-profit organization of professionals in the fields of medicine, dentistry and psychology who have an interest in the scientific and clinical aspects of hypnosis. ASCH supports education programs, research and scientific publication, cooperation among related professional societies, and the incorporation of hypnosis into clinical medicine and scientific research.

Services for the professional: Holds annual workshops and scientific meetings with accredited continuing education hours for most disciplines; conducts regional educational workshops at the basic and advanced levels; engages in legislative activity regarding the use and practice of hypnosis; offers certification including ASCH certification in clinical hypnosis and ASCH approved consultant in clinical hypnosis; conducts public relations activities; publishes a journal, newsletter and membership directory.

Services for the public: Offers referrals by region to selected member doctors, dentists, psychologists, and social workers with extensive hours of training in clinical hypnosis techniques (send self-addressed stamped envelope).

Publications: *The American Journal of Clinical Hypnosis*, quarterly, free to members; *The ASCH Newsletter*, periodic, free to members.

432. Institute for Research in Hypnosis and Psychotherapy (IRHP)

1991 Broadway, Suite 18B, New York, NY 10023
Telephone: 212-874-5290; Fax: 914-238-1422
Contact: Jack Adler, administrator

A postgraduate research and training institute chartered by the Board of Regents of the University of the State of New York. Supports hypnotherapy as a specialized treatment modality for a wide range of mental health and behavioral problems through research, the development of standards and procedures for advanced education in hypnosis, education, training and clinical services.

Services for the professional: Provides education and training; offers a clinical fellowship in hypnosis and hypnoanalysis; conducts ongoing research; provides clinical services (see The Morton Prince Mental Health Center of the Institute for Research in Hypnosis under Hypnotherapy—Treatment Centers/Referrals); offers certification in hypnotherapy and hypnoanalysis.

Services for the public: Provides information and referral service.

433. International Medical and Dental Hypnotherapy Association (IMDHA)

4110 Edgeland, Suite 800, Royal Oak, MI 48073
Telephone: 810-549-5594; Fax: 810-549-5421
Contact: Anne H. Spencer, Ph.D., founder and executive director

A membership organization promoting the therapeutic services of certified hypnotherapists in the medical and nonmedical treatment situation.

Services for the professional: Offers certification in hypnotherapy; publishes an annual international referral directory distributed to doctors, health care providers and the general public; provides a mentor program for new members; provides various marketing tools such as brochures, audiotapes and videotapes on hypnosis; offers training and examinations for specialty certifications; sponsors conferences and seminars; publishes a newsletter.

Services for the public: Provides a referral service to qualified hypnotherapists by geographic location; conducts seminars and workshops open to the public.

Publications: *Subconsciously Speaking*, bimonthly newsletter, free to members, $12 nonmembers.

434. National Society of Hypnotherapists (NSH)

2175 N.W. 86th Street 6A, Des Moines, IA 50325
Telephone: 515-270-2280
Contact: Dr. Kathie K. Wolfe, Ph.D., C.HT., executive director

A nonprofit membership organization promoting hypnotherapy as a distinct profession. Maintains high standards through certification and continuing education opportunities. Works to educate the general public on the practice of hypnotherapy.

Services for the professional: Provides a recognized certification examination; keeps members informed on the latest laws and regulations regarding the practice of hypnotherapy; sponsors an annual symposium.

Services for the public: Provides information on hypnotherapy and a referral service nationwide.

Publications: *National Society of Hypnotherapists Journal,* quarterly, free to members; *NSH Hypnosis Organization Directory,* $7.00.

435. The Society for Clinical and Experimental Hypnosis (SCEH)

6728 Old McLean Village Drive, McLean, VA 22101-3906
Telephone: 703-556-9222; Fax: 703-556-8729
Contact: Laura Degnon, executive assistant

A professional membership organization of psychologists, psychiatrists, dentists, medical doctors and social workers with an MSW, who practice, study, research, or teach hypnosis. The society's goals include education and training in hypnosis, communication through scientific meetings and publications, the establishment of practice guidelines, dissemination of information to the public and to public and private agencies, interdisciplinary cooperation, encouragement of scientific research in the field, and maintenance of a referral service.

Services for the professional: Conducts annual workshops and scientific programs in clinical and experimental hypnosis with university co-sponsorship (provides professional continuing education credits); provides information to professionals seeking a course of study in hypnosis; publishes a journal and newsletter.

Services for the public: Provides information to public inquiries on hypnosis; makes referrals to professional practitioners by geographic location.

Publications: *The International Journal of Clinical and Experimental Hypnosis,* quarterly, free to members, $54 (individual subscription), $101 (institutional subscription) (reviewed under Hypnotherapy—Journals and Newsletters); *The Society for Clinical and Experimental Hypnosis Newsletter,* quarterly, free to members.

Schools

436. Hypnosis Motivation Institute (HMI)
18607 Ventura Boulevard, #310, Tarzana, CA 91356
Telephone: 818-758-2747; 800-479-9HMI
Contact: Admissions Director

The only college of hypnosis in the United States to be accredited by the Accrediting Council of Continuing Education and Training, the institute offers a one-year, 720-hour program in clinical hypnotherapy. The program is comprised of six courses: Hypnosis 101, an introductory course; Hypnosis 201, which exposes students to a variety of hypnotherapy styles; Hypnosis 301, which teaches students how to apply the tools they have learned in the preceding classes to different areas of clinical application. In this class, every fourth lesson consists of actual therapies performed on clients in the classroom. Upon completion of this class, students are awarded a hypnotherapy diploma. The remainder of the program consists of courses in handwriting analysis, clinical applications and a clinical internship. Students who complete the entire program are eligible for certification as a hypnotherapist. Financial aid through federal loan and grant programs is available. Through the institute's extension school, the first three courses are also available as a correspondence course. Visa and MasterCard accepted for payment of correspondence course tuition. Both programs are appropriate for health care professionals as well as interested members of the lay public.

437. Infinity Institute International (III)
4110 Edgeland, Department 800, Royal Oak, MI 48073-2251
Telephone: 810-549-5594; Fax: 810-549-5421
Contact: Anne H. Spencer, Ph.D., founder

Offers forty-four-hour programs in basic hypnosis and advanced hypnosis, and a forty-eight-hour hypnoanalysis training program. All courses are held on weekends and are approved by the American Institute of Hypnotherapy and the International Medical and Dental Hypnotherapy Association. Completion of these programs qualifies students for certification with the International Medical and Dental Hypnotherapy Association. Throughout the year, the institute offers two-day specialty hypnosis workshops for continuing education. All courses are appropriate for those working in any aspect of the health care field. (See also chapter 5: Therapeutic Touch—Schools.)

438. Institute for Therapeutic Learning (ITL)
8631 21st Avenue N.W., Seattle, WA 98117
Telephone: 206-783-1838
Contact: Jack Elias, director

Offers a 150-hour course completed over six weekends, during a seventeen-day summer intensive session, or through a correspondence course, and leading to certification as an advanced clinical hypnotherapist. Such certification qualifies an individual for certification and membership as a clinical hypnotherapist with state, national and international professional associations. Also offers a 300-hour course leading to certification as a master clinical hypnotherapist. Customized continuing education programs and courses on a noncertification basis are also available.

439. The Milton H. Erickson Foundation, Inc. (MHEF)
3606 North 24th Street, Phoenix, AZ 85016-6500
Telephone: 602-956-6196; Fax: 602-956-0519
Contact: Jeffrey K. Zeig, director

Offers five-day programs for professionals with a minimum of a master's degree in a health/mental health field from a regionally accredited institution and for graduate students in the health/mental health fields in accredited programs. Three levels of training are offered: Fundamental training assumes no prior knowledge of or experience with Ericksonian hypnotherapy; Intermediate training explores in detail hypnotic application for specific clinical issues; the advanced intensive focuses on the process of Ericksonian therapy and resources of the therapist. Courses are approved for continuing education credits for physicians by the American Medical Association and for psychologists by the American Psychological Association. Visa and MasterCard are accepted for payment of fees.

Treatment Centers/Referrals

See Hypnotherapy—Organizations for referrals to individual practitioners.

440. Biofeedback Institute of Los Angeles
1450 10th Street, Suite 402, Santa Monica, CA 90491-2831
Telephone: 213-933-9451
See Biofeedback—Treatment Centers/Referrals.

441. Hypnosis Motivation Institute
18607 Ventura Boulevard, #310, Tarzana, CA 91356

Telephone: 818-758-2747; 800-479-9HMI

Founded in 1967 by Dr. John G. Kappas, HMI is a multidisciplinary clinic of hypnotherapy services treating a variety of problems and individual treatment goals. The clinic sees several hundred clients per week and has a clinic staff of over fifty therapists. A nonprofit program providing free hypnotherapy services through the clinical hypnotherapy program is also available.

442. The Morton Prince Mental Health Center of the Institute for Research in Hypnosis

1991 Broadway, #18B, New York, NY 10023
Telephone: 212-874-5290; Fax: 914-238-1422

This is the oldest nonprofit mental health center in the United States providing low-cost hypnotherapy for a variety of emotional and physiological disorders. It provides treatment programs in psychological and medical hypnosis for psychosomatic and sleep disorders, phobic reactions, allergic disorders, learning problems, obesity, anorexia nervosa, speech disorders, pain problems and addictive behaviors. The Morton Prince Center is the clinical arm of the Institute for Research in Hypnosis, a postgraduate research and training institute approved by the American Psychological Association for continuing education and chartered by the Board of Regents of the University of the State of New York. For the professional, the center offers fellowships in clinical hypnosis and hypnoanalysis leading to certification.

Imagery

Images are internal mental representations of external reality. These mental impressions use all the senses, seeing, hearing, smell, taste, touch and movement, and are used consciously for a specific purpose. There are various therapeutic forms of imagery, including guided visualization, progressive relaxation, desensitization, inner guide visualization, and others. Imagery is thought to operate by stimulating the autonomic nervous system, which affects physiological processes such as heart rate, the immune response, stress reactions, the gastrointestinal system, and the circulatory system. It may be used for pain control, stress reduction, depression, self-improvement, and in the healing of various diseases and conditions.

Organizations

443. International Imagery Association (IIA)
Post Office Box 1046, Bronx, NY 10471

A nonprofit international membership organization dedicated to the study and applications of mental imagery. Promotes a multidisciplinary approach, encourages communication on the uses and benefits of imagery and encourages imagery research. Organizes publication of books and periodicals on imagery.

Services for the professional: Provides education, training, and networking through local, national and international research, clinical and personal growth programs and conferences; holds division, chapter and state meetings on imagery; sells books and audiotapes; publishes a journal and newsletter.

Services for the public: Provides referrals to practitioners and information on imagery.

Publications: *Journal of Mental Imagery,* quarterly, $40.00 (subscription); *Imagery Today,* newsletter, free with membership; *Mental Imagery Abstracts: 1977-1989,* monograph, $25.00; *Imagery Bibliography (1977-1991),* monograph, $25.00.

Schools

444. Academy for Guided Imagery (AGI)
Post Office Box 2070, Mill Valley, CA 94942
Telephone: 415-389-9324, 800-726-2070; Fax: 415-389-9342
Contact: David E. Bresler, Ph.D., co-director; Martin L. Rossman, M.D., co-director

Offers a professional certification program in Interactive Guided Imagery, a 150-hour training program, given in six workshops over a twelve- to twenty-four-month period, consisting of workshop training, personal supervision and independent study. Also offers workshops in a variety of locations around the United States and a home study program in Interactive Guided Imagery. All programs are appropriate for medical, nursing and mental health professionals. Continuing education credits available for most professionals. Visa and MasterCard accepted for payment of fees.

Treatment Centers/Referrals

See Imagery—Organizations for referrals to individual practitioners.

Product Suppliers

445. Academy for Guided Imagery
Post Office Box 2070, Mill Valley, CA 94942
Telephone: 415-389-9324; 800-726-2070; Fax: 415-389-9342
Credit Cards: Visa, MasterCard

Sells books, conference tapes, audiotapes, videotapes, self-learning educational systems and related imagery products.

446. International Imagery Association
Post Office Box 1046, Bronx, NY 10471
See Imagery—Organizations.

447. Nightingale Knowledge
11053 Bel Aire Court, Cupertino, CA 95014
Telephone: 408-253-2770
See Relaxation/Meditation/Stress Reduction—Product Suppliers.

448. Whole Person Associates, Inc.
210 West Michigan, Duluth, MN 55802
Telephone: 218-727-0500; 800-247-6789; Fax: 218-727-0505
Credit Cards: Visa, MasterCard

Sells Julie T. Lusk's *Thirty Scripts for Relaxation, Imagery and Inner Healing.* For other products sold by this company, see Meditation/Relaxation/Stress Reduction—Product Suppliers.

Meditation/Relaxation/Stress Reduction

This group of therapies seeks to influence behavior, emotions, and attitudes through learned forms of mental concentration, deep relaxation, self-awareness, visualization and lifestyle change. It is an interdisciplinary field covering such areas as medicine, psychology, psychiatry, nursing, education, dentistry, physical and occupational therapy, and spiritual practice. These approaches have been used therapeutically both to help alleviate and manage stress-related symptomotology and illness such as headache, cardiovascular problems, gastrointestinal disorders and more, and to actively promote positive health and well-being.

Organizations

449. The American Institute of Stress (AIS)
124 Park Avenue, Yonkers, NY 10703
Telephone: 914-963-1200; Fax: 914-965-6267
Contact: JoAnn Ogawa, administrative assistant

A not-for-profit organization acting as a clearinghouse for information related to stress and disease and as an impartial and reliable resource for evaluating various stress-reduction strategies, programs and measurement methodologies.

Services for the professional: Maintains extensive current files on all aspects of stress research and provides reprints for a small cost; maintains a list of stress-reduction services with evaluation where possible; develops and coordinates conferences and symposia on stress-related topics for lay and professional audiences; publishes a newsletter.

Services for the public: Sells stress packets on specific stress-related topics ($35.00 minimum charge); provides expert witness services.

Publications: *The Newsletter of the American Institute of Stress,* monthly, free to members, $35.00 (subscription) (reviewed under Meditation/Relaxation/Stress Reduction—Journals and Newsletters).

450. International Stress Management Association (ISMA)
Institute for Stress Management
United States International University, 10455 Pomerado Road, San Diego, CA 92131
Telephone: 619-271-4300; Fax: 619-693-4669

A nonprofit international organization with professional members from the fields of dentistry, medicine, education, psychology, physical therapy, nursing, speech pathology, occupational therapy and human communication as well as the general public. Supports the acquisition and dissemination of knowledge on stress management, stress-related disorders and tension control strategies.

Services for the professional: Promotes the education of professionals and students and interdisciplinary scientific research in the field of stress management.

Publications: *International Journal of Stress Management,* quarterly, $18.50 (member subscription), $35.00 (nonmember subscription), $75.00 (institutional subscription) (reviewed under Meditation/Relaxation/Stress Reduction—Journals and Newsletters).

451. The Society of Behavioral Medicine (SBM)

103 South Adams Street, Rockville, MD 20850
Telephone: 301-251-2790; Fax: 301-279-6749

A multidisciplinary nonprofit organization of researchers and clinicians promoting the integration of behavioral and biomedical approaches to health and disease prevention. Members include physicians, nurses, clinical psychologists, epidemiologists, experimental psychologists, medical biologists and others.

Services for the professional: Holds an annual scientific meeting; disseminates technical information; provides information on training in behavioral medicine; educates the health professions and the public on developments in the field; publishes journals, annual meeting proceedings, and a newsletter.

Publications: *Annals of Behavioral Medicine,* quarterly journal, free to members, $135.00 (subscription) (reviewed under Meditation/Relaxation/Stress Reduction—Journals and Newsletters); *Mind-Body Medicine,* quarterly journal, $80.00 (individual subscription), $120.00 (institutional subscription) (reviewed under Meditation/Relaxation/Stress Reduction—Journals and Newsletters); annual meeting proceedings.

Schools

452. Stress Reduction Clinic (SRC)

Division of Preventive and Behavioral Medicine, University of Massachusetts, Department of Medicine, University of Massachusetts Medical Center, 55 Lake Avenue North, Worcester, MA 01655
Telephone: 508-856-2656; Fax: 508-856-1977
Contact: Saki F. Santorelli, Ed.D., director of professional training and development

Offers professional training programs at various locations across the United States through the Omega Institute (see also chapter 1: General—Schools). Conducted by Drs. Jon Kabat-Zinn and Saki Santorelli, programs vary in length from five to seven days and are intended to introduce health professionals to "mindfulness-based stress reduction training." Also offers a professional "internship" program at the stress reduction clinic, which provides health professionals the opportunity to train intensively in mindfulness meditation and, at the same time, spend time in the clinic and explore how mindfulness may be of use in one's own work.

Treatment Centers/Referrals

453. Biofeedback Institute of Los Angeles

1450 10th Street, Suite 402, Santa Monica, CA 90491-2831
Telephone: 213-933-9451
See Biofeedback—Treatment Centers/Referrals.

454. El Camino Hospital

c/o Community Health Education, Stress Reduction Clinic, 2500 Grant Road, Mountain View, CA 94039
Telephone: 415-940-7070; 408-223-4040

An eight-week educational program consisting of weekly two-and-one-half hour sessions and one all-day session in relaxation and awareness training and practice which is modeled on the Stress Reduction and Relaxation Clinic developed by Jon Kabat-Zinn, Ph.D., at the University of Massachusetts Medical Center. This is a wellness and stress-management program for healthy people as well as an adjunct to the medical management of chronic pain and stress-related disorders such as high blood pressure, cancer, fibromyalgia, arthritis, gastrointestinal disorders and others.

455. Deaconess Hospital

Division of Behavioral Medicine, Mind/Body Clinic, One Deaconess Road, Boston, MA 02164
Telephone: 617-632-9530; Fax: 617-632-7383

The behavioral medicine clinical programs treat patients with chronic illness or stress-related physical symptoms. Based on the latest findings in behavioral medicine, the programs combine conventional medical treatments with strategies that address the behavior and attitudes of the patient. Treatment includes the use of the relaxation response (a physiological state of deep relaxation), exercise/activity programs, nutrition, cognitive therapies to enhance coping skills, stress management, goal setting, and instruction in specific appropriate skills relative to the patient's condition. The programs are directed by Herbert Benson, M.D., Eileen Stuart, M.S., R.N, and Margaret Caudill, M.D., Ph.D. There are eleven clinical programs available: behavioral medicine general program for general stress-related symptoms; HIV+/AIDS; cancer; cardiac rehabilitation; chemotherapy and radiation therapy; chronic pain; cardiac risk reduction program for hypertension, diabetes and dyslipedemia; infertility; insomnia; IVF/GIFT; and pre-medical, surgical or radiological procedure program. All programs are conducted on an outpatient basis and most consist of one initial assessment, ten weekly two-hour visits, and one discharge assessment. In most cases medical insurance claims are submitted directly to the patient's insurance carrier as hospital outpatient medical clinic visits.

456. The Hart Institute

645 North Michigan Avenue, Suite 800, Chicago, IL 60611
Telephone: 312-493-HART; Fax: 312-493-4278 (call first)
Contact: Dr. Ariel Kerman, executive director

Dedicated to identifying, developing and mainstreaming cost-effective solutions to major health problems, the institute offers a variety of individual treatment programs. These include the HART Program, a biobehavioral treatment program to lower blood pressure without drugs, using deep relaxation, temperature feedback, stress management and lifestyle change; the heart disease reversal program, based on the work of Dr. Dean Ornish, incorporating stress management, low-fat diet, exercises, social support, relaxation, imaging, breathing and lifestyle changes; custom-designed mind body stress management programs, consisting of stress management and relaxation techniques and lifestyle changes; the behavioral medicine pain management program, based on the work of Margaret Caudell, M.D., and Jon Kabat-Zinn, Ph.D., including mindfulness awareness training, relaxation and cognitive behavioral strategies, exercise, and lifestyle changes; the positive interactions workshop, teaching verbal and nonverbal communication skills and problem solving. The institute, along with the Rush Corporate Health Center, conducts clinical and outcomes research and invites individual and corporate participation. The institute is headed by Dr. Ariel Kerman, Adjunct Faculty Member of the University of Chicago Hospital Academy. Dr. Kerman has a Ph.D. in clinical psychology and behavioral medicine. The medical director is Dr. Keith Berndston, Assistant Professor of Family and Preventive Medicine, Rush-Presbyterian-St. Luke's Medical Center.

457. Himalayan International Institute of Yoga Science and Philosophy (Himalayan Institute)

RR1 Box 400, Honesdale, PA 18431
Telephone: 717-253-5551; Fax: 717-253-9078
See chapter 6: Yoga—Treatment Centers/Referrals.

458. The Institute of Preventive Medicine

95 East Main Street, Denville, NJ 07834
Telephone: 201-586-4111

320 Belleville Avenue, Bloomfield, NJ 07003
Telephone: 201-743-1151

230 Silver Lake Road, Blairstown, NJ 07825
Telephone: 908-362-8446
See chapter 1: General—Treatment Centers/Referrals.

459. Life Transition Therapy, Inc.
100 Delgado Compound, Suite A, Santa Fe, NM 87501
Telephone: 505-982-4183
See chapter 1: General—Treatment Centers/Referrals.

460. Livingston Foundation Medical Center
3232 Duke Street, San Diego, CA 92110
Telephone: 619-224-3515; Fax: 619-224-6253
See chapter 1: General—Treatment Centers/Referrals.

461. Mind/Body Medicine
2440 East Fifth Street, Suite 110, Tyler, TX 75701
Telephone: 903-592-2202
Contact: Patricia Grelling, M.A., program director

This treatment program is directed to patients who have an illness that is created or complicated by stress, such as cardiovascular disease, migraine headaches, digestive disorders, back pain or asthma, or are coping with a stressful chronic or serious illness such as cancer. Mind/body medicine programs consist of ten-week sessions meeting once a week for two hours. The core program includes teaching and practicing the relaxation response, a technique based on years of research and clinical experience by Harvard Medical School, the University of Massachusetts Medical Center, and other leading medical schools and hospitals. Also included is instruction in the use of visualization, gentle stretching exercises, nutrition, and mind/body principles. The Optimal Living Program is a preventive program of stress-management strategies. Other programs are geared to hypertension, cardiac rehabilitation, back pain therapy, and the two-hour pre-surgery program. The mind/body medicine team consists of two M.D.s, an M.A. and a Ph.D. psychologist.

462. Preventive Medicine Research Institute
900 Bridgeway, Suite 1, Sausalito, CA 94965
Telephone: 415-332-2525; Fax: 415-332-5730
See chapter 1: General—Treatment Centers/Referrals.

463. Santa Cruz Medical Clinic

Stress Reduction Program, 2025 Soquel Avenue, Santa Cruz, CA 95062
Telephone: 408-458-5842

An outpatient program based on the mindfulness stress-reduction work of Jon Kabat-Zinn of the University of Massachusetts Medical Center, this eight-week training session in mindfulness-based meditation meets once a week for two hours. The program is appropriate for the management of daily life stress as well as a complement to the medical management of a variety of medical conditions including arthritis, heart disease, hypertension, AIDS, migraine headaches, panic and sleep disorders, fibromyalgia, and others.

464. Shealy Institute for Comprehensive Health Care

1328 East Evergreen, Springfield, MO 65803
Telephone: 417-865-5940; Fax: 417-865-6111
See chapter 1: General—Treatment Centers/Referrals.

465. The University of Massachusetts Medical Center

Division of Preventive and Behavioral Medicine, Stress Reduction Clinic, Department of Medicine, 55 Lake Avenue North, Worcester, MA 01655
Telephone: 508-856-2656; Fax: 508-856-1977

The stress reduction and relaxation program (SR and RP) at the University of Massachusetts Medical Center, an outpatient behavioral medicine clinic led by Jon Kabat-Zinn, Ph.D, is the oldest and largest hospital-based stress-reduction clinic in the United States. The eight-week course is intended as a complement to medical treatment for conditions such as heart disease, chronic pain, gastrointestinal disorders, high blood pressure, cancer, AIDS, fatigue, headaches, anxiety, panic, and other conditions. Referral from a physician or health care provider, including diagnosis, is required. The program consists of intensive training in mindfulness meditation and yoga and includes a pre- and postevaluation interview and twenty-seven hours of class time. It is offered in cycles three times a year in the fall, winter and spring. Registration begins two months prior to the beginning of each cycle. Also offered is a five-day stress-reduction retreat for health, stress and pain-related problems. Mindfulness practices are taught, including the body scan, sitting meditation, hatha yoga, walking meditation, and group discussions and presentations.

Product Suppliers

466. The Hart Institute

645 North Michigan Avenue, Suite 800, Chicago, IL 60611
Telephone: 312-493-HART; Fax: 312-493-4278 (call first)
Credit Cards: None

Sells HART biobehavioral treatment program audiotapes and workbooks. Discounts on large orders are available to clinic-based programs.

467. Nightingale Knowledge

11053 Bel Aire Court, Cupertino, CA 95014
Telephone: 408-253-2770
Credit Cards: None

Sells audiotapes containing relaxation and guided imagery programs. Tapes were developed by Nightingale Knowledge owner Eileen Durham, who is also a pediatric staff nurse and relaxation and imagery coordinator at Stanford University-affiliated Lucile Salter Packard Children's Hospital.

468. Stress Reduction Tapes

Post Office Box 547, Lexington, MA 02173
Credit Cards: None

Sells mindfulness meditation tapes, a series of audiotapes with Dr. Jon Kabat-Zinn designed to help develop or expand a personal meditation practice based on mindfulness.

469. Whole Person Associates, Inc.

210 West Michigan, Duluth, MN 55802
Telephone: 218-727-0500; 800-247-6789; Fax: 218-727-0505
Credit Cards: Visa, MasterCard

Sells stress and wellness materials which focus on the whole person: body, mind, spirit and relationships. Offerings include the well-known *Thirty Scripts for Relaxation, Imagery & Inner Healing,* other books, videotapes, audiotapes and related products on the topics of stress management, wellness and relaxation.

CHAPTER 8: SENSORY THERAPIES

Aromatherapy

Aromatherapy focuses on the therapeutic use of essential oils extracted from the leaves, stems, roots, flowers and other parts of aromatic plants. Essential oils are a potent form of herbal treatment and can be used to restore and enhance well-being of body, mind and spirit. Oils may be applied topically or inhaled, and are often used in massage and bodywork and other healing therapies. Essential oils may be used to treat digestive ailments, muscle pains, circulatory and respiratory problems, arthritis and other medical conditions.

Organizations

470. American Alliance of Aromatherapy (AAA)
Post Office Box 750428, Petaluma, CA 94975-0428
Telephone: 707-778-6762; Fax: 707-769-0868
Contact: Evan Parker

A not-for-profit professional membership organization for aromatherapy practitioners, manufacturers, retailers and distributors to share knowledge, encourage education, and promote ethical and fair business practices.

Services for the professional: Sponsors conferences; acts as a network for the exchange of information; publishes a newsletter and journal.

Services for the public: Provides referrals to aromatherapists by geographic location; provides information on aromatherapy.

Publications: *The International Journal of Aromatherapy*, quarterly, $30 (subscription) (reviewed under Aromatherapy—Journals and Newsletters); *American Alliance of Aromatherapy News Quarterly*, newsletter, free to members.

471. National Association for Holistic Aromatherapy (NAHA)
219 Carl Street, San Francisco, CA 94117
Telephone: 415-564-6785; Fax: 415-564-6799
Contact: Jeanne Rose, chair; Sara Hindman, editor

A membership organization dedicated to the research and maintenance of high standards of aromatherapy in the United States. Conducts research and product evaluations, sets standards of education and quality, promotes communication and public awareness, and participates in the maintenance of an independent National Aromatherapy Certification Board.

Services for the professional: Publishes a membership directory of professional aromatherapists; maintains a list of accepted aromatherapy schools; facilitates networking with other professionals; offers support from an advisory board.

Services for the public: Offers courses, lectures and classes; publishes a quarterly newsletter.

Publications: *Scensitivity,* quarterly newsletter, free with membership, $8/issue, $20 (subscription) (reviewed under Aromatherapy—Journals and Newsletters); monographs of groups of oils, published regularly.

Schools

472. Atlantic Institute of Aromatherapy (AIA)
16018 Saddlestring Drive, Tampa, FL 33618
Telephone: 813-265-2222; Fax: 813-265-1513
Contact: Sylla Sheppard-Hanger, director

Offers one-day and two-day introductory courses and a three-day advanced seminar. Upon successful completion of the three-day seminar and a written examination, the institute awards a certificate in aromatherapy. Also provides state-certified continuing education credits for licensed massage therapists. All classes are also available on a home-study basis.

473. Aromatherapy and Herbal Studies School (AHSS)
219 Carl Street, San Francisco, CA 94117
Telephone: 415-564-6785; Fax: 415-564-6799
Contact: J. R. Rose

Offers two correspondence courses to train the herbalist and aromatherapist: a thirty-six lesson basic course in herbal studies and an advanced course for the study of aromatherapy and related treatments. Graduates of the aromatherapy course receive a certificate of completion/aromatherapy specialty for fifty hours of advanced aromatherapy study. The course takes a holistic approach, emphasizing not only the oils themselves but the plants from which they come. Also offers beginning classes in herbalism and aromatherapy for the lay public. Jeanne Rose, the instructor and originator of the courses, is a well-known herbalist and aromatherapist. She has written several books and has been teaching and practicing in these fields for twenty-five years. She is also a supplier of essential oils and other aromatherapy products (see Aromatherapy—Product Suppliers). Publishes the newsletter, *AROMAtherapy 2037* (reviewed under Aromatherapy—Journals and Newsletters).

474. Aromatherapy Institute and Research (AIR)
Post Office Box 2354, Fair Oaks, CA 95628
Telephone: 916-965-7546
Contact: Victoria Edwards, owner

Offers two- , three- and five-day certification courses in aromatherapy in cities throughout the United States. Also offers classes at the institute's aromatherapy center in California. Topics covered include: aromatics and the immune system, creating formulas, chakra work with essences, meridian balancing with essential oils, and more.

475. Aromatherapy Seminars (AS)
1830 South Robertson Boulevard, #203, Los Angeles, CA 90035
Telephone: 310-838-6122; Fax: 310-838-2812
Contact: Joan Clark; Michael Scholes

Offers courses in aromatherapy on a home-study basis and "live" classes throughout the United States. With a strong emphasis on blending of essential oils, programs range from a one-day introduction to a five-day certification to a two-year advanced training. These courses are appropriate for anyone interested in aromatherapy, including members of the lay public as well as health care professionals. Aromatherapy Seminars is also a source of Aroma Vera products (see Aromatherapy—Product Suppliers) and publishes a quarterly newsletter, *Beyond Scents* (reviewed under Aromatherapy—Journals and Newsletters).

476. The Australasian College of Herbal Studies (ACHS)
Post Office Box 57, Lake Oswego, OR 97034
Telephone: 503-635-6652; Voice Mail: 1-800-48-STUDY; Fax: 503-697-0615
See chapter 2: Herbal Medicine—Schools.

477. International School of Herbal Cultures (ISHC)
(Herbal Essence, Inc.)

8524 Whispering Creek Trail, Fort Worth, TX 76134
Telephone: 817-293-5410
Contact: Judy Griffin, president and master herbalist
See chapter 2: Herbal Medicine—Schools.

478. The New England Center for Aromatherapy (NECA)
60 Myrtle Street, Suite #1, Boston, MA 02114
Telephone: 617-720-4585
Contact: Elizabeth Gray, president

Offers a ten-lesson correspondence course in holistic aromatherapy, leading to a certificate of completion in the art and science of aromatherapy. Included with the course are thirty sample essential oils and twenty-two drawings of plants used for essential oils.

479. The Pacific Institute of Aromatherapy (PIA)
602 Freitas Parkway, Post Office Box 6723, San Rafael, CA 94903
Telephone: 415-479-9121; Fax: 415-479-0119
Contact: D. Kurt Schnaubelt

Offers a correspondence course on aromatherapy covering every aspect of the field, from scientific data to traditional wisdom, and consisting of original material, reference information, worksheets and essential oil samples. International certification is available to those who successfully complete the course. Also publishes a free newsletter, *Inside Aromatherapy*, on a seasonal basis.

Treatment Centers/Referrals

See Aromatherapy—Organizations for referrals to individual practitioners.

Product Suppliers

480. Aphrodesia Naturals
62 Kent Street, Brooklyn, NY 11222-1517
Telephone: (In NY) 718-383-3677; (All others) 800-221-6898; Fax: 718-383-6618
Credit Cards: Visa, MasterCard, American Express

Sells aromaceutical oils, massage oils and aromatherapy-related products. Minimum order for wholesale is $100.

481. Aroma Vera

5901 Rodeo Road, Los Angeles, CA 90016-4312
Telephone: 310-280-0407; 800-669-9514; Fax: 310-280-0395
Credit Cards: Visa, MasterCard, American Express

Creates and sells essential oil products from safe, renewable resources. Oils are concentrated to save on bottling; they contain no animal ingredients and have not been tested on animals. Refills, large, and bulk sizes are offered to promote reuse and help further preserve resources. Also sells aromatherapy books, posters, aromatic music, health and beauty and related aromatherapy products.

482. Aromatherapy International

300 North Fifth Avenue, Suite 210, Ann Arbor, MI 48104
Telephone: 313-741-1617; Fax: 313-741-7109

3 Seal Harbor Road, Suite 735, Winthrop, MA 02152
Telephone: 617-846-0285; Fax: 617-846-5474

Telephone: 800-722-4377 (Orders only from either location)
Credit Cards: None

Sells aromatherapy oils certified as botanically and biochemically defined essential oils. Also sells glass diffusers, books and related aromatherapy products.

483. Blessed Herbs

109 Barre Plains Road, Oakham, MA 01068
Telephone: 800-489-HERB (4372); Fax: 508-882-3755
Credit Cards: Visa, MasterCard
See chapter 2: Herbal Medicine—Product Suppliers.

484. The Essential Oil Company

Post Office Box 206, Lake Oswego, OR 97034
Telephone: 503-697-5992; 800-729-5912 (Orders only); Fax: 503-697-0615
Credit Cards: Visa, MasterCard

Sells essential oils and massage oils in quantities ranging from one dram to one pound. Wholesale only.

485. Herbal Essence, Inc.

8524 Whispering Creek Trail, Fort Worth, TX 76134

Telephone: 817-293-5410
Credit Cards: None

Sells aromatherapy essential oils.

486. Jeanne Rose Aromatherapy
219 Carl Street, San Francisco, CA 94117
Telephone: 415-564-6785; Fax: 415-564-6799
Credit Cards: Visa, MasterCard

Sells aromatherapy kits for travel and first aid, stress relief, women's care, and meditation. Each kit contains essential oils and instructions for use. Also sells individual essential oils, books on aromatherapy, and other aromatherapy products.

487. Leydet Aromatics
Post Office Box 2354, Fair Oaks, CA 95628
Telephone: 916-965-7546
Credit Cards: Visa, MasterCard, Discover

A mail-order distribution service for essential oils, massage and body oils, healing formulas, products for aromatherapy classes, books, and related aromatherapy products.

Color and Light Therapy

These techniques use the therapeutic effect of light and color frequencies for healing on psychological and physical levels. Based on ancient knowledge and modern science, it is felt that the different wavelengths in light and color affect the human energy system and the physiological processes of the body. The application of various color and light techniques may be used to balance energy and promote healing of such varied conditions as cancer, stress, depression, fatigue and insomnia, and to maintain optimum health.

Organizations

488. Center For Environmental Therapeutics (CET)
Executive Office: Box 532, Georgetown, CO 80444
Telephone: 303-569-0910; Fax: 303-569-0910
Contact: Cynthia Neely, executive director

CET is a nonprofit research and educational organization dedicated to the promotion of scientific research and dissemination of information on environmental interventions for the problems of fatigue, insomnia, stress, SAD (seasonal affective disorder) and depression. Special areas of interest include light therapy, ionization, and sleep surfaces.

Services: Creates and monitors research projects on the development and evaluation of environmental therapies such as light devices, dawn/dusk simulators and high-density negative air ionization; serves as a source of public and professional information, maintaining a library of consumer and technical publications; maintains a list of companies which sell light units and ionizers.

Publications: *Personal Inventory for Depression and SAD Self Assessment,* $3.00; *SAD Information Packet,* includes a list of clinicians and research centers, $7.00; *Clinical Assessment Tools Packet for Clinicians,* $40.00.

489. Dinshah Health Society (DHS)

Post Office Box 707, Malaga, NJ 08328
Telephone: 609-692-4686
Contact: Darius Dinshah, president

An international nonprofit educational and scientific membership organization devoted to increasing public awareness of alternative healing methods, with emphasis on chromotherapy. Based on the work of Dinshah Ghadiali, who studied the effects of light and color in the human body.

Services: Provides information on chromotherapy.

Publications: *Let There be Light,* by Darius Dinshah, book, $12.00; *Spectro-Chrome Metry Encyclopedia,* Dinshah P. Ghadiali, $14.00; *My Spectro-Chrome,* Darius Dinshah, videotape, $13.00; newsletter, three or four per year, included with membership, and various other publications are available through the society.

490. The Mankind Research Foundation (MRF)

1315 Apple Avenue, Silver Spring, MD 20910
Telephone: 301-587-8686; Fax: 301-585-8959
See chapter 1: General—Organizations.

491. Society for Light Treatment and Biological Rhythms (SLTBR)

10200 West 44th Avenue, #304, Wheat Ridge, CO 80033
Telephone: 303-424-3697; Fax: 303-422-8894
Contact: Francine Butler, Ph.D., executive director

A not-for-profit international membership organization for both the professional and lay public fostering research, professional development and clinical applications of light therapy.

Services for the professional: Conducts an annual research and training conference; publishes a membership directory and a bulletin containing research articles and proceedings.

Services for the public: Offers an information kit on SAD (seasonal affective disorder) and light therapy; provides insurance information packets, $20.00, with letter of recommendation from the society, diagnostic summary and supporting clinical treatment papers; offers a SAD Information Packet, $7.00 (public information brochure), maintains a list of clinicians who accept patient inquiries and a complete publication list.

Publications: *Research Bulletin*, six times a year, free with membership, $20.00 (subscription); annual proceedings.

Schools

492. Light Therapy Education Service (LTES)
1055 West College Avenue, #107, Santa Rosa, CA 95401
Telephone: 707-525-4747

Offers classes in light therapy techniques. Also offers a practitioner referral service for interested patients.

Treatment Centers/Referrals

See Color and Light Therapy—Organizations for referrals to individual practitioners.

493. Clinical Chronobiology Program
Columbia-Presbyterian Medical Center, New York Psychiatric Institute, 722 West 168th Street, Unit 50, New York, NY 10021
Telephone: 212-960-5714; Fax: 212-960-2584

Conducts clinical research treatment trials with bright light therapy, high-density negative ionization therapy, and dawn/dusk simulation therapy. Emphasis on seasonal affective disorder (SAD), chronic fatigue syndrome (CFS), and delayed sleep phase syndrome (DSPS).

494. Light Therapy Education Service
1055 West College Avenue, #107, Santa Rosa, CA 95401
Telephone: 707-525-4747
See Color and Light Therapy—Schools.

Product Suppliers

495. Ott bioLight Systems, Inc.
28 Parker Way, Santa Barbara, CA 93101
Telephone: 805-564-3467; 800-234-3724; Fax: 805-564-2147
Credit Cards: Visa, MasterCard

Offers full-spectrum lights which provide the proper balance of color wavelengths needed to maintain a healthy body.

496. Samarco, Inc.
Post Office Box 153008, Dallas TX 75315-3008
Telephone: 214-421-0757; Fax: 214-428-4504
Credit Cards: Visa, MasterCard, American Express

Sells Roscolux color filters.

497. Tools for Exploration
4460 Redwood Highway, Suite 2, San Rafael, CA 94903
Telephone: 415-499-9050; 800-456-9887 (Orders Only); Fax: 415-499-9047
Credit Cards: Visa, MasterCard
See chapter 5: General—Product Suppliers.

498. Verilux, Inc.
Post Office Box 2937, Stamford, CT 06906-0937
Telephone: 203-921-2430; 800-786-6850; Fax: 203-921-2427
Credit Cards: Visa, MasterCard, American Express

Sells a variety of lighting products designed for healthy living, including full-spectrum fluorescent tubes, neodymium light bulbs, light boxes, fixtures and lamps.

Music Therapy

The field of music therapy addresses the therapeutic application of sound and music to health, education, rehabilitation, the creative arts, and personal and spiritual growth and development. It combines music with various psychological and medical therapeutic approaches to physical, behavioral, cognitive and emotional disorders. Specific applications in hospital, clinic, educational and private settings include stress management and pain relief, physical rehabilitation, psychological counseling and psychiatric treatment, special education, language development and substance abuse treatment. Throughout history, music has been thought to have healing effects, but it was not until the 1940s in the United States that music therapy became established as a recognized therapeutic modality. U.S. colleges now offer academic programs leading to bachelors, masters or doctoral degrees in music therapy, and it is an active and growing profession internationally.

Organizations

499. American Association for Music Therapy (AAMT)

1 Station Plaza, Ossining, NY 10562
Telephone: 914-944-9260; Fax: 914-944-9387
Contact: Katie Hartley Opher, executive director; Gary Hara, president

A nonprofit membership organization of individuals, agencies, schools, institutions, and businesses in the field of music therapy. The AAMT is involved with professional development, establishing and implementing standards of professional competence, encouraging and disseminating research through professional publications, creating an international network of music therapists, and promoting music therapy through legislative awareness, public education and the development of employment opportunities.

Services for the professional: Certifies individuals and approves university curricula; encourages professional communication through various publications; sponsors an annual conference; offers continuing education programs; provides job referrals; publishes membership directory.

Services for the public: Provides listing of AAMT-approved schools and referrals to AAMT professional members; fosters community awareness and public education of the goals and applications of music therapy.

Publications: *Music Therapy,* annual journal, $20 (individual subscription), $30 (institutional subscription) (reviewed under Music Therapy—Journals and Newsletters); subject and author index to AAMT journals, $25/individuals and institutions; *Tuning In,* quarterly newsletter, $19 (reviewed under Music Therapy—Journals and Newsletters); *Music Therapy International Report,* newsletter published every other year, $10.50; *AAMT Membership Directory,* annual, free to members; conference proceedings, $15.

500. Association for Music and Imagery, Inc. (AMI)

331 Soquel Avenue, Suite 201, Santa Cruz, CA 95062-2331
Telephone: 408-426-8937; Fax: 408-423-7230
Contact: James L. Rankin, executive secretary

An association for professionals trained in the Bonny Method of Guided Imagery and Music (GIM). Organizational goals include fostering the growth and recognition of GIM, serving as an educational resource, promoting research on the therapeutic benefits of GIM, and serving as the endorsing body for training programs in GIM.

Services for the professional: Provides networking; offers continuing education programs; sponsors an annual conference; maintains GIM mailing list.

Services for the public: Provides a directory of fellows of the association.

Publications: *AMI Newsletter*, free to members, $8.00 (subscription); *Journal of the AMI*, annual, $20 (individual subscription), $30 (institutional subscription), $15 (student subscription) (reviewed under Music Therapy—Journals and Newsletters).

501. The Georgiana Organization (GO)
Post Office Box 2607, Westport, CT 06880
Telephone: 203-454-1221; Fax: 203-454-3788
Contact: Peter Stehli, president

Promotes the practice of Auditory Integration Training (AIT), a form of music therapy utilized to improve comprehension and offer some relief of painful hearing. Acts as a center for the collection of teaching materials for AIT and as a repository for research studies on AIT and related therapies. Encourages the teaching and practice of AIT as well as research by the neuroscience research community on the technique. AIT treatment consists of twenty half-hour sessions at a rate of two per day over a ten-day period. A repetition of the course of treatment after six months may be indicated.

Services for the professional: Certifies professionals as AIT practitioners; maintains a referral list; will be teaching the method in the near future.

Services for the public: Provides information about AIT; maintains a list of certified practitioners nationally and internationally; sells books and copies of articles on AIT.

Publications: Sends out regular mailings of Annabel Stehli's newsletter; updates in the field of AIT; list of new practitioners, annual, $12.00.

Schools

The following organizations are involved with accrediting, certifying and/or establishing standards and qualifications for music therapy programs and music therapists: American Association for Music Therapy (914-944-9260), Certification Board for Music Therapists (602-297-9892, 800-675-CBMT), National Association for Music Therapy (301-589-3300), and National Association of Schools of Music (703-437-0700).

502. The Bonny Foundation (BF)

2020 Simmons Street, Salina, KS 67401
Telephone: 913-827-1497; Fax: 913-827-1497
Contact: Dr. Helen L. Bonny, director

Offers several levels of training in the Bonny Method of Guided Imagery and Music, a process which focuses on the conscious use of imagery arising in response to a formalized program of relaxation and classical music: a nineteen-hour introductory course which may serve as a prerequisite for further training; Level I training, a five-day, thirty-five-hour program which explores personal and transpersonal levels of consciousness; Level II training, a thirteen-day, ninety-hour hands-on training program in individual and group Guided Imagery and Music, leading to certification to practice Guided Imagery and Music in clinical settings. All trainings are approved by the Certification Board for Music Therapists for continuing education credits through the Therapeutic Arts Psychotherapy and Training Center.

503. Hahnemann University (HU)

Medical College of Pennsylvania, MS 905, Broad and Vine Streets, Philadelphia, PA 19102-1192
Telephone: 215-762-6924; Fax: 215-762-6933
Contact: Ronald E. Hays, director of creative arts in therapy education

Through the graduate school and the Department of Mental Health Sciences, Hahnemann University offers a master of arts (M.A.) in creative arts in therapy - music therapy, consisting of two years of academic course work and clinical experience. Also offered is a music therapy equivalency program, consisting of one year of music therapy courses followed by a six-month clinical internship. This program is appropriate for those who do not wish to pursue a master's degree but want to meet the requirements for registration or certification as a music therapist. The program is approved by the National Association for Music Therapy and the American Association for Music Therapy. Financial aid is available.

504. Immaculata College (IC)

Graduate Division, Immaculata, PA 19345-0500
Telephone: 610-447-4400, x3211, x3212; Fax: 610-251-1668
Contact: Sandra Rollison, assistant director of graduate admission

Offers a forty-credit graduate program leading to a master of arts degree in music therapy. The focus of the curriculum is research and study in the applications of music to health, education, business and day-to-day living.

The program is approved by the National Association of Schools of Music. A certificate in music therapy (CMT), approved by the American Association for Music Therapy, is also offered. Financial aid, in the form of federal grants, loan and work-study programs, is available. Visa and MasterCard accepted for payment of tuition.

505. Institute for Music, Health & Education (IMHE)
Post Office Box 4197, Boulder, CO 80306
Telephone: 303-443-8484; 800-490-4968; Fax: 303-443-0053
Contact: Don G. Campbell, founder and director

Offers several educational programs in the use of sound and music for health. The Therapeutic Sound School is a year-long program which meets quarterly, in which students learn about the use of sound and music for therapeutic uses, health and personal transformation. The independent study program is a correspondence course designed for those who wish to learn more about the applications of sound and music in education and health but are unable to travel to the institute. Each of the four courses takes approximately four months to complete; students may begin at any time, and no previous musical training is necessary. The institute also offers workshops, lectures and training programs throughout the year, conducted by Don Campbell, at various locations across the United States.

506. Molloy College (MC)
1000 Hempstead Avenue, Post Office Box 5002, Rockville Centre, NY 11571-5002
Telephone: 516-678-5000; 800-229-1020 (Admissions)
Contact: Wayne F. James, director of admissions

Offers a 137-credit undergraduate program in music therapy, leading to a bachelor of arts degree. This interdisciplinary program includes course work in music, psychology and music therapy, as well as field work and a 900-hour internship. The program is approved by the American Association for Music Therapy. Students who successfully complete the program are eligible to become certified music therapists and may take the national board certification examination given by the Certification Board for Music Therapists. A variety of federal and state financial aid programs and institutional and private grants and scholarships are available.

507. The Naropa Institute (NI)
2130 Arapahoe Avenue, Boulder, CO 80302
Telephone: 303-444-0202; Fax: 303-444-0410

Contact: Ina Russell, publicity director
See chapter 1: General—Schools.

508. New York University (NYU)

School of Education, Department of Music and Performing Arts Professions, 35 West Fourth Street, Suite 777, New York, NY 10012-1172
Telephone: 212-998-5424; Fax: 212-995-4043
Contact: Stan Greidus, director of enrollment management

Offers a master of arts and a doctor of arts degree in music therapy. The M.A. program varies in length from thirty-four credits to sixty credits, depending upon the student's experience and background. The doctoral program is designed for those professionals who already hold a master's degree in music therapy and have at least five years of experience in clinical practice. In addition, post-master's training in Nordoff-Robbins Music Therapy and the Bonny Method of Guided Imagery and Music are also offered. Both the master's and doctoral programs require an audition and are approved by the American Association for Music Therapy. Financial aid in the form of scholarships, loans, fellowships, assistantships and student employment is available.

509. Saint Mary-of-the Woods College (SMWC)

Conservatory of Music, Saint Mary-of-the-Woods, IN 47876-1009
Telephone: 812-535-5180; 812-535-5106
Contact: Tracy Richardson

Offers a bachelor of science degree in music therapy which includes courses in music therapy, psychology, and anatomy and physiology as well as field work and an internship. For those who already have a bachelor's degree in a music-therapy-related field, the college offers a music therapy certification program which is approved by the National Association of Schools of Music and the American Association for Music Therapy. A variety of scholarships and other student aid programs are available.

510. Temple University (TU)

Department of Music Educational Therapy, 012-00 Temple University, Philadelphia, PA 19122
Telephone: 215-204-8542; Fax: 215-204-4957
Contact: Dr. Cheryl Maranto, professor of music therapy

Offers a thirty-six-credit master's program in music therapy, consisting of sixteen credits in music therapy, fourteen credits in electives, and six credits in independent projects. The program's emphasis is on music in medicine and music psychotherapy. Auditions, either taped or live, are required for consideration for admission. Assistantships are available to individuals who will be full-time students with Philadelphia residency. Students may also apply for federal student loans.

Treatment Centers/Referrals

See also Music Therapy—Organizations for referrals to individual practitioners.

511. Nordoff-Robbins Music Therapy Clinic
26 Washington Place, 4th Floor, New York, NY 10003
Telephone: 212-998-5151; Fax: 212-995-4045
Contact: Carol M. Robbins, co-director

The clinic is located in the Department of Music and Music Professions, School of Education, New York University. It offers an outpatient treatment program for children, adolescents and young adults with various disabilities as well as an outreach program serving two special education centers. A wide range of disabling conditions are treated, including developmental delay, learning disabilities, autism, emotional disturbance, seizure disorders, aphasia, behavioral problems, sensory deficits, physical disabilities, multiple handicaps, and more. Clients are directly involved in the creation of music through singing, instrumental activities and movement either with a single therapist or a team approach. In addition to treatment, the clinic is an international training center in music therapy, conducts and publishes research, presents lectures, workshops and symposia to professional audiences, publishes musical and instructional materials and acts as an information dissemination center, providing consultant services, organizing seminars and workshops, and hosting professional visitors.

512. Shealy Institute for Comprehensive Health Care
1328 East Evergreen, Springfield, MO 65803
Telephone: 417-865-5940; Fax: 417-865-6111
See chapter 1: General—Treatment Centers/Referrals.

513. Sound Listening and Learning Center
2701 East Camelback Road, Suite 205, Phoenix, AZ 85016
Telephone: 602-381-0086; Fax: 602-957-6741
Contact: Billie M. Thompson, Ph.D., director

This treatment program is based on the Tomatis Method, a system of sound stimulation developed by the French ear, nose and throat specialist

Dr. Alfred Tomatis. This method is used to correct problems and enhance abilities. The center runs programs for children, adolescents, and adults to improve listening, language, and learning using the Tomatis Method, Accelerated Learning and other integrative methods. Treatment begins with an initial listening assessment and the development of an individualized program including listening to electronically filtered sounds of music and voice simulating the main phases of listening and communication development. The remainder of the program varies with individual needs. The goals are to improve the ability to communicate, learn and relate; improve motivation; discriminate and integrate phonetic sounds of language; train the ear and voice for speech, language and music; and prepare the ear to learn a foreign language as a native speaker would hear it. Problems addressed by the program include poor coordination, dyslexia, hyperactivity, attention deficit disorders, speech difficulties and depression.

514. Well-Springs Foundation, Ltd.

21 North Prospect Avenue, Madison, WI 53705
Telephone: 608-233-5188
Contact: Kay Ortmans Pawley, director and founder

The Well-Springs Program and Alignment Through Music (a massage to classical music originated by Kay Ortmans) are offered at various places internationally by certified Well-Springs facilitators as well as at the Well-Springs Discovery House in Wisconsin. The programs include evenings for movement and meditation, one-day workshops, weekend retreats, individual "Alignment" sessions and movement programs for conferences. In addition to the program, Kay Ortmans has produced a series of eight audiotapes for movement and nine videotapes for home and school use as well as an instructional training manual for facilitators and a booklet on the Well-Springs principles. All are available for purchase through the foundation. Professional certificate training courses are offered for facilitators at Well-Springs in Ben Lomond, California (408-336-8594) and Marion, South Carolina (803-423-6824). A massage certificate and previous experience in movement to music and in the channelling of healing energies are required.

Product Suppliers

515. Institute for Music, Health & Education

Post Office Box 4179, Boulder, CO 80306
Telephone: 303-443-8484; Fax: 303-443-0053

Credit Cards: Visa, MasterCard
Sells books, audiotapes and videotapes on music, health and education.

516. Music Is Elementary
Post Office Box 24263, Cleveland, OH 44124
Telephone: 800-888-7502
Credit Cards: Visa, MasterCard, American Express, Discover

Sells a variety of music therapy books, curriculum guides, conference proceedings and related products.

517. Well-Springs Foundation, Ltd.
21 North Prospect Avenue, Madison, WI 53705
Telephone: 608-233-5188

Sells a series of eight audiotapes for movement and nine videotapes, produced by Well-Springs Foundation founder and director Kay Ortmans. These materials are appropriate for home and school use. Also sells an instructional training manual for facilitators and a booklet on the Well-Springs principles.

PART II: BIBLIOGRAPHY

CHAPTER 9: GENERAL WORKS

Books

518. Altenberg, Henry E. *Holistic Medicine: A Meeting of East and West.* Tokyo and New York: Japan Publishing, 1992. 200 p. Biblio., index. $18.00. ISBN: 0-87040-876-3.

This book offers the reader an opportunity to learn more about alternative therapies that maintain health and promote healing. The author, a practicing psychiatrist for more than forty years, discusses traditional scientific medical practices and explores some alternative approaches to healing. Written in plain language, various aspects of these methods are discussed, including their early history and development, basic underlying principles, professional training and organizations, and current practice and developments in the field. Part I explores western healing methods including conventional medicine, herbal medicine, homeopathy and nutrition; Part II looks at eastern healing traditions such as Ayurveda and traditional Chinese medicine; Part III examines nonmedical healing techniques such as visualization and affirmations; Part IV looks ahead to the 21st century and discusses the incorporation of both eastern and western healing techniques for improved health in the decades ahead.

519. The Burton Goldberg Group. *Alternative Medicine: The Definitive Guide.* Puyallup, WA: Future Medicine Publishing, 1994. 1068 pg. Illus., index. $59.95. ISBN: 0-9636334-3-0.

This educational and informative book for the lay public and health care professionals provides an authoritative and extensive overview of alternative medicine therapies. The text is well researched and includes studies from leading medical journals as well as information from over four hundred prominent alternative health professionals. Part I is a background discussion of the future of medicine, describing the crisis in health care and the factors that contribute to illness and a return to health. Part II lists alphabetically forty-three alternative therapy modalities, approximately six to twelve pages each, covering a description and brief history of the modality, how it works (with illustrations where appropriate), the conditions benefited, a typical treatment, the future of the approach and a resource guide of organizations and recommended readings. "See" references to other related modalities are included. Explanations are clear, direct and well written with supportive research and commentary by experts in the fields. Part III presents specific health conditions by categories, from addictions through vision disorders. It includes a discussion of the disease, its causes and the various alternative medicine therapies appropriate to each specific condition, including their benefits and a description of the work of doctors studying or using the therapy. Self-care therapies that can be done at home and therapies that need professional care are described. Information, referrals and recommended readings follow. The next section is a quick reference to additional health conditions listed alphabetically, from abscess to wounds, with similar information provided. The book ends with a glossary of medical terms, illustrations of bodily systems with major parts labelled, an appendix on antibiotics and probiotics, and a single name and subject index with ample "See also" references. This is an excellent place to start to gain an overview of the field, an idea of specific therapeutic alternatives for varying conditions, and resources for further investigation.

520. Chopra, Deepak. *Quantum Healing: Exploring the Frontiers of Mind/Body Medicine.* New York: Bantam Books, 1989. 278 p. Biblio., index. $9.95. ISBN: 0-553-34869-8.

The author, a native of India who was trained in western medicine, explores the relationship between the physical and mental forces which comprise the healing process. Having seen cancer patients in his own medical practice who had completely recovered after being pronounced incurable, Dr. Chopra returned to India to learn about Ayurvedic medicine and its role in healing. According to Chopra, "in Ayurveda, a level of deep relaxation is the most important precondition for curing any disorder." This very readable book explains in nontechnical language how the body is controlled by neurological impulses originating in the brain and suggests that these impulses can be harnessed for their dynamic healing powers. Liberally interspersed with anecdotal information, a connection is made between Ayurvedic medicine and the developing field of psychoneuroimmunology.

521. Dienstfrey, Harris. *Where the Mind Meets the Body: Type A, the Relaxation Response, Psychoneuroimmunology, Biofeedback, Neuropeptides, Hypnosis, Imagery, and the Search for the Mind's Effect on Physical Health.* New York: HarperCollins, 1991. 154 p. Biblio., index. $10.00. ISBN: 0-06-092290-7.

This fascinating and original recounting of, and inquiry into, seven major pioneering approaches to understanding the mind's effect on the body sheds clarity on an area of study that is rarely illuminated in the larger sense. Through analysis and comparison of these seven approaches, Dienstfrey, founder and editor of the mind/body journal *Advances* and former in-house editor of the Institute for the Advancement of Health, seeks to demonstrate the variety of ways the mind affects the body. He proposes that only a mind intentionally used to affect the body can be the basis of a therapeutic mind/body medicine. Dienstfrey examines the work of Meyer Friedman and Ray Rosenmann in identifying the Type A personality, Herbert Benson's relaxation response, Neal Miller and biofeedback, Robert Ader and psychoneuroimmunology (PNI), Candace Pert and neuropeptides, Theodore Barber and hypnosis, and Gerald Epstein and imagery. He recounts in dramatic detail the thought and discovery processes these investigators underwent and the aspects of mind that lead to physiological changes they identified, including the emotional mind, the active mind, the conditioned mind and the aware mind. This book offers a thoughtful, stimulating, critical and authoritative look at the emerging subject of mind/body medicine.

522. Dossey, Larry. *Meaning and Medicine.* New York: Bantam Books, 1991. 286 p. Biblio., index. $12.50. ISBN: 0-553-07869-0.

Larry Dossey, physician, author, and scholar, has written a thought-provoking book on the relationship between mind, meaning (mind-set) and matter (the body). Drawing on the insights of philosophers, physicians, anthropologists, physicists and researchers, as well as many clinical stories from his medical practice, Dr. Dossey clearly illustrates how beliefs and emotions influence the body and offers a new empowering perspective with which to deal with illness and disease. Meaning is transformation is the message of this book. "Whatever external approaches we choose, disease has another side, which can be approached not through doing but through understanding. Illness contains an inner code by which it wants to 'say something'. . ." Examples of this code are given in various chapters such as "Getting Ahead and Getting Cancer." Dossey's approach to his material is balanced and scholarly, yet compassionate, taking the reader into a deeper and wiser understanding of the individual nature of life's challenges, adversities and possibilities.

523. *Healers on Healing.* Edited by Richard Carlson and Benjamin Shield. Los Angeles: Jeremy P. Tarcher, 1989. 203 p. $12.95. ISBN: 0-87477-494-2.

This anthology of thirty-seven essays by some of the world's leading thinkers, teachers and practitioners of healing has as its goal the uncovering of the common principles underlying all healing work. Many viewpoints are represented, from physicians and psychologists to metaphysical healers and shamans. In clear and simple language, complex aspects of healing are examined: what healing is and how it takes place, the role of attitudes and emotions, love as a healing force, and the role of spirituality in healing. The essays are organized according to three basic principles common to all healing: love as the healer, returning to wholeness, and the healer within. Among the contributors are Norman Cousins, Larry Dossey, Stephen Levine, O. Carl Simonton, Dolores Krieger and Louise Hay. With support, encouragement and gentleness, this book will orient the reader to the wider context of all healing, its basic nature, state of mind and emphasis on self-empowerment.

524. Kastner, Mark and Burroughs, Hugh. *Alternative Healing: The Complete A-Z Guide to over 160 Different Alternative Therapies*. La Mesa, CA: Halcyon Publishing, 1993. Biblio., index. 336 p. $15.00. ISBN: 0-9635997-1-2.

This basic introduction provides an extensive sampling of the alternative therapeutic modalities currently practiced in the United States. Useful as a reference work, the book describes 160 approaches, including background information on the development of the therapy, the underlying principles, a description of a session, benefits to be derived, and books and organizations related to the specific modality being discussed. Time has been taken to capture the unique flavor of each approach and personal stories relevant to the technique are included where appropriate. In addition, the authors provide a substantial list of resources, glossary of terms, in-depth index, list of appellations explaining a practitioner's credentials, and an up-to-date bibliography including otherwise hard to find material written by organizations and institutions explaining a particular modality. This is a useful book for anyone wanting to know more about the general field or a specific approach and serves both as an educational tool and a lead to further information.

525. Levine, Stephen. *Healing into Life and Death.* New York: Anchor Books, 1987. 290 p. $8.95. ISBN: 0-385-26219-1.

After many years of working with people who are seriously ill, Stephen Levine, well-known author and teacher, has written this wise and gentle book on healing mentally, physically and spiritually, on becoming whole. Using illness as a teacher, he advises developing what he calls "merciful awareness," paying attention, loving and forgiving as a means of diffusing fear, finding your truth, and healing through the power of the mind and heart. A detailed table of contents presents the various aspects of the healing process, including discussions of the nature of healing, techniques for healing the body/mind, letting the healing in, dealing with pain and grief, and much more. Interspersed throughout the book are different types of meditations (heart meditation, breath, forgiveness) to be practiced as tools for healing, each with a different and specific purpose. This is an in-depth, insightful and supportive teaching, guiding the reader into new ways of looking at both life and death.

526. Marti, James E. with Andrea Hine. *The Alternative Health and Medicine Encyclopedia.* Detroit: Visible Ink Press, 1995. 376 p. Biblio., index. $15.95. ISBN: 0-8103-8303-0.

Written in plain language, this work provides an excellent overview of a wide range of treatment modalities "designed to acquaint readers of different ages, backgrounds and interests with the major components of alternative medicine." Arranged in nineteen chapters, it addresses such therapies as acupressure, acupuncture, Ayurvedic medicine, biofeedback, botanical medicine, chiropractic, homeopathy, hypnosis, meditation, naturopathy, osteopathy, visualization and yoga. The various components of good health are discussed, and alternative treatments for specific conditions such as pregnancy, childbirth and infant care, heart disease, cancer, aging, stress-related disorders, and drug abuse are examined. References to the work of alternative medicine practitioners such as Herbert Benson, Deepak Chopra, Dean Ornish, Bernie Siegel, Dana Ullman and Andrew Weil are found throughout the book. Particularly useful is the list of resources found at the end of each chapter, including references, suggested readings, and relevant organizations.

527. Mills, Simon and Finando, Steven J. *Alternatives in Healing: An Open-Minded Approach to Finding the Best Treatment for Your Health Problems.* New York: New American Library, 1988. 240 p. Illus., index. $22.95. ISBN: 0-453-00629-9.

Intended to provide the reader with the information needed to make informed choices in health care, this book compares traditional western medicine with five alternative treatments: osteopathy, herbalism, homeopathy, acupuncture, and chiropractic care. Introductory chapters on each modality include illustrations and describe the principles, philosophy, and techniques of diagnosis and treatment. This is followed by chapters arranged by bodily systems which cover 250 medical conditions and alternative medical treatments for each one. Thirty case studies of common health problems are arranged in spreadsheets and examine how each treatment modality addresses each medical condition. Special sections are included on AIDS and cancer. Lists of names and addresses of important organizations in each health care treatment system are provided at the end of the book.

528. ***Mind Body Medicine: How to Use Your Mind for Better Health.*** Edited by Daniel Goleman and Joel Gurin.Yonkers, NY: Consumer Reports Books, 1993. 482 p. Biblio., index. $24.95. ISBN: 0-89043-580-4.

Editors Daniel Goleman, *New York Times* writer on health and human behavior, and Joel Gurin, *Consumer Reports* science editor, have compiled up-to-date and thoroughly researched information on what is currently known about the role of the mind in health and healing. Thirty-one leading American physicians, psychologists, and researchers have contributed authoritative chapters explaining, documenting and evaluating state-of-the-art scientific information in order to "sort out the truth about mindbody medicine" and help readers make intelligent, informed decisions about their health problems. The book is divided into five sections. Part I presents a general overview of the field, including scientific information on the mind's effect on the body and a review of what is established and what is currently being researched on the connection between mental and physical states. Part II explores the role of the mind in specific illnesses, including such diseases as cancer, diabetes, heart disease and arthritis. Part III describes and assesses various mind/body approaches based on research and clinical experience, including meditation, hypnosis, imagery and biofeedback. The last two sections discuss attitudinal aspects of this approach to health care, such as social support, stress management and becoming an active patient.

529. Moskowitz, Reed C. *Your Healing Mind.* New York: Avon, 1993. 304 p. $10.00. ISBN: 0-688-10461-4.

Mind/body medicine refers to a biochemical connection between the brain and the body in which the mind exerts power over the body to effect physiological changes and restore good health. Reed, the founder of New York University's Stress Disorders Medical Services Program, uses case histories from his work to discuss his experiences in treating a variety of ailments with mind/body techniques. Consisting of three parts,"Health," "Happiness," and "Healing," specific methods are provided for addressing a range of medical conditions such as allergies, high blood pressure, and eating disorders. Case histories are followed by discussions of techniques that restore the body to health and well-being.

530. Moyers, Bill. *Healing and the Mind.* New York: Doubleday, 1993. 369 p. Illus., index. $25.00. ISBN: 0-385-46870-9.

As an outgrowth of personal experience and in response to the growing popularity of alternative medicine, author Bill Moyers, the well-known television journalist and editor, produced the television series, "Healing and the Mind," and wrote this companion work by the same name. The issue of how thoughts and feelings influence health is explored, as is the healing connection between the mind and the body. Moyers talked with physicians, scientists, therapists and patients to determine the meaning of health and sickness and the relationship between the mind and the body in healing. He traveled to China to experience a culture whose model of human health incorporates western practices with traditional Chinese medicine. This book is arranged in five parts: "The Art of Healing," "Healing From Within," "The Mind/Body Connection," "The Mystery of Chi," and "Wounded Healers." Each section is comprised of articles written by professionals who are leaders in their respective fields.

531. ***New Choices in Natural Healing:*** *Over 1,800 of the Best Self-Helf Remedies from the World of Alternative Medicine.* Edited by Bill Gottlieb with Susan G. Berg and Patricia Fisher. Emmaus, PA: Rodale Press, 1995. 687 p. Illus., index. $27.95. ISBN: 0-87596-257-2.

This high-quality reference work is one of many by the editors of Prevention Magazine Health Books. Arranged in three complementary parts, each part is also valuable standing alone. Part I contains very readable discussions of sixteen therapeutic modalities, including information on history, uses, acquiring appropriate products and locating practitioners. Part II addresses 160 common ailments and provides a brief overview of each condition, information on symptoms which may indicate a problem requiring the attention of a medical doctor, and explanations of how the appropriate therapies discussed in Part I can promote healing. At the end of Part II is a section which clearly illustrates techniques for using acupressure, massage, reflexology, relaxation and yoga. For each of the therapies discussed, Part III provides information on organizations, books and products, as well as a list of degrees currently awarded for educational programs.

532. Null, Gary. *Healing Your Body Naturally: Alternative Treatments to Illness.* New York: Four Walls Eight Windows, 1992. 328 p. Index. $16.95. ISBN: 0-941423-66-2.

Based upon interviews with qualified health care practitioners from all over the world and more than twenty-five years of personal research, Null, a well-known health and fitness advocate, author, and radio personality, has written a book on various alternative therapies which have been proven useful in improving the health of many people. All of these therapies are nontoxic, generally noninvasive, and administered by qualified practitioners. A great deal of information is provided on sources for a broad array of treatment options, and includes discussion of some of the political issues involved in the acceptance of alternative treatments by conventional medical practitioners. Organized by broad ailments (mental illness, heart disease, cancer, diabetes, etc.), the book includes case histories demonstrating the success of these alternative therapies. Also included are chapters devoted to nutrition and chelation therapy, and a glossary of relevant terminology.

533. Olshevsky, Moshe; Noy, Shlomo; and Zwang, Moses, with Robert Burger. *The Manual of Natural Therapy: A Succinct Catalog of Complementary Treatments.* New York: Facts on File, 1989. 372 p. Biblio., index. $24.95. ISBN: 0-8161-1243-1.

The authors, each of whom is a specialist in a particular area of alternative medicine, provide detailed information on a variety of alternative treatment modalities. No preference for any particular therapy is expressed; rather the authors explain that many of these therapies will work together in treating various medical conditions and may be used in conjunction with conventional medical treatments. Arranged in chapters by bodily system (digestive, respiratory, immune, circulatory, etc.), each chapter opens with symptoms of the illnesses found in that section. For each medical condition, symptoms are listed, followed by appropriate alternative treatments, their recipes, and recommended dosages as appropriate. A lengthy, though not current, bibliography arranged by subject is included at the back of the book. The appendix provides information about diets, vitamins, hypnosis, orthomolecular therapy, yoga, and Chinese medicines, as well as a list of suppliers of foods and vitamins.

534. O'Regan, Brenda and Hirshberg, Carlyle. *Spontaneous Remission: An Annotated Bibliography.* Sausalito, CA: the Institute for Noetic Sciences, 1993. 719 p. $49.00. ISBN: 0-943951-17-8.

This huge research undertaking is published by the Institute for Noetic Sciences, a nonprofit research foundation, educational institution and membership organization studying mind/body health and consciousness. Written by Brenda O'Regan, Vice President for Research for the Institute, and Carlyle Hirshberg, Senior Research Associate and Project Manager of the Remission Project, it represents the collection of the largest electronic database of medically reported cases of spontaneous remission of cancer and other diseases (over 35,000 articles from more than 860 international medical journals). The book contains 1,385 of these references with annotations including abstracts and case histories for over 430 case reports. Remission, the spontaneous disappearance or reduction of disease, is categorized into four types by the authors: remission with no allopathic treatment, remission with inadequate medical treatment, remission with a complex of traditional and alternative treatment, and miraculous remission which is sudden and complete with no medical treatment. This impressive book is organized according to the International Classification of Diseases and is divided into three major sections. Part I covers the remission of cancer, with each of ten chapters reporting on a different cancer site. Case reports are organized chronologically, with the earliest dating from the 1800s to the most current. Part II presents the remission of diseases other than cancer with nine chapters organized by different bodily systems. Part

III has four appendices and an addendum and provides historical perspective via review articles, psychological and spiritual reports, clinical and experimental studies and analysis of cases associated with infection or fever. The addendum cites 286 bibliographic citations found since completion of the publication in 1990. It is hoped by the authors that the study of spontaneous remission will uncover information on how the human body can cure itself or heal at will and how to support that process.

535. Pelletier, Kenneth. *Mind as Healer, Mind as Slayer.* New York: Delta/Seymour Lawrence, 1977. 368 p. Biblio., index. $12.00. ISBN: 0-8446-6093-0.

This classic 1977 work remains a relevant and authoritative exposition on stress, its role in human illness, and strategies for disease prevention. Kenneth Pelletier, senior clinical fellow at Stanford University School of Medicine and author of over 200 professional journal articles on behavioral medicine and psychoneuroimmunology (PNI), has written an extremely well documented, in-depth and objective account of the field of mind/body medicine based on clinical and research information. Early sections deal with the nature of stress from a physiological point of view as well as the types of life events that trigger stress reactions. Subsequent sections include profiles of different personality types and highly specific illnesses, such as cancer, migraine and rheumatoid arthritis. Finally, practical methods of controlling stress are presented, examining meditation, autogenic training, visualization and biofeedback as holistic strategies for maintaining health and treating disease. Dr. Pelletier wrote an updated, extensive preface in 1992 addressing the new findings in the fields of behavioral medicine and PNI since 1977 and defining promising new areas of research.

536. ______. *Sound Mind, Sound Body: A New Model for Lifelong Health.* New York: Simon & Schuster, 1994. 319 p. Biblio., index. $23.00. ISBN: 0-671-77000-4.

A compelling argument for the connection between state of mind and good physical health is made in this work by the author of *Mind as Healer, Mind as Slayer.* Dr. Pelletier, a well-known professional in the field of mind/body medicine, puts forward a definition of good health which, rather than addressing the absence of disease, encompasses the psychological aspects of health, including outlook, values, and spiritual well-being. Using research he has conducted on more than fifty prominent individuals, Pelletier links the role of their spiritual and psychological states of mind to their physical state of health, and discusses the role of altruism in attaining and maintaining good health. For anyone with an interest in mind/body medicine, this book is a "must read."

537. Rogo, D. Scott. *New Techniques of Inner Healing.* NY: Paragon Press, 1992. 248 p. Biblio. $12.95. ISBN: 1-55778-492-2.

This book consists of eleven interviews with well-known professionals in the field of inner healing. Originally published individually in *Science of Mind* magazine, these "conversations" were conducted with such notable practitioners as Deepak Chopra, Louise Hay, and Kenneth Pelletier. Each piece is preceded by a brief biographical sketch and collectively grouped under three headings. "Ways to Better Living" consists of four interviews that explore the relationship between mind and body; "Ways to Spiritual Growth" contains four interviews which examine spiritual healing; and "Ways to Holistic Health" consists of three interviews that discuss religious and personal growth. Three additional articles on spiritual healing written by the author are also included, as is an annotated bibliography listing books on stress management, personal growth, overcoming disease, therapeutic touch, and other topics discussed in the book.

538. Siegel, Bernie. *Peace, Love and Healing: Bodymind Communication and the Path of Self Healing: An Exploration.* New York: Harper and Row, 1989. 259 p. Biblio., index. $12.00. ISBN: 0-06-091705-9.

This clear and encouraging book by Dr. Bernie Siegel, practicing physician, teacher and author, seeks to bring insight to the process of illness through understanding its message to the self, through attitudinal changes, and through openness to the truth. Speaking from personal experience, case stories, and examples from the medical literature, Siegel explains the physiological basis of mind-altering processes such as meditation, hypnosis and visualization, and the effect of emotions like joy, love and optimism on the body and healing. He describes how to communicate with the body/mind, receiving messages from your inner self through your symptoms, dreams, symbols and drawings and sending messages back through your feelings, words, visualization and relaxation techniques. Siegel provides mental exercises throughout the book to clarify the meaning of one's illness on a deep level of consciousness and practice healing and self love. Bibliographic references, a reading list and resource lists of audiotapes and videotapes provide leads to further relevant information.

539. Sinclair, Brett Jason. *Alternative Health Care Resources: A Directory and Guide.* West Nyack, NY: Parker Publishing, 1992. 498 p. Index. $12.95. ISBN: 0-13-156522-2.

Writing expressly to make available to the general public information on all aspects of alternative health care, the author evaluates almost 400 self-help groups, organizations, journals, magazines and newsletters which provide services relating to such issues as treatments, disease-prevention and health-related issues. Organized alphabetically, the book covers a wide range of health conditions such as AIDS, eating disorders, environmental illness, and Parkinson's disease. Within each chapter, information is arranged alphabetically by resource, giving background data and information about what each resource offers.

540. ***The Visual Encyclopedia of Natural Healing:*** *A Step-by-Step Guide to Solving 100 Everyday Health Problems.* Edited by Alice Feinstein. Emmaus, PA: Rodale Press, 1991. 423 p. Illus., index. $26.95. ISBN: 0-87857-928-1.

This self-care guide is designed to help the reader make informed health care decisions. Topics covered span the spectrum from simple common ailments to life-threatening medical conditions, and include such problems as allergies, burns, heart disease, poison ivy, and varicose veins. Organized alphabetically by ailment, the book contains extensive illustrations and easy-to-follow instructions for each condition's natural healing methods. Techniques discussed and illustrated include acupressure, herbal remedies and relaxation, to name a few. Intended as a reference guide, the book encourages the reader to seek medical care for any serious medical problems.

541. Weil, Andrew. *Natural Health, Natural Medicine: A Comprehensive Manual for Wellness and Self-Care.* Boston: Houghton Mifflin Co., 1990. 356 p. Biblio., index. $10.95. ISBN: 0-395-49340-4.

A complete guide to preventive health maintenance, this book includes suggestions for self-treatment of many common ailments, using methods described as safe, natural, effective and relatively inexpensive. The author, a practicing physician who incorporates the use of natural remedies in his own work, addresses the general reader in a straightforward, easy-to-read style. Emphasizing the self-responsibility of the patient for good health and well-being, he presents basic information about achieving and maintaining a healthy lifestyle, offers natural treatments that can be used by the layperson, and provides detailed recommendations for the use of home remedies to treat a large number of common ailments. Where appropriate, recommendations for using allopathic treatments simultaneously are included. Listings of suggested readings are provided at the end of many of the chapters. Appendices include names and addresses of organizations that can provide referrals to nonallopathic practitioners and companies from which recommended materials can be ordered.

542. ______. *Health and Healing.* Boston: Houghton Mifflin Co., 1988. 296 p. Biblio., index. $9.95. ISBN: 0-395-36200-8.

Winner of the American Health Book of the Year Award and the Medical Self-Care Book Award, Dr. Weil draws on his experience as a medical researcher, teacher, and Harvard-trained practicing physician to elucidate the nature of health and healing. The differences between conventional allopathic medicine and alternative medicine and the broad spectrum of alternative healing methods are described. Written in a warm, easy-to-read style, the book analyzes concepts of health and presents ten principles of health and illness that are meant to inform choices on the selection of healing methods. Various alternative healing approaches, including homeopathy, chiropractic, Chinese medicine and osteopathy, are described, providing information on their history, underlying theory, why they work, allopathic criticism of the practices, and response to that criticism from the point of view of that particular approach. This is a well-researched and authoritative overview of health and healing, with the strengths and weaknesses of both allopathic medicine and alternative medicine evaluated in an objective and balanced way. A detailed index adds to the usefulness of this book.

543. ______. *Spontaneous Healing: How to Discover and Enhance Your Body's Natural Ability to Maintain and Heal Itself.* New York: Alfred A. Knopf, 1995. 309 p. Biblio., index. $23.00. ISBN: 0-679-43607-3.

In this highly readable book, Dr. Weil, Director of the Program in Integrative Medicine at the University of Arizona in Tuscon and Harvard-trained physician, primarily orients the lay reader to the ability of the body to heal itself, an approach to maintain wellness, and strategies to enhance the body's capabilities during illness. He also analyzes what he sees as necessary changes in the present-day health care environment in terms of attitudes, medical education, and research in order to broaden the scope of medical care offered to the public. Weil articulates in a clear and down-to-earth manner the basis of natural healing and the differences between the western model of scientific technological medicine and the eastern model of health enhancement and healing. The book is arranged in three parts. Part I presents nine case histories of healing through natural, noninvasive means, many of which were considered incurable by the medical profession. He explains how these reflect the normal workings of our internal healing systems, how each system operates, and the role of the mind in healing, as far as is currently understood. Part II explores common obstacles to healing such as lack of energy, poor circulation, toxins, etc., and their effect on our bodily systems. He then suggests practical means for enhancing the body's internal healing processes, such as diet, tonics, activity and rest, and a thoughtful and well-paced eight-week work program to create a healing lifestyle. In Part III, Weil provides guidelines for deciding on appropriate treatment in case of illness, for discerning what will do the most good and the least harm, when conventional medical treatment is advisable and in which circumstances it is least effective. He illustrates these points with eleven case histories of various conventional and natural treatments for a variety of diseases such as asthma, rheumatoid arthritis, and HIV infection. Fifteen common alternative medical practices and the conditions they may be effective in treating are decribed. In addition, Weil suggests seven basic strategies to adopt when dealing with a condition to be healed, requiring an involved and personally responsible attitude on the part of the patient. Examples are given of broad categories of illnesses such as allergy, cardiovascular disease and digestive diseases with general recommendations for dietary changes, vitamin supplementation, herbal treatments, alternative medical treatments and mind/body interventions as appropriate. Guidelines for cancer management are explored in more depth. A short appendix provides useful contact information for organizations and product suppliers in the field. Overall, this is a balanced approach to the issue of health care, validating areas where conventional medical treatment is effective and appropriate, and offering sound, common-sense guidelines to help people understand the pivotal role of their natural healing system, how to support it, how to evaluate which alternative therapies are helpful for particular conditions, and how to play an active role in one's health care management.

544. Wilen, Joan and Wilen, Lydia. *Live and Be Well: New Age and Age-Old Folk Remedies.* New York: HarperPerennial, 1992. 324 p. Biblio., index. $10.00. ISBN: 0-06-096563-0.

Appropriately titled, this book is evenly divided between such New Age remedies as color therapy, gem therapy, visualization and affirmations, and a wide variety of age-old remedies. Overall, it provides easy-to-use solutions for a range of medical ailments such as fatigue, headaches, hemorrhoids, herpes, motion sickness, and ulcers. The table of contents contains an alphabetic arrangement by condition, and the final chapter on well-being provides information on products, services and books.

545. Wood, Matthew. *The Magical Staff: The Vitalist Tradition in Western Medicine.* Berkeley, CA: North Atlantic Books, 1992. 209 p. Biblio. $14.95. ISBN: 1-53643-127-9.

Sponsored by the Society for the Study of Native Arts and Sciences, this work looks at the forerunners of and historical connections between early movements representing the western vitalist tradition in medicine. Thus it is more than just a history of the antecedents to later thought and practice. It offers an opportunity to return to some of the early wisdom on mind, spirit and matter that has been overshadowed by rationalistic, technological thinking in medicine. Wood examines the lives, writings and works of eight great practitioners: Paracelsus, Hahnemann, Kent, Bach, Scudder, Burnett, Rademacher, and Beach, representing folk medicine, alchemical healing, herbalism, vitalism, homeopathy, flower essences, eclecticism and medicine of the spirit. Chapters provide background on the contribution and perspective of each man, a biographical profile, and an explanation of his important ideas and contributions to medicine. It is a clearly written, informative and colorful work offering not only factual perspective but the flavor of the man and the *gestalt* out of which his ideas arose. Highly appropriate for the lay reader as well as the health professional, it is a well researched book providing an interesting bibliography of both current works and historical writings dating back to the 1800s.

546. ***World Medicine:*** *The East West Guide to Healing Your Body.* Edited by Tom Monte and the Editors of *EastWest Natural Health.* New York: Jeremy P. Tarcher/Perigee Books, 1993. 340 p. Illus., biblio., index. $15.95. ISBN: 0-87477-733-X.

This book examines five different systems of healing: traditional Chinese medicine, Ayurveda, homeopathy, naturopathy, and Greek medicine, and compares them with the treatment methods of conventional western medicine, focusing on how each system approaches the concept of good health and illness. Arranged in four major parts, this work first explores the theoretical principles underlying each of these healing methods, and then moves on to discuss the body's organs, senses and systems from the perspective of each of these modalities. Written in plain language, this very readable book is enhanced by clear illustrations. Monte has written numerous books on health and the environment. He is the former editor of *Nutrition Action* (a publication of the Center for Science in the Public Interest) and an associate editor of *EastWest Natural Health,* a leading publication on natural health and personal growth.

Journals and Newsletters

547. ***Advances: the Journal of Mind-Body Health.*** Kalamazoo, MI: John E. Fetzer Institute. v.1, no.1, 1983. Quarterly. $39.00 (individual subscription), $79.00 (institutional subscription), $19.00 (students and retirees subscription). ISSN: 0741-9783.

Published by the Fetzer Institute, a nonprofit educational organization promoting research and the dissemination of information on scientifically tested mind/body health care approaches, this prestigious journal is edited by Harris Diestenfrey. Contributors and editors include prominent educators, clinicians, researchers, and scientists at major U. S. institutions. This eighty-page journal is designed for health professionals and general readers interested in prevention, treatment and enhancement of health from a mind/body perspective. Each issue offers discussion of recent research and new directions, abstracts of current research findings, reviews of books, letters, and a calendar of forthcoming meetings. Topics covered have included psychoneuroimmunology, the scope of unconventional medicine, psychosocial interventions and cancer, the well-being movement, spontaneous remission, and the mind and the immune system. Articles are authoritative, well documented, and stimulating. Subscriber benefits include a supplemental cumulative index with the winter issue as well as the Fetzer Institute Report detailing research, education and programs of the institute.

548. ***Alternative and Complementary Therapies.*** New York: Mary Ann Liebert. v.1, no.1, 1994. Bimonthly. Adv. $91.00 (individual subscription), $122.00 (institutional subscription). ISSN: 1076-2809.

This new journal is geared to health care practitioners, presenting practical and current information on a wide range of alternative therapies. Hoping to provide practitioners with authoritative information on which to evaluate and possibly integrate alternative therapies into their practices, the publisher sees this as a way to facilitate bridging the gap between allopathic and alternative practice. Ten feature articles per issue cover such areas as chiropractic, biofeedback, dietary supplements, homeopathy, acupuncture and oriental medicine, chelation therapy and alternative treatments for specific medical conditions. Also included in each issue is a news section on medical findings, the pharmacist's corner, reviews of books, journals, videotapes, audiotapes, and patient materials, listings of upcoming conferences and training seminars, and a bibliography of current relevant journal literature on alternative medicine. Articles are written by health care practitioners and medical writers, with senior medical advisors including Dr. Joseph E. Pizzorno, President of Bastyr University, and Nicholas Gonzalez, M.D. Articles are balanced, well- researched, substantive, and readable, and contain short resource lists as leads to further information and bibliographical references. This journal provides well- rounded reporting on the world of alternative medicine, from the Office of Alternative Medicine, to alternative medicine on the Internet, to the individual health practitioner.

549. ***Alternative Therapies in Health and Medicine.*** Aliso Viejo, CA: InnoVision Communications. v.1, no.1, 1995. Bimonthly. $48.00 (individual subscription), $120.00 (institutional subscription). ISSN: 1078-6791.

This prestigious new journal is edited by Larry Dossey, M.D., and has a distinguished and extensive editorial and advisory board. It serves as a vehicle for disseminating information on the practical use of alternative therapies for prevention, treatment and health promotion. The journal publishes scientific research and other disciplined inquiry methods as well as theoretical articles on alternative medicine in general and various therapeutic approaches such as traditional Chinese medicine, homeopathy, energy medicine and others. Each issue contains an OAM (Office of Alternative Medicine) report providing the latest information from the OAM, news on developments in alternative medicine, a section of original papers, interviews with leaders in the field, and columns discussing various issues such as the history of homeopathic medicine, society and alternative medicine, and public policy. Also included are abstracts from leading medical journals giving the major data from research studies including objectives, design, setting, participants, procedure, outcome measures, results and conclusions, as well as a section on book reviews, a directory of academic centers and a conference calendar. The journal hopes to bridge the gap between alternative and conventional medicine, leading to an integration in health care policy and practice.

550. ***A. M.*** **(renamed: *Complementary and Alternative Medicine at the NIH*).** Bethesda, MD: Office of Alternative Medicine, National Institutes of Health. v.1, no.1. 1993. Bimonthly. Free.

The Office of Alternative Medicine, National Institutes of Health, publishes this short newsletter reporting on its activities. It includes administrative news, announcements and descriptions of grants awarded, and a calendar of alternative medicine meetings and events. Literature reviews and summaries of articles originally published in other journals are also included.

551. ***American Health:*** *Fitness of Body and Mind.* New York: RD Publications. v.1, no.1, 1982. Ten times a year. Illus., adv. $17.97 (subscription). ISSN: 0730-7004.

This is a well-known general health magazine covering a wide range of issues from the simple to the complex in a way that is accessible to the lay reader. The emphasis is on prevention. Subjects covered include nutrition, mental health, environmental issues and specific medical conditions. Six feature articles plus twenty regular departments provide the reader with current health facts and trends.

552. ***Brain/Mind.*** *A Bulletin of Breakthrough.* Los Angeles: Interface Press. v.1, no.1, 1975. Monthly. Illus., adv. $45.00 (subscription). ISSN: 1072-3927.

Published by Marilyn Ferguson, author of *The Brain Revolution,* this publication documents research activities on the subject of consciousness. Coverage is interdisciplinary and includes the fields of neuroscience, psychology, medicine, physics and related disciplines. Regular features include reports of current research, book reviews, interviews, and listings of upcoming workshops, symposia and other events. Though written in a fairly readable style, this bulletin's subject matter is clearly most appropriate for professionals in those sciences which deal with the brain and consciousness.

553. ***The Choice.*** Chula Vista, CA: Committee for Freedom of Choice in Medicine, c/o American Biologics. v.1, no.1, 1975. Quarterly. Illus., adv. $16.00 (subscription, includes membership).

This consumer publication covers integrative medicine, metabolic therapy and degenerative diseases. It regularly reports on legislative, court and governmental actions, developments in cancer research and treatment, news on various other diseases such as Alzheimers, arthritis and AIDS, dietary questions, research studies, the pharmaceutical industry, and new books and journals. The magazine serves as a watchful eye, and while many articles report basic news and findings from around the world, the perspective is generally one of monitoring the powers-that-be in medicine, advocacy of natural medicine approaches, and aggressively keeping people informed. There is no table of contents, and the format resembles a newsletter, with many short bulletins on different topics interspersed among half-page articles. A great deal of information is presented in each fifty-page issue and the writing is direct, clear and easy to understand. The large board of consultants and contributors are all doctors from the U.S. and around the world.

554. ***Citizens for Health Report.*** Tacoma, WA: Citizens for Health. v.1, no.1, 1992. Bimonthly. Free with membership. ISSN: 1062-1245.

This newsletter provides timely coverage of federal and state legislative and governmental developments relating to alternative medicine and freedom of choice issues. There are regular reports on the progress of Citizens for Health political activities and pending issues, and of actions taken by governmental agencies, courts, state licensing boards, congress, and other organizations' advocacy efforts. The articles are short and direct, covering the basic factual information, although from one point of view only, and providing names and numbers for reader follow-up if appropriate. Also included are reviews of books and journals on alternative health. The layout is clear and easy to read. Each newsletter of approximately twenty-five pages contains a good deal of relevant information for people interested in the safeguarding and promotion of natural medicine from a political/activist point of view.

Complementary and Alternative Medicine at the NIH. See entry no. 550.

555. ***Consumer Reports on Health.*** Yonkers, NY: Consumers Union. v.1, no.1, 1989. Monthly. $24.00 (one-year subscription), $38.00 (two-year subscription). ISSN: 1044-3193.

The Consumers Union, a nonprofit organization established in 1936 to provide consumers with information and advice on health issues, goods, services and personal finance, publishes this newsletter for the lay public. It covers recent health and medical findings, news on diet, nutrition and exercise, and views of leading doctors and medical experts on health and preventive care. Issues consist of regular departments including Mind/Body Update, Fitness Update, Nutrition Update, Medical Update, Office Visit, and On Your Mind (a question and answer section addressed to Consumers Union's medical and dental consultants). Several feature articles cover subjects in more depth, providing background on a topic, reviewing research, and including useful charts of information such as the efficacy and risk factors of various birth control devices. Articles are clearly written, unbiased, and informative. This newsletter is a general consumer health publication, not exclusively devoted to alternative medicine.

556. ***H & N: Healthy and Natural.*** Sarasota, FL: Measurement and Data Corporation. v.1, no.1, 1994. Six times a year. Illus., adv. $18.00 (one-year subscription), $32.00 (two-year subscription), $45.00 (three-year subscription). ISSN: 1079-4530.

This two-part magazine for the lay public consists of *Healthy and Natural News* and *Healthy and Natural Journal.* The news magazine is a resource guide to natural health and environmental products, including supplements and remedies, natural and organic foods, books, courses and education, natural body care products, health devices and buyer's guide surveys on different topics listing manufacturers and distributors, product descriptions and prices where available. Part II contains approximately twenty short two- to four-page feature articles on natural health issues, consumer activism, and the environment by authoritative health practitioners, writers and teachers. Examples include Steve Halpern on music and health, Deepak Chopra on mind/body medicine, and Roy Upton on herbs. Articles are clearly written, informative and interesting. Although the presentation is cluttered and a bit confusing, this publication provides a great deal of information of interest to the public on a wide variety of natural health topics.

557. ***Harvard Women's Health Watch.*** Palm Coast, FL: Health Letter Associates. v.1, no.1, 1994. Monthly. $24.00 (subscription). ISSN: 1070-910X.

Harvard Medical School publishes this eight-page newsletter which interprets current medical information for the lay reader. The newsletter reports on issues relative to women's health, such as menopause and alternatives to hormone replacement, conquering incontinence, PMS, cosmetic surgery, and estrogen. It reports studies from leading medical journals and provides a balanced presentation of the latest thinking and options available. Articles supply background information on a topic including causes, diagnostic procedures, risk reduction strategies and other suggestions for management. A question-and-answer section is included as well as short reports on research studies such as pesticides and breast cancer risk and low-fat diets and skin cancer.

558. ***Health.*** San Francisco, CA: Time Publishing Ventures. v.1, no.1, 1969. Seven times a year. Illus., adv. $24.00 (subscription). ISSN: 1059-938X.

Covering all general health maintenance, this consumer health magazine features regular departments on food, fitness, mind, self-image, healthy cooking, and vital signs, which provides brief reports on various health issues. Approximately six feature articles, three to six pages in length, discuss topics such as the cancer vaccine, tips on walking, and the health aspects of metal pots and pans.

559. ***Health Facts.*** New York: Oryx Press. v.1, no.1, 1976. Monthly. $21.00 (subscription). ISSN: 0738-811X.

This six-page health newsletter is published by the Center for Medical Consumers in New York City, a nonprofit consumer health organization promoting informed health care decision making. It summarizes recent research published in leading medical journals such as the *New England Journal of Medicine* and the *Journal of the National Cancer Institute.* Each issue has one feature-length article on a different topic such as the great cholesterol myth and the pros and cons of clinical trials. Reporting is well researched, balanced and critical.

560. ***Health Freedom News.*** Monrovia, CA: The National Health Federation. v.1, no.1, 1955. Ten times a year. $36.00 (individual subscription), $24.00 (senior citizen subscription). ISSN: 0749-4742.

Published by the National Health Federation, a nonprofit organization supporting natural health education and freedom of choice in health care, this consumer health publication contains approximately ten feature articles covering medical topics such as mammograms, nutritional information, research findings, medical politics and particular herbs and foods. Regular departments include legislative updates, letters, book reviews, health notes, classifieds, and an advertisers' list. The perspective is skeptical toward the medical establishment and government health care information and practice.

561. ***Health Waves.*** Syosset, NY: The New Center for Wholistic Health Education & Research. v.1, no.1. 1994 . Three times a year. Illus. Free.

This newsletter provides information about the activities of the New Center for Wholistic Health Education & Research, a school and treatment center which offers a holistic nursing program and provides a wide range of treatment services. In addition, the newsletter covers current issues in alternative medicine, including legislative activities, health insurance, mind/body medicine, and the use of a variety of alternative therapies such as acupuncture, T'ai Chi, bodywork, etc. Each issue also contains a calendar of the center's events.

562. ***Holistic Health Directory and Resource Guide.*** Brighton, MA: New Age Journal. Annual. Adv. $5.95 or as part of a subscription to *New Age Journal.* ISSN: 0746-3618.

Published annually by *New Age Journal,* this 200-page directory covers over 100 categories of complementary and holistic health. It includes information on different modalities including descriptions and health benefits, and a listing of over 7,000 practitioners by geographic locations. Also included is a resource guide for education and professional training, health spas and retreats, information and referral services, meditation teachers and centers, miscellaneous resources, professional associations, publishers, audiovisual materials, and beauty and skin care information. Introductory sections give overall advice on holistic health care including choosing a practitioner, a guide to common credentials, alternative medical insurance, book reviews, conferences, and self-care health promotion strategies.

563. ***Holistic Medicine.*** Raleigh, NC: American Holistic Medical Association. v.1, no.1, 1978. Quarterly. Adv. Free to members, $30.00 (subscription). ISSN: 0898-6029.

The magazine of the American Holistic Medical Association (AHMA) covers the latest developments in holistic medicine, AHMA news, book reviews, news releases and upcoming events including U.S. conferences, workshops and training programs. Approximately five feature articles per issue cover such topics as a Chinese perspective on chronic fatigue, the essence of energy-based medicine, bioenergetic technique, the wet cell appliance, and a holistic approach to sinus problems. Articles are written by medical doctors and others associated with holistic organizations and centers.

564. ***Journal of Advancement in Medicine.*** New York: Human Sciences Press. v.1, no.1, 1988. Quarterly. $62.00 (individual subscription), $195.00 (institutional subscription). ISSN: 0894-5888.

A scientific journal for health care professionals interested in innovative advances in medical science, this journal focuses on nutritional/preventive medicine. Special emphasis is placed on less well-known and nontraditional methods of diagnosis and treatment that are safe and effective. The editors and editorial board are composed primarily of M.D.s and Ph.D.s.

Included are case reports, research studies, opinion pieces, letters to the editor, abstracts of reports and studies, and book reviews. Articles contain abstracts and references. The journal runs approximately sixty pages per issue.

565. ***The Journal of Alternative and Complementary Medicine:*** *Research on Paradigm, Practice, and Policy.* New York: Mary Ann Liebert. v.1, no.1, 1995. Quarterly. $89.00 (individual subscription), $120.00 (institutional subscription). ISSN: 1075-5535.

This peer-reviewed journal focuses on research in nontraditional medical therapies including clinical trials, observational and analytical reports, and information on how to design research studies. The journal's editor-in-chief is Marc S. Micozzi, M.D., Ph.D., Director of the National Museum of Health and Medicine, and senior editors are Fredi Kronenberg, Ph.D., Director of the Richard Rosenthal Center for Alternative and Complementary Medicine at Columbia University College of Physicians and Surgeons, and Kim A. Jobst, M.A., M.R.C.P, of the University of Oxford. According to the editors, the intention of this journal is to serve as a resource for medical researchers, scientists and practitioners of both alternative and allopathic medicine and provide a forum for discussion, communication, and investigation. The journal includes editorials and commentaries, philosophical analyses, reports of research studies, case reports, abstracts from symposium, reports on annual meetings of various societies, political issues, and an ongoing list of alternative medicine courses taught at U.S. medical schools. Articles are scientifically and academically rigorous (one article contained a 149-item bibliography of books and journals) and run from four to twenty pages. They are well written, thought provoking, informative and clear.

566. ***Let's Live.*** Los Angeles, CA: Hilltopper Publication. v.1, no.1, 1933. Monthly. Illus., adv. $19.95 (subscription). ISSN: 0024-1288.

For over sixty years this consumer health magazine has covered the field of alternative and preventive medicine. Topics covered are varied, with approximately twelve feature articles per issue on such subjects as meditation, homeopathy, reflexology, chiropractic, health vacations, healthy cooking and the like. Regular departments include sections on herbs, exercise, natural beauty, staying healthy and others. This is a good all around health magazine, easy to read, full of practical information, responsible in its reporting, and entertaining. Articles are written by health writers and practitioners, and an expert advisory board includes Dana Ullman on homeopathy, Hal Huggins on dentistry and David Hoffmann on herbs.

567. ***Natural Health:*** *The Guide to Well-Being* (Formerly: *EastWest: Journal of Natural Health and Living; EastWest Journal*). Brookline, MA: Natural Health Ltd. Partnership. v.1, no.1, 1971. Bimonthly. Illus., adv. $24.00 (subscription). ISSN: 0816-2751.

This popular journal provides the latest information on alternative approaches to health and includes articles on such topics as alternative medicine, holistic health, natural foods, mind/body techniques, personal growth, and folk medicine. Each issue contains five feature articles as well as a range of regular departments covering news and updates, resource guides, recipes, book reviews, home remedies, etc. With an advisory board consisting of well-known authorities in the field (e.g., Andrew Weil, Harris Dienstfrey), and contributions from experts in specialized areas of alternative health, this journal presents articles which are informative, straightforward, and readable.

568. ***NaturalPET.*** Trilby, FL: National Animal Health Alliance. v.1., no.1., 1992. Bimonthly. Illus., adv. $20.00 (one-year subscription), $34.00 (two-year subscription), free with $35.00 membership. ISSN: 1080-3076.

This alternative pet care magazine focuses on preventive, natural approaches to pet health and grooming. It investigates and reports on the effects of commercial foods, chemicals, and medications on an animal's health and covers holistic approaches including home remedies, nutritional approaches to disease, tooth care and preventive dentistry, supplementation, and alternatives to vaccination. Each issue has five to six feature articles and three regular columns including readers' questions to a veterinarian, Linda Tellington-Jones, on animal training and touch therapy, and a column on animals' emotional health. Articles are clearly written and practical, giving precise instructions on specific pet care issues, signs and symptoms of disease, treatment recommendations and prevention information. The magazine has veterinary and herbology advisory boards, and articles are written by veterinarians, health writers, educators, breeders and holistic animal care practitioners.

569. ***New Age Journal*** (Formerly: *New Age; New Age Magazine*). Watertown, MA: New Age Publishing. v.1, no.1 1974. Bimonthly, with additional special issue published each winter. Illus., adv. $24.00 (subscription). ISSN: 0746-3618.

Although not exclusively devoted to alternative medicine, this popular journal on holistic living provides a wealth of information on health-related issues. Five feature articles are found in each issue, and a special section presents a series of articles exploring one particular subject in greater depth. Regular departments cover various aspects of natural living. A large mail order guide to products, services, resources, and alternative educational programs and careers is found at the back of each issue. The editorial board includes Joan Borysenko and George Leonard, two leading figures in the field of mind/body medicine. Feature articles draw upon the talents of such noted individuals as Dr. Bernie Siegel, author of many books on alternative medicine.

570. ***Noetic Sciences Review.*** Sausalito, CA: Institute of Noetic Sciences. v.1. no.1, 1986. Quarterly. Free to members. ISSN: 0897-1005.

Published by the Institute of Noetic Sciences, a prestigious research foundation, educational institution and membership organization, this journal serves as a forum for the communication of diverse ideas related to the study of the mind and consciousness. Writers include prominent scientists, philosophers, teachers and scholars such as Jean Houston, Stanislov Grof and Joan Borysenko. Approximately six feature articles per issue run from five to seven pages long, many with bibliographical references. These are stimulating theoretical discussions, offering insights, analyses and conceptual frameworks for important ideas in the area of consciousness. Regular departments include an editor's letter, research highlights from institute projects and various symposia, book reviews, and a description of the institute's travel programs.

571. ***Prevention.*** Emmaus, PA: Rodale Press. v.1, no.1., 1950. Monthly. Illus., index, adv. $19.97 (subscription). ISSN: 0032-8006.

One of the earliest magazines to promote consumer health information, *Prevention*'s reporting is intended to inform the reader on issues relating to the prevention of illness and the enhancement of a healthy lifestyle. Published by Rodale Press, known for its thorough and objective coverage of medical issues, *Prevention* maintains an advisory board consisting of experts in the fields of medicine, psychology, pharmacology and consumer health. Each issue is comprised of three lengthy features, eight to ten shorter articles on such subjects as fitness, nutrition, and hygiene, and six regular departments on health news and updates. With a strong consumer health orientation, this magazine sees its role as educator of the public and consumer advocate.

572. ***Spectrum:*** *The Wholistic News Magazine.* Belmont, NH: Spectrum Universal Corp. v.1, no.1, 1988. Six times a year. Illus., adv. $18.00 (subscription). ISSN: 1049-9075.

With a strong public interest and consumer health orientation, *Spectrum* is a news digest that primarily provides highly current, condensed articles on health information appearing in other authoritative print sources. These sources are listed at the end of each article to direct readers to the original, complete printed information. Each issue has seven broad topics consisting of approximately eight articles each. Topics include healing, medicine, mind and spirit, food and nutrition. One lengthy feature article presents a timely health issue, such as an interview with Dr. Ralph Moss, Executive Advisor to the National Institutes of Health's Office of Alternative Medicine, on alternative medicine and cancer treatment. Articles are clearly written, straightforward, and informative.

573. ***Townsend Letter for Doctors.*** Port Townsend, WA: Jonathan Collin, M.D. v.1, no.1, 1983. Ten times a year. Illus., adv. $42.00 (yearly subscription), $77.00 (two-year subscription), $27.00 (student subscription).

This magazine serves as an informal forum for doctors of all disciplines including medical doctors, doctors of naturopathy, osteopathy, chiropractic, podiatry and other health professionals with an interest in natural medicine. Topics covered include iridology, medical politics, homeopathy, natural hygiene, environmental medicine, acupuncture, nutrition and supplementation, herbs, phytotherapy and more. Original articles, reviews of research with commentary, case studies, an extensive letters to the editor section, book and journal reviews, and a calendar of annual conferences and meetings make this 100 + page magazine a good source of current information on a wide variety of topics. Some articles include references and suggested readings and all are clearly written, many appropriate for the lay public as well as the health professional. All areas of alternative medicine are covered here, including the more controversial treatments such as chelation, orthomolecular medicine, electrical medicine and alternative cancer therapies.

574. ***University of California at Berkeley Wellness Letter.*** Palm Coast, FL: Health Letter Associates. v.1, no.1, 1984. Monthly. $24.00 (subscription). ISSN: 0748-9234.

From the School of Public Health, UC Berkeley, this eight-page newsletter addresses wellness from a broad perspective including environmental medical issues, nutrition, fitness, stress management and various medical conditions. Regular sections include wellness facts, a buying guide, wellness tips, questions and answers, and myths. Each issue contains a centerpiece feature article such as full sun protection and the truth about stretching exercises. Other shorter articles report on various issues such as heel pain, pap tests, a constructive approach to worry, and bursitis, giving background information, prevention and treatment tips, and suggestions. Reporting is authoritative, practical and balanced.

575. ***World Research News.*** Sherman Oaks, CA: World Research Foundation. Quarterly. $15.00 (subscription).

This twelve-page newsletter reports on the latest medical information, both traditional and alternative, internationally. Short articles cover research reported in worldwide medical journals with an emphasis on alternative medicine, such as magnetic fields and osteoporosis, and foot reflexology and diabetes. Two longer feature articles cover various topics such as alternative treatment for depression. Also included are reader letters describing their experience with alternative medicine treatment for various conditions and an extensive book review section.

CHAPTER 10: SYSTEMS OF MEDICINE

Ayurvedic Medicine

Books

576. Chopra, Deepak. *Perfect Health.* New York: Harmony Books, 1991. 327 p. Illus., biblio., index. $13.00. ISBN: 0-517-58421-2.

Written by an accomplished physician in both western and eastern medicine as well as the author of several pioneering books of international renown, *Perfect Health* introduces the reader to a 5,000-year-old Indian system of preventive medicine and health called Ayurveda, "the science of life." Calling for a total shift of perspective, the basic principle of Ayurvedic medicine is that the mind influences the body on the deepest level of being, the level of quantum physics, making perfect health within our control if we understand and practice the principles involved. In a clear, encouraging, and easily understandable manner (despite the complexity of the concepts), Dr. Chopra provides a practical guide to this mind/body approach to health. Part I explains and identifies the body type classifications of Ayurveda. Part II explores how the mind directs the body and discusses techniques to open the channels of body/mind communication and healing. Part III delineates and illustrates specific exercises, diets, and daily and seasonal routines for each body type to restore balance and strengthen the body/mind connection.

577. Frawley, David. *Ayurvedic Healing: A Comprehensive Guide.* Salt Lake City, UT: Passage Press, 1989. 368 p. Illus., biblio., index. $18.95. ISBN: 1-878423-00-2.

A recognized expert on ancient Vedic wisdom and author of several books on Ayurveda, yoga and herbology, Dr. Frawley has written a thorough and authoritative book on Ayurveda, the ancient system of natural medicine of India. This comprehensive source serves both the beginner and those seeking highly specific information and a depth of approach. The first section describes the theory and principles of this medicine, including the six tastes and three major mind/body natures, as well as the therapies used to treat imbalances for each type of constitution. Section II explores the diagnosis and treatment of over eighty diseases, organized by bodily systems, from digestive system disorders to mental disorders. The last section on Ayurvedic treatments is a detailed description of specific remedies covering both classical and modern formulas, oils, aromatherapy, herbs, spiritual remedies and yoga. Frawley's goal is clearly to inform and instruct. He includes a very detailed table of contents, a bibliography, three herbal glossaries (western, Ayurvedic and Chinese), an English and Sanskrit glossary, and a general and herbal index.

578. Ranade, Subhash. *Natural Healing Through Ayurveda.* Salt Lake City, UT: Passage Press, 1993. 238 p. Biblio., index. $11.95. ISBN: 1-878423-13-4.

Originally prepared for students of the Certificate of Proficiency Course in India and revised and edited for western audiences by Dr. David Frawley, this book presents a systematic and thorough introduction to the study and understanding of Ayurveda. Dr. Ranade, renowned doctor and teacher, discusses all aspects of Ayurveda. Part I covers the overall Ayurvedic approach to health and includes historical and philosophical information on the foundations of the system; the basic conceptual principles covering the humors, the five elements and seven constitutional types; the Ayurvedic approach to optimal health through daily, seasonal and ethical regimens; and the three pillars of life (food, rest and sexual energy). Part II delineates the methods of treatment and includes important chapters on the Marma points (Ayurvedic pressure points), the channel systems, and the interrelationship of yoga and Ayurveda. Information on nutrition, fasting, herbal remedies, exercises, breathing and cleansing are all discussed as preventive and curative measures. A Sanskrit glossary, herb medicine glossary and Ayurvedic treatment regimen for obesity are included in the appendices, and many charts and diagrams present material in an easy-to-use format. This is a clearly written and straightforward guide to the study of a complex, highly evolved system of living and maintaining health.

Journals and Newsletters

579. ***Ayurveda Today.*** Albuquerque, NM: The Ayurvedic Institute. v.1, no.1, 1988. Quarterly. $3.50/issue, $25.00 (subscription with membership).

This fifteen-page journal, more closely resembling a newsletter, is published by the Ayurvedic Institute, directed by Dr. Vasant Lad. Issues contain two substantive feature articles covering aspects of Ayurveda such as a detailed introduction to Ayurveda and its therapeutic techniques and discussion of various medicinal plants in the traditional Ayurvedic pharmacopeia. Regular departments include Ayurvedic cuisine with recipes, household herbs used for healing, and sections on the institute's course offerings and Dr. Lad's teaching itinerary. This is a useful source of information for the student and layperson interested in the Ayurvedic approach to health.

Chinese Medicine/Acupuncture

Books

580. Beinfield, Harriet and Korngold, Efrem. *Between Heaven and Earth: A Guide to Chinese Medicine.* New York: Ballantine Books, 1991. 432 p. Illus., biblio., index. $12.00. ISBN: 0-345-37974-8.

Written by two well-known American acupuncturists and educators in eastern medicine, this readable and comprehensive guide keeps the western lay reader clearly in mind. It covers both the philosophical and practical aspects of Chinese medicine, exploring how it works, why it works, and what readers can do to promote balance and health in their lives. Part I presents the theoretical basis for this system of medicine, explaining the concepts of the Tao, yin-yang, five phase theory and the method of diagnosis, and clearly differentiates between the eastern and western approaches to health. Part II corresponds to the second vital area of Chinese medicine: five phase theory westernized into five phase types for self-understanding. Providing many charts and illustrations, Part III is devoted to the three main forms of therapy aimed at promoting the self-care of the reader: acupuncture, Chinese herbs, and herbal food. With its glossary, bibliography, reading lists, and referral and resource lists, this book offers a complete introduction to the Chinese approach to medicine.

581. Eisenberg, David with Thomas Lee Wright. *Encounters with Qi: Exploring Chinese Medicine.* New York: Penguin Books, 1985. 254 p. Illus., index. $10.00. ISBN: 0-14-009427-X.

During his trips to China between 1977-1985, Dr. Eisenberg, clinical research fellow at the Harvard Medical School and the first U.S. medical exchange student to the People's Republic of China, studied Traditional Chinese Medicine from QiGong masters, including acupuncture, massage and herbal therapies. His book reflects an open yet skeptical look at Chinese medicine, examining the basic concept of Qi ("vital energy") and its use in healing, relieving pain and curing disease. Questions of what western medicine can learn from this system of health that is thousands of years old and what aspects should be investigated and integrated into western medical practice are explored. Using personal stories and case histories in an anecdotal style that is readable and entertaining, Eisenberg presents a balanced and objective view of nonwestern medicine and of the areas where the interrelationship of both eastern and western medical thought may be highly beneficial.

582. Fulder, Stephen. *The Tao of Medicine: Ginseng and Other Chinese Herbs for Inner Equilibrium and Immune Power.* Rochester, VT: Healing Arts Press, 1990. 328 p. Illus., biblio, index. $12.95. ISBN: 0-89281-388-1.

The use of ginseng and other traditional Oriental remedies to promote good health and longevity are examined in this book. Not a "how-to" book, it is written from a scientific viewpoint and provides basic information on the responsible use of such medicines. Fulder, who holds a Ph.D. in pharmacology, provides background on how he became interested in this subject and his first tentative steps toward experimentation with Oriental "harmony" herb remedies. A history of the use of some of these herbs and a hypothesis for their more widespread use in the future are offered. General concepts of oriental medicine are explored, and the properties of these harmony remedies to encourage health and vitality are examined. Although approached scientifically, this book is written in plain language accessible to the general reader. Extensive references are provided and the appendix contains general recommendations for the use of ginseng by the interested reader.

583. Gaeddert, Andrew. *Chinese Herbs in the Western Clinic: A Guide to Prepared Herbal Formulas Indexed by Western Disorders & Supported by Case Studies.* Dublin, CA: Get Well Foundation, 1994. 245 p. Biblio., index. $15.95. ISBN: 0-9638285-0-9.

As the title indicates, this book, arranged alphabetically by western ailment, provides information on appropriate herbal treatments for a wide variety of disorders. Each chapter also includes recommended herbs listed by English and Pinyin names, and case studies which expand upon the proper use of these herbs. The book opens with a very readable introduction to Chinese herbal medicine, and includes information on major energy imbalances, Chinese herbal preparations, and Chinese dietary therapy. Appendices include discussions of Chinese herbal treatments for chronic digestive disorders, chronic fatigue immune deficiency syndrome, and HIV. A table of formulas provides easy access to the different herbal treatments discussed. Written primarily for health care practitioners and students, the book provides a good overview of the use of Chinese herbs in healing.

584. Hin, Kuan. *Chinese Medicine and Acupressure.* New York: Bergh Publishing, 1991. 250 p. Illus. $15.95. ISBN: 0-930267-08-7.

Stating that "prevention is the core of Chinese medicine," Dr. Hin, an internationally known physician, describes the methods and benefits of

Chinese massage, acupressure, moxibustion and Inhea, a special method of healing. Written in a style that is accessible to the westerner, the book also conveys the sense of serenity and balance that characterize Chinese philosophy. Hin discusses the basic principles of Chinese medicine, teaches the eight components of daily massage, and explains the use of acupressure to treat fifty common ailments. Instruction is given through text and well-drawn and well-labeled illustrations which clearly indicate the location of the various acupoints along the meridians or energy pathways of the body. All these techniques have as their goal maintaining or reestablishing the free flow of energy through the body. With Chinese line drawings interspersed throughout the text, Hin reinforces the lessons of balance, harmony and flow that represent not just a therapeutic intervention but a total way of being that is the basis of the Chinese view of health.

585. Liu, Da. *The Tao of Health and Longevity.* New York: Shoots Star, 1994. 203 p. Illus., biblio. $9.95. ISBN: 1-56924-900-8.

Da Liu, a noted author and practitioner of T'ai Chi Ch'uan, provides an introduction to the concept of Taoism. Included are historical information, Taoist philosophy, an explanation of T'ai Chi Ch'uan techniques and their effect on the various systems of the body, and descriptions of other alternative therapies. Instructions and illustrations are provided for exercises which can be used by people of all ages and backgrounds to prevent physical deterioration and promote good health to an advanced age. Focusing not only on physical techniques, the book also emphasizes the importance of the spiritual component of T'ai Chi Ch'uan in promoting longevity. A holistic approach to good health and long life is offered, incorporating T'ai Chi exercises, Taoist philosophy, good nutrition and a peaceful lifestyle.

586. Manning, Clark A. and Vanrenen, Louis J. *Bioenergetic Medicines East and West: Acupuncture and Homeopathy.* Berkeley, CA: North Atlantic Books, 1988. 269 p. Biblio., index. $12.95. ISBN: 1-55643-017-5.
See Homeopathy—Books.

587. Reid, Daniel P. *The Complete Book of Chinese Health and Healing.* Boston: Shambhala, 1994. 484 p. Illus., biblio., index. $27.50. ISBN: 0-87773-929-3.

Written for a general audience, this book, arranged in five parts, presents the traditional Chinese approach to good health and longevity. Part I, "The Roots," explains such Taoist concepts as the Three Treasures of Life, Yin and Yang, the Four Foundations of Health and the Five Energies. Part II, "The Branches," discusses at length the Three Treasures: body, mind and spirit. Part III, "The Fruits," explores key elements in a long and healthy life. Part IV, "The New Hybrids: Grafting East and West," looks at approaches that combine modern western medical techniques with traditional eastern medical therapies. Part V, "Precious Prescriptions: Harvesting the Tree of Health," offers tonic medicines, therapeutic food recipes and Chinese herbal remedies. Appendices contain information on traditional Chinese medicine schools and products and a brief list of books for further reading. Overall, this clearly written, very readable book provides an excellent introduction to the subject of traditional Chinese medicine. The author has studied this subject for many years and has written two other books on this topic: *Chinese Herbal Medicine* (reviewed below) and *The Tao of Health, Sex and Longevity*.

588. ______. *Chinese Herbal Medicine*. Boston: Shambhala, 1992. 174 p. Illus., biblio., index. $20.00. ISBN: 0-87773-397-X.

The practice of Chinese medicine goes back more than 5,000 years. According to the author, "it remains the world's oldest, safest and most comprehensive system of medical care, developing as dynamically today as throughout its long history." In order to draw the attention of western readers to the benefits of this ancient practice, Reid has researched ancient Chinese sources and sought out contemporary Chinese experts for information on this subject. Introductory chapters provide a historical framework, while subsequent chapters cover the principles of Chinese medicine, herbal descriptions, and herbal prescriptions for a select list of ailments. Color illustrations for identifying herbs are found throughout the text.

Journals and Newsletters

589. *Qi: The Journal of Traditional and Eastern Health and Fitness*. Chantilly, VA: Insight Graphics. v.1, no.1, 1991. Quarterly. Illus, adv. $18.95 (subscription). ISSN: 1056-4004.

This journal explores the various aspects of eastern medicine, from the practical to the pure theoretical. Areas covered include Chinese medicine, acupuncture, meditation, eastern philosophies, yoga, diet, herbs and T'ai Chi. Issues contain four feature articles and various departments including news information, a section on herbology, book reviews, a calendar of events, and a listing of professionals across the country. While writing is geared for the western lay reader, some background in eastern philosophy and practice would be useful.

Herbal Medicine

Books

590. Bach, Edward and Wheeler, F. J. *The Bach Flower Remedies.* New Canaan, CT: Keats Publishing, 1952. 148 p. $9.95. ISBN: 0-87983-193-6.

This classic presentation of Dr. Bach's work is three books in one: *Heal Thyself: An Explanation of the Real Cause and Cure of Disease, The Twelve Healers and Other Remedies*, both by Bach, and the *Bach Remedies Repertory* by F. J. Wheeler, M.D. These books are a compilation of theory and practical information. Edward Bach (1886-1936) developed a specialized branch of herbal medicine using only nonpoisonous wildflowers to treat disease on an energy level before it becomes manifest in the body. *Heal Thyself* is a treatise on the nature of disease (the result of "conflict between soul and mind") and cure ("removing those basic factors which are its primary cause"). Disease is seen as preventable and curable ("the personality without conflict is immune to illness"). *The Twelve Healers* offers the practical knowledge of this natural system of healing. Thirty-eight different psychological states are described under seven headings (fear, uncertainty, insufficient interest in present circumstances, loneliness, oversensitivity to influences and ideas, despondency or despair, and over-care for the welfare of others), with the original twelve remedies asterisked. The method of preparation and dosage are described. Dr. Wheeler's book follows the basic premise that the remedies treat the mood and temperament of the patient, as it is these disharmonies (fears, anxieties, worries, etc.) that lead to disease. A repertory of remedies is given that provides a more detailed breakdown of moods and their corresponding remedies. The reader then refers back to *The Twelve Healers* for a full description of the remedy recommended. The book concludes with indexed references to the remedies, giving each one and the pages in which it appears in all three books.

591. Bisset, Norman Grainger. *Herbal Drugs and Phytopharmaceuticals: A Handbook for Practice on a Scientific Basis.* Boca Raton: CRC Press, 1994. 556 p. Illus, biblio., index. $179.95. ISBN: 0-8493-7192-9.

This translation of the original German edition by Max Wichtl is written primarily for pharmacists, physicians, herbalists, botanists, chemists and manufacturers. It provides scientifically based information on 181 herbal drugs arranged by Latin names with references to their English language Pharmacopoeias as is appropriate and standard license number if it exists. Each drug monograph contains a color illustration and description of its features for identification; the plant source with scientific name, common English name, plant family and picture of the source; synonyms in English, Latin, German and French; origin, including main exporting countries;

constituents of the drug with quantitative data and pharmacopoeial requirements if possible; indications for use divided into scientifically based therapeutic use and folk medicinal application; side effects; preparation; prepared herbal remedies; phytomedicines describing the drug's use in the manufacture of prepared remedies; authentication information including microscopic examination and TLC test methods; current adulteration information; storage instructions; and literature citations for data verification, mostly from the German periodical literature. An initial section covers general concerns, issues and information on herbal drugs. An index provides lists of indications by system disorder (such as gastrointestinal disorders), noting the type of action, relevant herbs by order of importance and a listing of applicable folk medicinal herbs. In addition there is an author index for the specific drug monographs and a subject index of monograph titles and botanical names. This authoritative text serves as a standard for professional medical and pharmaceutical education and clinical use.

592. Castleman, Michael. *The Healing Herbs: The Ultimate Guide to the Curative Power of Nature's Medicine.* Emmaus, PA: Rodale Press, 1991. 436 p. Illus., biblio., index. $26.95. ISBN: 0-87857-934-6.

This well-organized book, arranged in two parts, discusses 100 herbs used in traditional healing. Part I presents important background information, including the history of herbal healing, preparation and storage of herbal treatments, and overall safety considerations for the use of herbs. Part II profiles these commonly used medicinal herbs, providing history, folklore, medicinal use and, where available, scientific research results on the benefits and hazards of each herb. Three ready-reference tables at the back of the book arrange the herbs by medical condition, by type of healing action and by other uses.

593. Gladstar, Rosemary. *Herbal Healing for Women.* New York: Simon & Schuster, 1993. 303 p. Illus., biblio., index. $12.00. ISBN: 0-671-76767-4.

Pointing out the fact that women have been using herbs to restore and maintain health and vitality for thousands of years, Rosemary Gladstar has written a clear, comprehensive, easy-to-understand guide to the use of herbs for women. Detailed information is provided on the preparation of herbal teas, oils, salves, ointments, tinctures, liniments, pills and capsules. In sections on adolescence, the childbearing years, pregnancy and childbirth, and the menopausal years, the author provides instructions for the use of herbs to treat common and not-so-common ailments. Acne, menstrual irregularities, endometriosis, fertility and infertility, problems in pregnancy and menopause are some of the conditions addressed, with herbal recipes offered for each. A *materia medica* contains more than two dozen herbs that are especially useful for women. Appendices include an annotated bibliography of herb books for beginners and women, general books on women's health, and books on health in general; resource guides of herbal suppliers, newsletters and educational programs; and a questionnaire which assists women in designing a personal health program. The author, founder of the California School of Herbal Studies and current owner of SAGE (see chapter 2: Herbal Medicine—Schools, and Herbal Medicine—Product Suppliers) has drawn upon her more than twenty years of experience as an herbalist to write a warm, thorough, and intelligent work.

594. Green, James. *The Male Herbal: Health Care for Men & Boys.* Freedom, CA: The Crossing Press, 1991. 267 p. Biblio., index. $12.95. ISBN: 0-89594-458-8.

This unique book has been written to allow men to achieve the independence gained from taking responsibility for one's own health and well-being. Based upon information drawn from the experiences of holistic health care practitioners and medical herbalists, it fills a gap in the literature by providing herbal health care information for males. The author provides some background and historical information as well as the basics of selecting herbs and techniques for preparing herbal remedies. Noting that men tend not to seek help for their medical disorders, specific male medical problems and appropriate treatments for general health care are discussed. Details about the properties of many of the herbs noted in the book are arranged alphabetically by herb. The bibliography, listing of herb books, schools, journals, tools and organizations, and a glossary at the end of the book are particularly useful. The author is co-director and a teacher at the California School of Herbal Studies (see chapter 2: Herbal Medicine—Schools), and has led workshops in eco-plant harvesting, herbal medicine-making, and traditional herbal therapies.

595. Hallowell, Michael. *Herbal Healing: A Practical Introduction to Medicinal Herbs.* Garden City, NY: Avery Publishing, 1994. 191 p. Illus., index. $12.95. ISBN: 0-89529-604-7.

For those with little or no background in the field of herbal medicine, this basic guide takes a comprehensive approach to the subject. The book is arranged in three parts, each of which can be used independently of the other two sections. Part I contains basic information on medicinal plants, their collection and storage. Also included are simple methods of preparing herbal medicines and an extensive glossary of terms. In Part II, plant identification and poisonous plants are discussed, and a concise herbal provides botanical information, therapeutic uses, and dosage for each plant. Part III includes listings of herbal colleges, correspondence courses and suppliers, and a brief, annotated list of books on herbalism. Appendices contain valuable information on dosages, weights and measures, and common medical abbreviations. Clear, carefully drawn, black-and-white illustrations of various plants are interspersed throughout the text. For those interested in learning about medicinal plants, this book is an excellent place to start.

596. Hoffmann, David. *An Herbal Guide to Stress Relief.* Rochester, VT: Healing Arts Press, 1991. 192 p. Illus., biblio., index. $9.95. ISBN: 0-89281-426-8.

David Hoffmann, a practicing herbal consultant and author of several books on herbalism, examines the concept of stress—what it is, how the body responds to it on both physiological and psychological levels, and the association between stress and illness. Approaching the subject from a holistic perspective with an emphasis on the use of herbs, various therapies (body work, herbal treatments, meditation, diet, etc.) for the control of stress are explored. General instructions are provided for the preparation of both fresh and dried herbal remedies used to relieve stress and tension, followed by a chapter devoted to commonly used herbs. Information is included on dosages, indications, beneficial herbal combinations and preparations. The book contains a selective bibliography of books on herbs and general advice; however, the bibliography does not appear to have been updated since the publication of the 1987 edition of this book.

597. ______. *An Elders' Herbal: Natural Techniques for Promoting Health and Vitality.* Rochester, VT: Healing Arts Press, 1993. 266 p. Illus., biblio., index. $14.95. ISBN: 0-89281-396-2.

Written to address the health care needs of those in their fifties, sixties and beyond, this book emphasizes practical information regarding the use of herbal therapies which focus on wellness and prevention as opposed to disease. Each chapter presents a different system of the body (pulmonary, upper respiratory, endocrine, etc.) and discusses the common effects of aging, how to encourage wellness, and specific herbal remedies for that particular system. Also included is a chapter on the preparation of herbal remedies and a *materia medica* for older adults. Information in the *materia medica* includes botanical name, parts used, actions, indications, preparation and dosage. Useful addresses for both medical and nonmedical organizations for seniors and a bibliography of herbal and general health materials provide the reader with leads to further information.

598. Hutchins, Alma R. *A Handbook of Native American Herbs.* Boston: Shambhala Publications, 1992. 256 p. Illus., index. $10.00. ISBN: 0-87773-699-5.

The author, a practitioner of herbal medicine for more than thirty years, has written an abridged version of her well-known previous work, *Indian Herbology of North America* (see below). This book contains detailed descriptions of 125 of the most useful medicinal plants commonly found in North America, along with directions for a range of uses, remedies for common ailments, and notes on the herbal traditions of other cultures. Arranged alphabetically, entries include such common medicinal plants as slippery elm and aloe, and common kitchen herbs such as thyme and parsley. For each entry, common names, features, medicinal part, solvent, bodily influence and, where appropriate, internal dosage, external applications and homeopathic clinical applications are included.

599. ______. *Indian Herbology of North America.* Boston: Shambhala Publications, 1973. 382 p. Illus., biblio, index. $17.00. ISBN: 0-87773-639-1.

This classic work in the field of medical herbalism covers Indian herbology of the United States and Canada and contains information on more than 200 medicinal plants found in these two countries. The author studied and worked with herbalist N. G. Tretchikoff and based her book on information compiled by him over several decades. Encyclopedic in scope, each entry lists common names and identifies significant features of each plant, as well as medicinal parts, solvents, and influence on the body. Uses of herbal medicines are discussed and dosages are provided. Where appropriate, information is also given on the uses of these plants by other cultures. An annotated bibliography is included at the back of the book, though, given the dates of publication, many of the listed works may be difficult to find. Nonetheless, this is a valuable resource for practicing herbalists.

600. Murray, Michael T. *The Healing Power of Herbs: The Enlightened Person's Guide to the Wonders of Medicinal Plants.* Rocklin, CA: Prima Publishing, 1992. 246 p. Illus., biblio., index. $12.95. ISBN: 1-55958-138-7.

To address what the author refers to as a "dearth of information in the area of botanical medicine which is accessible to the intelligent lay person," Murray has taken a scientific approach to the subject of herbs. Careful to define technical terms to promote understanding of the concepts being discussed, he offers concise and understandable clinical recommendations combined with scientific information from the peer review literature. An overview of botanical medicine, including historical background and prospects for the future, is followed by discussions of some common food herbs and herbal tonics. The remainder of the book is arranged in chapters by broad ailments (e.g., liver disorders, heart and vascular systems, urinary tract disorders, etc.) with selected herbs to address these conditions. Each chapter provides a general description of the ailments, followed by a discussion of the chemical composition, history and folk use, pharmacology, dosage and toxicology of each herb.

601. Nuzzi, Debra. *Pocket Herbal Reference Guide.* Freedom, CA: Crossing Press, 1992. 138 p. Biblio., index. $5.95. ISBN: 0-89594-568-1.

As the title suggests, this is a pocket-sized guide to the many uses of herbal medicines. The author, a certified master herbalist with more than twenty years experience in the field of herbal medicine, provides background information on herbology as well as information on the historical use of herbs. General information on herbs is provided in the first chapter, in a simple question/answer format, and is followed by chapters on herbal preparations and herbal formulations. A chapter on common complaints refers the reader back to the appropriate formulations. Also included are a section on the preparation of poultices and other natural therapies, a very brief *materia medica,* and information on dosages. Though far from comprehensive, this is a handy information guide to the many uses of herbal medicines.

602. Tierra, Lesley. *The Herbs of Life: Health & Healing Using Western & Chinese Techniques.* Freedom, CA: Crossing Press, 1992. 250 p. Illus., biblio., index. $14.95. ISBN: 0-89594-498-7.

In this clearly written guide to the use of herbs for achieving and maintaining good health, the author identifies five factors which she considers essential to a healthy life: breathing exercises and contemplation, exercise, diet, lifestyle and natural medicines. While all five factors are addressed, this book focuses on natural herbal medicines. Organized in three sections, each part is devoted to a distinct aspect of herbal medicine. Part I provides an overview of herbs and their use in healing and includes discussions of energetic and symptomatic uses of herbs, the energy of illness, herbal properties, plant chemistry, and herbal families and formulas. Extensive information on individual eastern and western herbs, including properties, dosages and precautions, is also found in this section. Part II explores the process of health and healing and includes recipes for herbal remedies which can be prepared at home and herbal therapies which can be used at home. Part III covers the harvesting, preparing and storing of herbs and provides instructions for making healing tools. Also found here is valuable information on how to shop for herbs and what to include in an herbal medicine kit. Among the appendices is a very useful chart of symptoms and their appropriate remedies. The author, an herbalist and licensed acupuncturist, has written a well-organized resource which will be of use to those just beginning to learn about medicinal herbs as well as to more experienced herbal practitioners.

603. Tierra, Michael. *American Herbalism: Essays on Herbs and Herbalism by Members of the American Herbalist Guild.* Freedom, CA: Crossing Press, 1992. 321 p. Biblio. $15.95. ISBN: 0-89594-540-1.

A compilation of essays from presentations of the First American Herbalist Guild symposium supplemented by other articles by American herbalists, this book brings together writings representing the most current and sophisticated thinking on herbs and herbalism. Essays cover five major topics: an historical perspective from prehistoric times to modern use; profiles of three great American herbalists; specific herbal traditions and practices; specific illness and treatment protocols; and issues in the practice of herbalism. A well-rounded bibliography of books, newsletters, databases, and foreign journals and newsletters, as well as an appendix listing herb schools, correspondence courses and societies, confirms this as a book for readers with a serious theoretical or practical interest in the field of herbology.

604. Tyler, Varro E. *The Honest Herbal: A Sensible Guide to the Use of Herbs and Related Remedies.* New York: Pharmaceutical Products Press, 1993. 375 p. Biblio., index. $15.95. ISBN: 1-56024-287-6.

Tyler, a well-known authority on herbs and their uses and author of several other publications on the subject, has written a very accessible guide which provides the reader with factual information on the appropriate uses of more than 100 commonly available herbs and related remedies. Introductory chapters offer an objective presentation of the pros and cons of using herbal remedies and background on their regulation. Chapters are arranged alphabetically by common name, with each devoted to discussion of a single herb. Each chapter follows a similar format: a brief description of the herb, including physical characteristics and proper nomenclature, a discussion of its therapeutic uses (both actual and purported), and easy-to-understand information on the chemical properties which cause it to work. Chapters conclude with the author's personal evaluation of each herb's efficacy, and a list of scientific references to which the reader can turn for further information. A final section contains a useful chart, arranged by each herb's common name, which summarizes the part of each plant used, the herb's primary uses, and its probable effectiveness and safety. Overall, this is an excellent source of balanced information which enables the reader to make informed decisions on the safe and effective use of herbs.

Journals and Newsletters

605. ***AHA Quarterly.*** Nevada City, CA: American Herb Association. v.1, no.1, 1981. Quarterly. Adv. $20.00 (subscription).

This well researched newsletter for medical herbalists and the general public searches approximately forty medical journals, thirty international herb-related publications, twenty-eight major magazines and newspapers, and the MEDLINE computer database of the National Library of Medicine to provide the most current information on herbs internationally. Issues are substantive in both size (approximately twenty pages) and content, containing profiles of particular herbs, herb news, international news, legal issues, book reviews, herbal case studies, information on organizations and resource directories, environmental and aromatherapy news, short reports on different remedies and diseases treated with herbs, and a classified section. The sources for news items and reports are cited after each abstract so the complete original article can be read. Advertisements for herbal schools, conferences, products and books are included. Editorial consultants include educators, botanists, biochemists, pharmacists, medical herbalists and researchers in the field of herbal medicine.

606. ***Flower Essence Society Newsletter.*** Nevada City, CA: Earth Spirit, Inc. Annual. Free with society membership.

Approximately thirty pages, this newsletter is full of useful information on the therapeutic effects of flower essences. Case studies and practitioner reports from around the world on various herbs, plants and botanicals provide detailed information on their uses and the treatment of various conditions. Also included are reviews of books, tapes and photographs, news reports on related issues, and educational programs, conferences and the like.

607. ***The Herb Companion.*** Loveland, CO: Interweave Press. v.1, no.1, 1988. Bimonthly. Illus., adv. $21.00 (one-year subscription), $38.00 (two-year subscription). ISSN: 1040-581X.

This beautifully illustrated magazine covers all aspects of the use of herbs for the lay reader, including healing, cooking, fragrance, gardening and herbal education. Each issue focuses on a particular topic such as urban herbs, herbs in history, and herbs for the garden, and contains eight in-depth feature articles and nine regular departments. These include letters, notes from regional herb gardeners, kitchen table, a profile of a particular herb, a calendar of upcoming events such as festivals, classes, lectures, workshops and conferences, and review of books. The articles, about six pages long, are written in a warm, lively manner and are replete with information, tips, useful charts and inviting illustrations. This is a wonderful source of information and pleasure.

608. ***Herb Gatherings:*** *The Newsletter For The Thymes*. Lafayette, IN: Nelson Graphics. v.1, no.1, 1993. Bimonthly. Illus., adv. $15.00 (subscription). ISSN: 1070-6682.

This general interest herbal newsletter offers articles on a broad range of herb-related topics, including a feature in each issue entitled "Herbs to Soothe and Heal." From time to time, this publication also includes articles focusing on the work of organizations that promote the medicinal use of herbs as a therapeutic modality. A small number of classified and display ads are also included as well as recipes for herbal healing and a listing of herb-related events. Written in an easy-to-read style, this newsletter is appropriate for anyone with an interest in herbs.

609. ***Herb Quarterly.*** San Anselmo, CA: Long Mountain Press. v.1, no.1, 1979. Quarterly. Illus., adv. $6.00/issue, $24.00 (one-year subscription), $45.00 (two-year subscription). ISSN: 0163-9900.

This "folksy" magazine is written and edited by individuals who have a love of herbs. Aimed at general audiences, the publication contains informative articles written in clear, easy-to-understand language. Issues include pieces on aromatherapy, tonic herbs, and herbal therapies for anxiety. Information on history and folklore as well as resource lists of books and products appear regularly. Letters to the editor, "Potpourri," "Herbal Updates" regarding conferences, seminars, workshops, etc., book reviews, recipes for both edible and medicinal preparations, and readers' advertisements are included in every issue. Michael Castleman, author of several books on herbal medicine, is a contributing editor.

610. ***HerbalGram.*** Austin, TX: American Botanical Council and Herb Research Foundation. v.1, no.1, 1979. Quarterly. Illus. $25.00 (subscription). ISSN: 0899-5648.

Although this publication does not exclusively focus on herbal medicine, it does provide very good coverage of this therapeutic modality. For example, issues have focused on European phytomedicines and traditional herbal medicine of India, Tibet, China, Africa, Japan and Polynesia. Regular departments include "Herb Blurbs," which contains brief items on various aspects of herbs; "Media Watch," which reviews herb-related articles in other publications; "Research Reviews," which briefly summarizes the results of current research; "Access," which lists publications, organizations and other resources of interest; as well as conference reports, market reports, book reviews, letters, a calendar of events, and classified advertising. This well-written journal contains beautiful full-color illustrations, and with Dr. Andrew Weil among its contributing editors, is an excellent source of information on herbal medicine.

611. ***Medical Herbalism:*** *A Clinical Newsletter for the Herbal Practitioner.* Portland, OR: Bergner Communications. v.1, no.1, 1989. Quarterly. Adv. $29.00 (subscription).

This professional journal regularly publishes results of scientific research, case studies, and reviews of current books, tapes and software relating to herbal medicine. Articles on the use of herbs in healing are well-researched, and pieces on related therapeutic modalities are also included. Past issues have included articles on the use of herbs to treat such conditions as hypertension, depression, liver disease, urinary tract infections and menopause, and on profiles of the use of dandelion, licorice, echinacea and other herbs. With its summaries of and commentaries on articles published in selected international journals, this is an important resource for medical herbalists.

612. ***Protocol Journal of Botanical Medicine.*** Harvard, MA: Herbal Research Publications. v.1, no.1, 1995. Quarterly. $96.00 (subscription).

This peer-reviewed publication offers well-researched articles appropriate for both clinical and educational use. Therapeutic protocols on various disorders such as urinary tract infections, allergies, diabetes, etc., are discussed, and the links between western allopathic medicine and naturopathy, Ayurveda and Chinese medicine explored.

Homeopathy

Books

613. Castro, Miranda. *The Complete Homeopathy Handbook: A Guide to Everyday Health Care.* New York: St. Martin's Press, 1990. 253 p. Index. $14.95. ISBN: 0-312-06320-2.

More than just a "how-to" book of homeopathic treatments, this well-written book provides a range of information on homeopathic remedies the author considers safe and effective. Castro reviews the history and principles of homeopathic medicine, and the "do's and don'ts" of prescribing homeopathic treatments. Separate sections on internal and external remedies, arranged alphabetically by formal name, provide the reader with general information about each remedy and instructions for its use in treating various conditions. An index of symptoms at the end of each section refers the reader to the appropriate remedies. Separate chapters contain case studies providing examples of how to use these remedies and details on the kinds of ailments covered by this book. Appendices include a glossary of terms and a listing of homeopathic treatments to be included in a first aid kit. This book is appropriate for beginners as well as for those who have had some exposure to this modality.

614. Coulter, Harris L. *Homeopathic Science and Modern Medicine: The Physics of Healing with Microdoses.* Berkeley, CA: North Atlantic Books, 1980. 170 p. Biblio. $9.95. ISBN: 0-913028-84-3.

Originally written as a three-part article for the *Journal of the American Institute of Homeopathy,* this definitive book is designed for the professional and lay reader who wants a deeper understanding of the foundations of homeopathy, how and why it works, its place in medical therapeutics, and the scientific basis of the practice. Dr. Coulter, considered the outstanding historian of homeopathic medicine, begins by describing the basic principles of homeopathy, including the general rather than local nature of disease, the organism's capacity to respond to environmental stimuli, and the importance of symptoms prior to physical signs of disease. Based on these principles, Coulter shows how Dr. Hahnemann (1775-1843), the originator of homeopathy, developed the cure through similars. He then describes the program of provings undertaken by Hahnemann, considered to be the homeopathic contribution to medicine and the basis of the homeopathic method of practice. Other basic concepts are enumerated, including the patient's hypersensitivity to similar medicine, the principle of the infinitesimal dose, the single remedy, and Hering's Law and chronic disease. Coulter clarifies both the differences and similarities between homeopathic and allopathic medicine, adding clarity and perspective to a controversy long mired in prejudice and misunderstanding. The text is extensively referenced throughout, citing books and articles by eminent scientists in the field. Although a scholarly work, it is also a very clear and readable account of the history, foundation and place of homeopathy in modern medicine. Three appendices present homeopathic dilutions, a sample of the case-taking process conducted by a homeopath, and a discussion of clinical trials in homeopathy and allopathic medicine.

615. Grossinger, Richard. *Homeopathy: An Introduction for Skeptics and Beginners.* Berkeley, CA: North Atlantic Books, 1993. 162 p. Biblio., index. $12.95. ISBN: 1-55643-165-1.

Though the title of this work might lead one to believe that this is a basic, "how-to" book, in reality it is more of a theoretical work. This well-researched book provides a good deal of information on the historical origins and scientific basis of homeopathy and its principles and methodology, and thoroughly discusses the rise and fall and rise again of homeopathy's popularity in North America. Readers looking to glean some background information on homeopathy will be well-served by this work.

616. Kruzel, Thomas. *The Homeopathic Emergency Guide: A Quick Reference Handbook to Effective Homeopathic Care.* Berkeley, CA: North Atlantic

Books & Homeopathic Educational Services, 1992. 366 p. Illus., index. $16.95. ISBN: 1-55643-123-6.

This practical book, written by a naturopathic doctor, summarizes the common symptoms of a wide range of medical conditions and their homeopathic treatments. Arranged alphabetically by disorder, its forty sections cover everything from abdominal inflammations to wounds and fractures. Each section begins with a brief description of the condition and then discusses appropriate homeopathic remedies for each, with remedies arranged alphabetically within each section. The author is careful to point out that this is not a comprehensive work, and that it includes only common symptoms and indications for each remedy. An appendix containing flow charts for selected conditions and two separate indexes, one by symptom, one by remedy, make it easy to find the information one may be looking for. This valuable guide is appropriate for use by homeopathic practitioners for ready reference or in situations where lack of time is a concern, and for use by allopathic physicians who would like to incorporate homeopathic treatments into their practices.

617. Lockie, Andrew. *The Family Guide to Homeopathy*. New York: Prentice Hall, 1989. 463 p. Illus., index. $24.95. ISBN: 0-13-306994-X.

Making the basic assumption that the less serious the medical condition, the more logical it is to apply nontoxic therapies first, Lockie has written a guide for homeopathic alternatives to allopathic medicine. Intended to be comprehensive, it provides a general overview, followed by information on the use of remedies, and a section on medical conditions. Medical conditions are arranged in chapters by bodily systems or parts, with ailments listed alphabetically within each chapter. A notable feature of these chapters is the use of symbols indicating when it is necessary to consult a physician. The appendix includes a discussion of the overall physical and mental conditions under which sixty commonly used homeopathic remedies should be administered.

618. Manning, Clark A. and Vanrenen, Louis J. *Bioenergetic Medicines East and West: Acupuncture and Homeopathy.* Berkeley, CA: North Atlantic Books, 1988. 269 p. Biblio., index. $12.95. ISBN: 1-55643-017-5.

Bioenergetic medicine is defined as an holistic approach, one which views health in terms of the well-being of the whole person. This book explores the commonalities and differences of two such systems of medicine, acupuncture and homeopathy. A chapter on the history of bioenergetic research offers brief biographies of important individuals who have studied bioenergy, from Huang Ti, the purported founder of Chinese medicine, to present-day physicians, scientists and researchers. Homeopathy and acupuncture are each discussed separately, then followed by an examination of cases which use either homeopathic or acupuncture methodologies. Fourteen select disharmony patterns are then assessed from a homeopathic perspective and compared with the Chinese medicine perspective. In this interesting and important work, the authors, both trained acupuncturists, present clear explanations of both systems of medicine which can be easily understood by health care professionals and the lay public.

619. Moskowitz, Richard, M.D. *Homeopathic Medicines for Pregnancy and Childbirth.* Berkeley, CA: North Atlantic Books & Homeopathic Educational Services, 1992. 288 p. Biblio., index. $14.95. ISBN: 1-55643-137-6.

This useful work offers homeopathic remedies for common ailments encountered during pregnancy, childbirth and the postpartum period. Part I provides an overview of homeopathy, including the Law of Similars, provings, the homeopathic *materia medica,* and homeopathic remedies. Part II consists of an abbreviated *materia medica,* with case presentations which illustrate the twenty-five remedies discussed. Part III examines common problems which can occur during pregnancy, labor and delivery, and the postpartum period, and offers remedies for each condition and sample cases as appropriate. The author, a past president of the National Center for Homeopathy, has been a homeopathic practitioner for more than twenty years and has attended hundreds of pregnancies. Although he has written this book primarily for the lay public, it is also a valuable resource for homeopathic practitioners, midwives and obstetricians.

620. Ullman, Dana. *Discovering Homeopathy: Medicine for the 21st Century.* Berkeley, CA: North Atlantic Books, 1991. 277 p. Biblio., index. $12.95. ISBN: 1-55643-108-2.

This solid introduction to the science and art of homeopathy is written by Dana Ullman, award-winning author, founder and president of the Foundation for Homeopathic Education and Research and major contributor to the increased public and professional awareness and acceptance of homeopathy in the United States. In Part I, Ullman explains the basic concepts underlying homeopathic practice and provides a history of the field. A major contribution is the review of homeopathic research consisting of double blind research experiments, clinical trials on animals, and laboratory evidence of the biological effects of microdoses, all thoroughly documented in the references at the end of chapter three. Part II discusses the clinical areas in which homeopathic treatment is effective, including pregnancy and labor, pediatrics, women's health, infectious disease, allergic conditions, chronic disease, sports medicine, psychological problems and dentistry. Although specific remedies are mentioned for various conditions, this section is not a guide to therapeutic use but an overview of the scope of homeopathy in treating disease and enhancing health. Part III is a useful resource for finding additional information on homeopathy and includes listings of homeopathic manufacturers, organizations, schools and training programs, self-care books, finding a practitioner and more. Everything about this book is authoritative, easy to use, clear and well done, from the excellent index, quality resource lists, and consistent documentation to the knowledgeable, balanced and highly readable presentation of ideas and information.

621. ______. *Homeopathic Medicine for Children and Infants.* New York: J. P. Tarcher/Perigee Books, 1992. 256 p. Biblio., index. $9.95. ISBN: 0-87477-692-9.

Written by a noted educator and author in the field of homeopathic medicine (*Discovering Homeopathy: Medicine for the 21st Century;* co-author of *Everybody's Guide to Homeopathic Medicine*), this book addresses the need for safe, effective alternatives to conventional medicine for the treatment of children and infants, without discounting the value of allopathic medicine. Part I provides an overview of homeopathy, including basic principles, limitations and risks. Part II contains information on when and how to use homeopathic medicines. Part III is an alphabetical listing of common ailments, accompanied by the most appropriate homeopathic remedies for each one. Part IV provides detailed descriptions of each of these remedies. Part V discusses common homeopathic remedies available commercially. Appendices include a guide to homeopathic medicines and their pronunciation, sources of homeopathic products and services, and a recommended reading list. For parents seeking an alternative to conventional medical treatment for their children, this well-organized work is an excellent source of information.

622. Weiner, Michael and Goss, Kathleen. *The Complete Book of Homeopathy.* Garden City Park, NY: Avery Publishing, 1989. 299 p. Biblio., index. $9.95. ISBN: 0-89529-412-5.

Intended to be a comprehensive source of information on homeopathic medicine, this book provides the reader with background on the philosophy, principles and practice of homeopathy. An overview of various homeopathic remedies arranged alphabetically is provided, followed by case studies which illustrate the use of some of these treatments. Also included are a discussion of homeopathic treatments as first aid for minor ailments, and a chapter of commonly asked questions and answers about this field. The closing chapters provide a look at the history of this treatment modality and its possible impact in the years to come. Suggestions for further reading and lists of homeopathic physicians and sources of homeopathic supplies are found in the appendices.

Journals and Newsletters

623. ***The American Homeopath.*** Plymouth, MN: The North American Society of Homeopaths. v.1, no.1, 1994. Annual. Adv. $20.00 (subscription).

This is a truly international journal of classical, professional homeopathy presenting cured cases, new *materia medica* information, homeopathic philosophy, medical politics, letters to the editor, book reviews, and interviews with doctors and other professionals important in the field of homeopathy, such as Dr. Edward C. Whitmont and Julian Winston. The journal contains approximately ten feature articles, five interviews and five case reviews and runs a little over 100 pages. Articles are interesting, clearly written and informative and serve to unify the homeopathic community by including contributions from leading homeopaths and homeopathic organizations from around the world.

624. ***Biological Therapy: Journal of Natural Medicine.*** Albuquerque, NM: Menaco Publishing. v.1, no.1, 1983. Quarterly. Adv. $3.50/issue, $10.00 (subscription). ISSN: 0773-2661.

This scholarly journal contains feature articles and reports of current research on a variety of therapies including homeopathy, naturopathy and nutrition. Most pieces begin with an abstract; some contain charts and footnotes. The address of the author is given at the end of each article. Brief alternative medicine news items and descriptive annotations of books distributed by Menaco Publishing appear regularly.

625. ***Homeopathy Today.*** Alexandria, VA: National Center for Homeopathy. v.1, no.1, 1989. Monthly, except for combined July/August issue. Adv. Free with National Center for Homeopathy membership. ISSN: 0886-1676.

This monthly newsletter covers current activities in the field of homeopathy. Legislation, listings of homeopathy in the media, the treatment of specific ailments, and interviews with or profiles of noted homeopaths are all regular features. A calendar of events lists upcoming classes and seminars. Articles are accepted for consideration from National Center for Homeopathy members.

626. ***Journal of the American Institute of Homeopathy.*** Glenco, CO: American Institute of Homeopathy. v.1, no.1, 1907. Quarterly. Adv. $45.00 (subscription). ISSN: 0002-8967.

A peer-reviewed scientific journal for physicians practicing homeopathy, this journal contains original manuscripts, feature articles, research reports, news articles, "Homeopathic Grand Rounds" case studies, short case reports for a "Clinical Snapshots" section, seminar reports and position papers. Also included are book reviews and letters to the editor. Articles contain abstracts, key words and references where applicable and are written by American and international homeopaths.

627. *Resonance.* Seattle, WA: International Foundation for Homeopathy. v.1, no.1, 1979. Bimonthly. Adv. $35.00 (subscription, includes membership).

Resonance covers all aspects of classical homeopathy for the lay and professional homeopath. It includes regular sections on homeopathic pediatrics, veterinary homeopathy, homeopathy for women, homeopathic dentistry, and homeopathic education. Also included are a book review section, letters to the editor, and homeopathic news, developments and articles of general interest in the field. Contributions are made by doctors of medicine, naturopathy, homeopathy, dentistry, and veterinary medicine.

628. *Simillimum.* Portland, OR: Homeopathic Academy of Naturopathic Physicians. v.1, no.1, 1988. Quarterly. Adv. $35.00 (free with membership).

Published by the Homeopathic Academy of Naturopathic Physicians, this journal is for the practicing homeopath. Each issue contains a variety of cases, *materia medica,* practical information, and philosophical discussions by leading international homeopaths. The articles are detailed, substantive, clearly written and authoritative. The journal runs over 100 pages per issue.

Naturopathy

Books

629. Murray, Michael. *Natural Alternatives to Over-the Counter and Prescription Drugs.* New York: William Morrow and Company, 1994. 383 p. Index. $25.00. ISBN: 0-688-12358-9.

A welcome addition to the literature of natural medicine, this book discusses the limitations and side effects of prescription and over-the-counter medications, and the natural remedies which can be used in place of those drugs. Most of the alternatives discussed can be purchased in supermarkets and health food stores. Section I discusses the present state of health care in America and the role of the drug companies in the prescription of drugs to treat illness. Section II covers common ailments and provides general information about each condition, a description of the drugs usually used for treatment, their benefits and side effects, and natural alternatives to these drugs. Section III focuses on maintaining good health and includes guides to nutritional supplements and medicinal herbs.

630. Murray, Michael T. and Pizzorno, Joseph E. *An Encyclopedia of Natural Medicine.* Rocklin, CA: Prima Publishing, 1991. 622 p. Illus., biblio., index. $18.95. ISBN: 1-55958-091-7.

This self-care guide is designed to help readers make informed decisions about their health. Topics covered span the spectrum from simple common ailments to life-threatening medical conditions, and include such problems as allergies, burns, heart disease, hiccups, poison ivy, and varicose veins. Organized alphabetically by ailment, the book contains extensive illustrations and easy-to-follow instructions for each condition's natural healing methods. Techniques discussed and illustrated include acupressure, herbal remedies and relaxation, to name a few.

631. Polunin, Miriam and Robbins, Christopher. *The Natural Pharmacy.* New York: Collier Books, 1992. 144 p. Illus., biblio., index. $18.95. ISBN: 0-020-36041-X.

This well-organized and informative guide to over 230 natural healing substances provides both an historical and practical perspective. Part I is an A-Z of nature's medicine chest, detailing the history of medicine from ancient civilization to twentieth-century western medicine. Basic methods and ingredients used in the key healing systems of Chinese herbalism, homeopathy, Indian medicine, herbal medicine and orthodox medicine are highlighted. Part II is an alphabetical full-color photographic catalog of medicinal ingredients ranging from the common to the exotic, and their page number location in the Reference Guide section. This alphabetical Reference Guide provides detailed, encyclopedic profiles of each ingredient appearing in the A-Z section. Part III is a "how-to" on preparing the various forms of herbal remedies from infusions to poultices. A table of everyday ailments and their common remedies, with dosage information, as well as a glossary, bibliography and index help make this an easy-to-use and useful source on natural medicine.

632. Scott, Julian. *Natural Medicine for Children.* New York: Avon Books, 1990. 191 p. Illus., index. $12.95. ISBN: 0-380-75876-8.

Written for parents who want to ensure their children's good health with natural remedies, this book provides a guide to herbs, homeopathy, massage and other forms of alternative medicine. Not intended as a replacement for conventional medical care, its purpose is to provide the reader with an understanding of the child's health and offer alternative therapies which can be used independently or in conjunction with conventional medical treatments. Part I discusses causes and patterns of ill health and presents background information on natural medicine. Part II provides general information on various natural remedies such as homeopathy, massage and herbal medicines, all of which are offered as treatments in Part III. Part III consists of a classified arrangement of childhood medical conditions, arranged under the broad categories of respiratory ailments, childhood diseases, digestive problems and skin conditions. A list of natural medicines for the home medicine cabinet, resources for further reading and additional information are found in the appendices. The author is an experienced practitioner of natural medicine, specializing in herbal remedies and acupuncture, particularly as they are applied to the treatment of children.

633. Scott, Julian and Scott, Susan. *Natural Medicine for Women.* New York: Avon Books, 1991. 191 p. Illus., biblio., index. $12.95. ISBN: 0-380-76381-8.

A complete compendium of natural medicine for women, the focus of this book is on self-help strategies for maintaining health and treating illness. This is a practical and useful guide covering a broad scope of therapies. Presented in a sensitive and visually appealing way, the book is replete with instructive photographs, drawings and charts, a detailed table of contents, and an index which includes both the scientific and common names of herbs. Section I is a general introduction to the subject of natural medicine, covering the concept of energy, energy imbalances, and patterns of ill health. Section II presents various natural therapies including herbal medicine, homeopathy, meditation, exercise and relaxation. Included are herbal and homeopathic *materia medica* and illustrated exercise routines on three levels of difficulty. Section III is a guide to treating specific ailments such as conditions associated with menstruation, pregnancy, menopause and osteoporosis. Each ailment is covered thoroughly, giving symptoms, physical causes, emotional aspects and prevention, and includes three to five suggestions for different therapies appropriate to that condition. A bibliography of books as well as a list of suppliers, organizations and societies is included.

Journals and Newsletters

634. ***Journal of Naturopathic Medicine.*** Norwalk, CT: Journal Management Group. v.1, no.1, 1990. Quarterly. $65.00 (subscription). ISSN: 1047-7837.

The peer-reviewed scientific journal of the American Association of Naturopathic Physicians, this journal publishes original research, philosophy and practical information for the practicing naturopath. Sections include research reviews, original research, letters, news and reviews, special topics, and a clinical arts series covering clinical applications, technique and analysis. Periodic roundtable discussions offer varying perspectives on the treatment of different diseases. Articles are written primarily by naturopaths, chiropractors and osteopaths.

CHAPTER 11: MANIPULATIVE THERAPIES

Books

635. Epstein, Donald M. with Nathaniel Altman. *The Twelve Stages of Healing: A Network Approach to Wholeness.* San Rafael, CA: New World Library, 1994. 256 p. Biblio. $12.95. ISBN: 1-878424-08-4.

Dr. Epstein is the founder of Network Chiropractic, an approach to healing based on a twelve-stage model of evolution of consciousness. In this book he systematically explains the process by first defining each stage, describing its nature and purpose, and demonstrating how to move through each rite of passage by adopting the appropriate perspective and the use of specific healing exercises and self statements. This is a broad conceptualization of the process underlying all healing independent of any specific therapeutic modality, representing a movement in the individual toward integration and wholeness. It is a guidebook for both the lay person as well as physicians, chiropractors, bodyworkers and therapists involved in the healing process. Written in a clear, direct and supportive manner, the book includes many examples from myths, fairy tales and anecdotal material from Epstein's practice and experience to clarify and simplify the concepts he presents. It is a challenging yet affirming point of view that draws upon the wisdom of both ancient and modern thought to provide a unified vision of the process of healing.

636. Moore, Susan. *Chiropractic.* Boston: Charles E. Tuttle, 1988. 96 p. Illus. $12.95. ISBN: 0-8048-1831-2.

Part of a series of consumer guides to various areas of holistic health entitled Tuttle Alternative Health, this practical introduction to chiropractic covers the basics. An opening section discusses the history, philosophy and methodology of chiropractic treatment in a clear and concise manner. A description of how chiropractic is used to treat various conditions throughout the body and what it cannot treat follows, as well as its applicability to children, pregnant women, senior citizens and sports problems. Moore then presents a visit to the chiropractor, describing the diagnostic process, treatment, including manipulative and nonmanipulative techniques, and reactions that can be expected. This step-by-step explanation details exactly what occurs at each part of the process. An overview of the course of chiropractic care explores issues relative to the duration and course of treatment. A self-help section presents useful advice on posture, exercise, diet and work-related issues. This is an excellent introduction for the lay public, answering basic questions on chiropractic, demystifying the subject, and teaching anatomical and functional concepts in a simple and effective manner.

637. Redwood, Daniel. *A Time to Heal: How to Reap the Benefits of Holistic Health.* Virginia Beach, VA: A.R.E. Press, 1993. 251 pg. Biblio., index. $12.95. ISBN: 0-87604-310-4.

Dr. Daniel Redwood, a well-known chiropractor and writer on alternative medicine, has written an easy-to-read, personal and down-to-earth introduction to chiropractic care and other holistic healing perspectives for the lay reader. He presents the rationale and overall approach of the "new medicine" with its emphasis on the whole person, self care, and health maintenance techniques through natural therapies and basic healthful living strategies. The book is organized into three main sections. The first is a collection of case studies from his practice and his own story, which introduce the reader to the basic approach of chiropractic, some of the specific techniques used in the therapy and why, and the underlying assumptions growing out of the commitment to addressing the mental, physical, emotional and spiritual aspects of the patient. The second section presents specific background on the chiropractic profession, its theoretical perspective, a review of the important scientific research on the approach, and an introduction to the Edgar Cayce readings on manipulative medicine, diet, the energy centers of the body and more. The final section is a practical tool enabling the reader to begin some of the work of self care including diet and nutrition, exercise and yoga (with an illustrated step-by-step routine), meditation and relaxation, and visualization, affirmations and prayer. Both the benefits and some of the methods of these practices are described. A useful bibliography covering major, relatively current works on the topics discussed in the book is provided for the reader's further study.

638. Upledger, John E. *Your Inner Physician and You.* Berkeley, CA: North Atlantic Books, 1991. 163 p. Illus. $12.95. ISBN: 1-55643-148-1.

In this lively recounting of the discovery and development of craniosacral therapy and SomatoEmotional Release, Dr. Upledger describes how he got "hooked" on this new bodily system and the therapies that evolved. Through the use of many fascinating case histories and anecdotal material, he leads the reader on the unfolding journey he took from his first accidental experience with the craniosacral system through his varied experiences of its use on patients with headaches, hyperactivity, dyslexia, spinal cord injury, spasticity, ruptured disc problems, brain function disorders and more. He then introduces the basic underlying principles of the work and the techniques used, such as therapeutic imagery and dialogue, intention and touch, the use of healing energy, tissue memory, energy cyst release and SomatoEmotional release. Written in an engaging and conversational style throughout, the book concludes with a description of the anatomy of the craniosacral system, information on how an evaluation and treatment are done, and a question and answer section aimed at the general reader. This is an inviting and highly accessible book that conveys with enthusiasm the possibilities inherent in this natural approach to healing.

Journals and Newsletters

639. ***The AAO Journal:*** *A Publication of the American Academy of Osteopathy.* Indianapolis: American Academy of Osteopathy. v.1, no.1, 1991. Quarterly. $25.00 (subscription).

This publication of the American Academy of Osteopathy (AAO) serves as a vehicle for disseminating information on issues relating to osteopathic medicine. Aimed at an audience composed of health care professionals, students of osteopathic medicine, and those with an interest in this field, the journal publishes reports of clinical and applied research, case studies, and articles about practical applications of osteopathy, as well as book reviews, relevant news items and letters to the editor, and a calendar of events. Manuscripts are accepted primarily from AAO members, osteopathic college faculty, residents, interns and students attending osteopathic colleges, and are reviewed by the journal's editorial board.

640. ***Journal of the American Chiropractic Association.*** Arlington, VA: American Chiropractic Association. v.1, no.1, 1930. Monthly. Illus., adv. $24.00 (member subscription), $80.00 (nonmember subscription), $3.00 (student subscription). ISSN: 0744-9984.

Published by the American Chiropractic Association and formerly entitled the *National Chiropractic Association Journal* and the *ACA Journal of Chiropractic,* this journal serves as a forum for discussion of issues related to chiropractic care. Approximately twelve feature articles report on chiropractic procedures, treatment protocols, case reports, research studies, related developments in other fields, issues relevant to office practice, and governmental activities related to health care in general and chiropractic in specific. Articles are two to four pages in length and contain an author biography and references, with some articles providing abstracts and key terms. Departments include letters to the editor, news updates, a calendar of events, a section on practice ideas, book reviews, an opinion piece, and council reports and college news. Though the writing style is clear and accessible, the content of the journal makes it most appropriate for those studying or practicing chiropractic or related subjects.

641. ***The Journal of the American Osteopathic Association.*** Chicago, IL: The American Osteopathic Association. v.1, no.1, 1901. Monthly. $50.00 (subscription), $15.00 (single copy). ISSN: 0098-6151.

The official publication of the American Osteopathic Association, this professional journal contains a variety of features which vary from issue to issue as well as regular departments. Offerings include original studies, review articles, special communications, clinical practice topics, case reports, medical education discussions, editorials, letters to the editor, research abstracts from AOA conferences, and federal updates on timely health topics. Articles range from three to six pages and provide abstracts, keywords, references and the address of the author for correspondence. The journal addresses the clinical, research and educational concerns of the osteopathic physician as well as briefings on new products and services, listing of new members, a home continuing medical education quiz, reviews of books, software programs and videotapes, and an advertiser's index.

CHAPTER 12: BODYWORK

Acupressure/Shiatsu

Books

642. Bauer, Cathryn. *Acupressure for Everybody: Gentle, Effective Relief for More than 100 Common Ailments.* New York: Henry Holt, 1991. 144 p. Illus., biblio., index. $11.95. ISBN: 0-8050-1579-5.

Written by a certified acupressure practitioner and author of *Acupressure for Women,* this "how-to" book presents the reader with information on the use of acupressure for the relief of over 100 common ailments and injuries. Detailed information on pressure points is accompanied by clear illustrations indicating the location of these points on the body. Also included are individual chapters on treating children, the elderly, and the disabled, as well as a chapter on other natural therapies which may be used in conjunction with acupressure. A resource list of products, books and periodicals round out this very accessible, well-written book.

643. Gach, Michael Reed. *Acupressure's Potent Points: A Guide to Self-Care for Common Ailments.* New York: Bantam Books, 1990. 251 p. Illus., index. $15.95. ISBN: 0-553-34970-8.

The author, who is the founder and director of the Acupressure Institute in Berkeley, California, has written a very readable work which provides a wealth of information on acupressure. Part I provides the reader with an overview of this healing art; Part II, arranged in chapters by ailment, discusses the potent points which will provide relief from each ailment, and offers detailed instructions on how best to apply pressure to the relevant points. Numerous illustrations and photographs complement the easy-to-follow instructions and help make this a very accessible book for a general audience.

644. Goodman, Saul. *The Book of Shiatsu: The Healing Art of Finger Pressure.* Garden City Park, NY: Avery Publishing Group, 1990. 215 p. Illus., index. $12.95. ISBN: 0-89529-454-0.

Founder of the International School of Shiatsu, Saul Goodman has written a clear, well-thought-out introduction to the practice of shiatsu. Through the use of simple analogies to common sense knowledge and experience, this straightforward presentation easily bridges the gap between the western mind and the eastern approach to healing. The book begins with a discussion of the fundamental principles of shiatsu, describing its approach to health, the human energy system, patterns of energy, five phase theory and the nervous system's role in the process. Goodman then orients the reader to the spirit of the work, such as centering, surrender and service, that move the reader beyond technique to enhance the quality and effectiveness of a treatment. The heart of the book contains experiential exercises to develop the necessary skills and awareness for the practice of shiatsu and then presents an entire full body shiatsu session. This section is extensively illustrated with clear, useful photographs and drawings demonstrating each movement of the treatment. The system of oriental diagnosis is presented with detailed charts coordinating physical appearance, organs, related conditions, causes, and physical and emotional expression. This is a well- written book by an experienced teacher who knows what people need to know, how to present it clearly, and how to inspire his readers toward self-development and quality work.

645. Jarmey, Chris and Tindall, John. *Acupressure for Common Ailments.* New York: Simon & Schuster, 1991. Illus., index. 95 p. $11.95. ISBN: 0-671-73135-1.

Appropriate for use by beginners as well as more advanced students, this self-help book provides clear instructions for the application of thumb and finger pressure to relieve symptoms of common health problems. Part I presents an overview of oriental medicine, including discussion of the causes of disease and basic information on treatment techniques. Part II, arranged in chapters by broad medical categories (e.g., respiration, digestion, nervous system), provides instructions and illustrations on which pressure points to treat for each given ailment. The authors encourage the reader to seek professional medical care as appropriate, noting that, although the book is intended to provide relief for common ailments, the services of a skilled medical practitioner may be required for more serious health problems.

646. Liechti, Elaine. *Shiatsu: Japanese Massage for Health and Fitness.* Health Essentials Series. Rockport, MA: Element, 1992. 122 p. Illus., biblio., index. $8.95. ISBN: 1-85230-318-2.

Shiatsu, a Japanese word meaning "finger pressure," uses physical pressure and stretches the body's energy pathways to encourage physical and spiritual health. This book presents information on the nature of shiatsu treatment sessions and on the similarities and differences between this treatment and other types of bodywork. Case studies provide a representative sample of the kinds of "imbalances" which may be treated with shiatsu, and illustrations and written instructions demonstrate techniques for applying this therapy. Advice on finding a reputable shiatsu practitioner and seeking training in this field can be found at the end of the text.

647. Lundberg, Paul. *The Book of Shiatsu.* New York: Simon and Schuster, 1992. 191 p. Illus., biblio., index. $14.95. ISBN: 0-671-74488-7.

Paul Lundberg, teacher and founder of the Shiatsu College in England, has written a clear and very readable introduction to the theory and practice of shiatsu. This form of bodywork uses gentle hand pressure to promote health by improving the state of ki (the Japanese equivalent to chi or qi), the life force which flows through the energy pathways in the body. A good background is provided through detailed description of the basic principles of oriental medicine (yin yang, ki, the five elements), preparing the beginner with an understanding of the underlying concepts and broad context of the work. Through text and beautiful illustrations which convey both technique and feeling, the proper mental approach to a session is described and a simple shiatsu routine plus three more advanced ones are presented. Further chapters cover the functions of each organ and the symptoms associated with them, the system of oriental diagnosis, and self-help exercises for the reader to apply. An appendix supplies a listing of resource organizations for further study and training.

648. Yamamoto, Shizuko and McCarty, Patrick. *Whole Health Shiatsu: Health and Vitality for Everyone.* New York: Japan Publications, 1993. 303 p. Illus., index. $23.00. ISBN: 0-87040-874-7.

By incorporating macrobiotic diet, breathing, exercise and shiatsu, Whole Health Shiatsu is a therapeutic approach which focuses on eliminating harmful toxins in the body and restoring the body's resistance to disease. In this book, Yamamoto, who developed this treatment modality, and McCarty, a certified shiatsu instructor and practitioner and co-director of the East-West Center for Macrobiotics, provide the reader with a framework for restoring and maintaining good health and vitality. Dr. Benjamin Spock has written the foreword for this book. Its five chapters are written in a very readable style and are enhanced by clear, sometimes entertaining illustrations. The basic functions of thinking, breathing, eating, moving, sleeping and interrelating are discussed, and how best to adjust one's lifestyle to promote healing of imbalances in these areas and maintaining health are explored. The basic premises of oriental medicine are presented, and information on Whole Health diagnosis is provided. Practical exercises and methods of treating patients are accompanied by groups of instructive photographs. This is a valuable book for anyone interest in learning about shiatsu's role in healing.

Journals and Newsletters

649. *Healthways.* Eureka, CA: International Macrobiotic Shiatsu Society. v.1, no.1, 1987. Three times a year. $25.00 (subscription). ISSN: 0898-9251.

This ten-page newsletter covers general issues on health and disease, herbs, foods, specific shiatsu topics, a news section, and a schedule of macrobiotic shiatsu events. Articles include such topics as the nature of illness, natural progesterone, and treating complex problems with acupoint therapy. Articles are written by Shizuko Yamamoto, whose readings form the basis of Macrobiotic Shiatsu, various shiatsu instructors and practitioners, and the editor Patrick McCarty, director of the East-West Center and the International Macrobiotic Shiatsu Society.

Applied Kinesiology

Books

650. Holdway, Ann. *Kinesiology: Muscle Testing and Energy Balancing for Health and Well-Being.* Rockport, MA: Element, 1995. 120 p. Illus., biblio., index. $9.95. ISBN 1-85230-433-2.

Part of the Health Essential Series of consumer books on natural therapies, this clear and compact introduction offers basic information on what kinesiology is, how it works and what it does. A thorough history of the technique is provided, from its beginnings in the work of chiropractor George Goodheart in the 1960s through its further development and the various branches of kinesiology in practice today. Methods utilized are explained using simple analogies, illustrations, reference to concepts from traditional Chinese medicine theory, and basic anatomical, neurological and structural information. A section entitled "Helping Yourself" describes some simple practices to relieve pain and stress and enhance health, vitality and balance. Holdway briefly describes a variety of other natural therapies and how they can be used in conjunction with kinesiology to increase their effectiveness. She provides a substantial list of worldwide kinesiology organizations and a useful bibliography of current and classic works relevant to the field. This excellent and very readable introduction will educate its audience on the practice and purpose of kinesiology, how it fits in with a natural approach to health maintenance, and where to go to pursue a professional or therapeutic interest in the field.

Hellerwork

Books

651. Heller, Joseph and Henkin, William A. *Bodywise.* Berkeley, CA: Wingbow Press, 1991. 260 p. Illus., biblio., index. $13.95. ISBN: 0-914728-73-3.

Joseph Heller, first president of the Rolf Institute and founder of Hellerwork in 1978, has co-written a good introduction to bodywork in general as well as a clear explanation of Hellerwork. Part I, called Knowledge of the Body, presents basic concepts of the body / mind approach emphasizing self-awareness, the split between ourselves and our bodies, and the reality of body, mind and spiritual wholeness. He teaches fundamental concepts such as unconscious patterning, energy, gravity and harmony through simple exercises, analogies, stories and metaphors that are easily accessible to the lay reader and useful for the professional as well. He then presents the elements that form the core issues of bodywork: the body's malleability, movement, balance, structure, function and alignment. A broad discussion divides the field of bodywork into four major perspectives with categorization and brief discussion of some of the major modalities in practice today: energetic (yoga and acupuncture); mechanical (Alexander, Trager, Feldenkrais, chiropractic, osteopathy and rolfing); psychological (the work of Wilhelm Reich and Alexander Lowen); and integrative (martial arts practices and Hellerwork). While this categorization seems highly subjective and even inaccurate in certain aspects, it may prove to be useful in some regards. Part II describes the basic approach of Hellerwork and the eleven Hellerwork sessions by bodily system and function, providing anatomical, structural and psychological information for each system. The book is a clear, well thought out and effective orientation to the goals and possibilities of bodywork as a means to understanding one's body and achieving greater ease, balance, aliveness and relief from pain, stress and discomfort. The authors provide a useful bibliography of important and classic works by such authors as Ida Rolf, Alexander Lowen, Frederick Perls, Mabel Elsworth Todd, Lulu Sweigard and Wilhelm Reich, although it does not appear to have been updated since the original publication in 1986.

Massage

Books

652. Mitchell, Stewart. *Massage: A Practical Introduction.* Rockport, MA: Element, 1992. 138 p. Biblio., index. $8.95. ISBN: 1-85230-386-7.

Stewart Mitchell, massage therapist, teacher and director of a massage training school in England, offers a basic primer to the theory and practice of massage. Written in a clear and straightforward fashion, this book touches on all the important aspects needed to introduce the beginner to this popular form of natural therapy. With the help of well-drawn and plentiful illustrations, the book provides instructions on basic massage of the various parts of the body and a sampling of techniques for specific conditions, such as shiatsu for the shoulders. Mitchell covers special massage for the treatment and prevention of common injuries and offers a section on self-massage as first aid for conditions from constipation to menstrual pain. A unique teaching tool, found in the appendix, contains drawings of the skeleton front and back and individually numbered drawings of muscles to be cut out and placed on the appropriate area on the skeleton according to detailed instructions and anatomical information. A glossary of terms used in massage is provided as well as a list of recommended readings and an index.

653. Prevention Magazine Health Books. *Hands-on Healing: Massage Remedies for Hundreds of Health Problems.* Edited by John Feltman. Emmaus, PA: Rodale Press, 1989. 448 p. Illus., biblio., index. $17.95. ISBN: 0-87857-966-4.

This comprehensive overview of hands-on therapies by the editors of Prevention Magazine Health Books is a well-researched, authoritative and accurate reference tool written in an easy-to-understand, conversational style. The authors thoroughly cover the field of bodywork, starting with a discussion of the power of touch itself and the connection between touch and well-being. The main portion of the book is an impressive directory of bodywork modalities, arranged alphabetically, each containing a variety of information including description of a session, background theory, applications, glossary of terms, history, bibliographies and resource lists. Special techniques for relieving neck, shoulder, back, leg and foot pain are presented with extensive detailed illustrations to assist the reader in learning the art of hands-on healing. This highly informative book concludes with a user's guide of resource lists covering such areas as products, instructional videotapes, spas and bodywork tools.

654. Thomas, Sara. *Massage for Common Ailments.* New York: Simon & Schuster, 1988. 95 p. Illus., biblio., index. $9.95. ISBN: 0-671-67552-4.

Preventing and treating illness with massage therapy is the focus of this book, although some information on the use of shiatsu is included as well. The author, a teacher and practitioner of massage, describes how to use touch to assist the body's natural healing processes, emphasizing those methods particularly useful for treating ailments resulting from daily stress. Instructions for basic massage strokes and shiatsu techniques, accompanied by clear illustrations, are followed by discussion of the use of these skills to provide relief for a range of common health problems such as indigestion, arthritis, headaches and muscle sprains.

Journals and Newsletters

655. *Massage.* Davis, CA: NOAH Publishing. v.1, no.1, 1985. Bimonthly. Illus., adv. $20.00 (subscription). ISSN: 1057-378X.

This is a journal devoted to disseminating information on the art and science of massage and the importance of therapeutic touch in achieving and maintaining good health. With the increasing focus on wellness as opposed to illness in this country, *Massage* fills an important niche by giving the reader an understanding of the breadth and depth of this field. Physical, emotional, spiritual and holistic aspects of massage therapy and bodywork are explored in four feature articles each month. Numerous regular departments provide such information as reviews of current books, music, videotapes and products; reports on the activities of various massage and bodywork associations; a calendar of events; and listings of schools, centers and training programs.

656. *Massage & Bodywork Quarterly.* Evergreen, CO: Associated Bodywork & Massage Professionals. v.1, no.1, 1992. Quarterly. Illus., adv. $15.00 (subscription). ISSN: 1066-9337.

The official publication of the Associated Bodywork & Massage Professionals provides coverage of such modalities as massage therapy, reflexology, Trager, Therapeutic Touch, shiatsu, acupressure and more. Articles are written by professionals in their respective fields. Although aimed at massage and bodywork professionals, this publication is also appropriate for those with an interest in these areas. Regular features include listings of classes, seminars, training programs, educational resources, letters to the editor, and current news items.

657. *Massage Therapy Journal.* Evanston, IL: American Massage Therapy Association. v.1, no.1., 1946. Quarterly. Illus., adv. $20.00 (subscription). ISSN: 0895-0814.

This publication of the American Massage Therapy Association (AMTA) covers a wide range of bodywork-related topics including craniosacral therapy, massage techniques, physiological ailments, government affairs, and more. The journal has a staff of contributing writers and also considers materials submitted by others. Pieces are written to appeal to a general audience as well as to bodywork professionals. Regular features include letters to the editor, book reviews, a "Members' Marketplace," which offers products at reduced prices to AMTA members, and a directory of schools with AMTA-accredited or -approved massage training programs. Its extensive coverage of the field and long publishing history make this journal a "must read" for those with an interest in massage therapy.

Reflexology

Books

658. Carter, Mildred and Weber, Tammy. *Body Reflexology: Healing at Your Fingertips.* West Nyack, NY: Parker Publishing, 1994. 343 p. Illus., index. $9.95. ISBN: 0-13-299736-3.

In this revised and updated edition of Carter's 1983 work, the authors discuss the use of reflexology to relieve pain and stress, improve circulation and restore the flow of energy to the systems and functions of the body. Easy-to-follow instructions are provided for massaging the reflexes on certain parts of the body to bring natural and speedy relief from a variety of chronic and acute aches and pains. Reflexology treatment for such conditions as asthma, back pain, headaches, kidney and bladder ailments and carpal tunnel syndrome are addressed, as is the use of this modality for maintaining good health of specific bodily systems. Basic reflexology techniques are demonstrated through the use of diagrams and photographs. Mildred Carter is a leader in the field of reflexology who has written several books on the subject; her daughter and co-author is a certified reflexologist and teacher who has studied with her mother for more than thirty years.

659. Dougans, Inge with Suzanne Ellis. *Reflexology: Foot Massage for Total Health.* Rockport, MA: Element, 1991. 122 p. Illus., biblio., index. $8.95. ISBN: 1-85230-218-6.

This book discusses the role of reflexology in activating the body's natural healing, including its role in reducing stress and improving circulation and nerve function. A brief history of reflexology is presented, along with an overview of reflexology treatment. Instructions on how to administer this therapy are accompanied by numerous diagrams which are intended to assist the reader in using reflexology at home. A bibliography and sources of further information are included at the back of the book.

660. Norman, Laura with Thomas Cowan. *Feet First: A Guide to Foot Reflexology.* New York: Simon & Schuster, 1988. 335 p. Illus., index. $14.00. ISBN: 0-671-63412-7.

Written in a very readable style, this book describes reflexology and the uses of this natural healing method to alleviate a range of conditions. Norman, a certified reflexologist and founder of the Laura Norman Reflexology Program, acknowledges that reflexology does not cure conditions but rather allows the body's immune system and healing properties to function more effectively. Reflex points are described; easy-to-follow directions accompanied by clear and simple illustrations are provided for basic and advanced reflexology techniques. A Table of Common Conditions, arranged alphabetically, describes each condition and the appropriate reflex points which should be worked.

Rolfing

Books

661. Rolf, Ida. *Rolfing and Physical Reality.* Edited by Rosemary Feitis. Rochester, VT: Healing Arts Press, 1990. 215 p. Illus., biblio. $12.95. ISBN: 0-89281-380-6.

Based on the original writing of Rolf entitled "Ida Rolf talks about Rolfing and Physical Reality," this book offers both the insights and unique creative and human perspective of Dr. Rolf herself as well as the context of her work through Rosemary Feitis' substantial introduction. The reader learns the historical and ideological placement of the work and is introduced to a way of looking at the physical and psychological components of man that offers much to ponder. Feistis, through her long association with Rolf and the human potential movement, chronicles Rolfing's early influences and development. The remainder of the book presents short discrete sections by Rolf in which she comments on the nature of her work, its basic assumptions relative to bodily structure, gravity and energy, comparisons with other manipulative approaches, and philosophical perspectives on a variety of relevant topics. The book is not a formal presentation of the work, but rather communicates the essence of its founder and the thought processes that have made Rolfing an important system of structural bodywork. It will inform students of all approaches to bodywork, those interested in receiving Rolfing, and the reader open to exploring the wisdom inherent in understanding the body's place in human development.

CHAPTER 13: ENERGY MEDICINE

General

Books

662. Brennan, Barbara Ann. *Light Emerging: The Journey of Personal Healing.* New York: Bantam Books, 1993. 341 p. Illus., biblio., index. $22.50. ISBN: 0-553-35456-6.

The author of the best-selling *Hands of Light* and an internationally known healer, teacher and scientist offers a new perspective on health and healing that embraces the concept of a human energy field which affects one's health. Part I provides an overview of healing, with some historical and scientific background as well as clear explanations of the importance of the four levels of creative energies—physical, auric, haric and core star—in the healing process. The author puts forth a holographic model as a means of restoring and maintaining one's physical and spiritual health. Part II describes healing techniques and the role of the healer. Part III examines the seven stages of the healing experience by the patient and the seven levels of the healing process. Part IV provides a framework which can assist in the design of a personal health plan. Part V focuses on the effect of healthy relationships on one's physical health and well-being. Part VI looks at the spiritual components of the healing process. Both black-and-white and color illustrations liberally interspersed throughout the text enhance and clarify the concepts presented.

663. Chin, Richard. *The Energy Within: The Science Behind Every Oriental Therapy from Acupuncture to Yoga.* New York: Marlowe, 1995. 204 p. Illus. $12.95. ISBN: 1-55778-349-7.

Richard Chin, medical doctor and doctor of oriental medicine, identifies the basis of all eastern healing: energetics, the science of energy. Stating that western, ancient Chinese and ancient Indian views all share the common belief that the world is comprised of energy, Dr. Chin explains in a clear, down-to-earth manner the principles of energetic healing, the three levels of human energy and the internal energy systems or channels. He describes how keeping one's energy balanced and flowing is the key to health and well-being. Using cases from his own practice, Chin illustrates how specific energy blocks create certain illnesses and how a variety of chronic ailments (diabetes, cancer, back pain) can be treated using energetic techniques. Practical exercises in visualization for learning to contact and control your energy are described, featuring a thirty-minutes-a-day, thirty-day regimen to maximize energy and prevent illness.

664. Gerber, Richard. *Vibrational Medicine: New Choices for Healing Ourselves.* Santa Fe, NM: Bear & Co., 1988. 559 p. Illus., biblio., index. $16.95. ISBN: 0-939680-46-7.

In this theoretical work, Dr. Gerber explains the principles behind the therapeutic practices of many alternative medicine modalities. Citing studies and papers by scientists, scholars and psychics, this is a well-documented and in-depth look at the energy-based systems underlying the mind/body approach to health and illness. Appropriate for the professional and sophisticated lay reader, complex information is presented in a thoughtful manner by summarizing key points at the end of each chapter, employing ample diagrams and charts, and by repeating references throughout the text to earlier and related material. Gerber's basic premise is that we are shifting from a mechanical "Newtonian" view of the body and health to an energy-based "Einsteinian" model. Early chapters document the history of the present drug/surgery model of treatment and the subsequent development of an electromagnetic therapeutic approach. Remaining chapters describe in detail the human energy system and relate these concepts to ancient healing practices such as acupuncture and various other treatment modalities including homeopathy, gem therapy, flower remedies and energy healing. This is an interesting, densely written attempt at reconciling science and metaphysics, placing the current state of healing in historical perspective and pointing the way to the evolution of a new system of mind/body medicine. A detailed index, table of contents, glossary and recommended reading list assist in the handling of technical language and in guiding the reader to specific information and further study.

665. Shealy, C. Norman and Myss, Carolyn. *The Creation of Health: The Emotional, Psychological and Spiritual Responses that Promote Health and Healing.* Walpole, NH: Stillpoint Publishing, 1993. 390 p. Biblio. $14.95. ISBN: 0-913299-94-4.

This clearly written and balanced view of health and illness and their underlying causes speaks with the voices of both traditional and holistic medicine. Realistically assessing the differences yet viewing these two approaches as ultimately complementary, Dr. Shealy, co-founder of the American Holistic Medical Association, and Carolyn Myss, international lecturer in human consciousness, introduce the reader to the role of the human energy system in creating dis-ease and health. Eight major dysfunctional patterns leading to significant stress on the body/mind are outlined, including unresolved life issues, negative belief patterns, lack of humor, and loss of meaning in one's life. Healing is viewed not as a cure but as a process of transformation. Through case histories, Shealy offers traditional diagnosis, while Myss provides intuitive diagnoses of the root causes of various illnesses (such as heart disease, stroke, cancer, acute and chronic disease and emotional disorders) based on her analysis of the individual's energy system. A final discussion on how to create health includes good nutrition, exercise and a healthy mental attitude attuned to the spiritual aspect of life.

666. ***Spiritual Healing.*** Compiled by Kunz, Dora. Wheaton, IL: Quest Books, 1995. 333 p. Biblio., index. $12.00. ISBN: 0-8356-0714-3.

Compiled by Dora Kunz with a forward by Dolores Krieger, pioneers in the development of Therapeutic Touch, this book is a collection of articles that appeared in various journals, books and conferences. All are explorations on healing, its basic nature, when and how it works, and the spiritual, energetic and psychological components of the process. The contributors include widely known practitioners, innovators, and teachers such as Larry Dossey, Ira Progoff, Elmer and Alyce Green, Janet Macrae, Erik Peper, Bernard Siegel, and more. These are well-thought-out, thought-provoking essays that clarify broader, widely discussed theories on healing and offer more unusual perspectives such as energy fields and their clinical implications. The ideas discussed are complex, and the reader would do well to have some background in spiritual, metaphysical and psychological systems of thought.

667. Weinman, Ric A. *Your Hands Can Heal: Learn to Channel Healing Energy.* New York: Dutton, 1988. 131 p. Biblio. $10.00. ISBN: 0-14-019361-8.

This practical and down-to-earth guide is based on the author's workshops on channeling inner energy for healing illness and enhancing positive health. Weinman presents three main methods for channeling this energy: sourcing from above, sourcing from the earth and sourcing from the heart. Many exercises, such as working with colors, words, memories and the mind set of unconditional love, are simply and clearly described to prepare the reader to develop these new skills. In addition, various models of the human energy system are explained, including the chakras, acupuncture, homeopathy and yoga, with techniques supplied to help master the art of aura balancing (a way to clear and balance the energy systems of the body). The essence of this book encourages the reader to allow the energy flow to happen by getting out of the way, being the vehicle and hooking up to the source.

Journals and Newsletters

668. ***Subtle Energies:*** *An Interdisciplinary Journal of Energetic and Informational Interactions*. Golden, CO: International Society for the Study of Subtle Energies and Energy Medicine. v.1, no.1, 1990. Three times a year. $50.00 (subscription).

Written for clinicians, researchers and theoreticians interested in all forms of energetic and informational interactions in biological systems, this refereed journal documents scientific observations and controlled experiments in subtle energies and energy medicine. It contains general papers on new developments in the field, current research problems and techniques, experimental clinical and theoretical papers, reports of preliminary research results, personal perspectives of distinguished contributors, correspondence, technical comments, and book and software reviews. Articles are detailed and lengthy with abstracts, key words and references. The editors and advisory board are predominantly M.D.s and Ph.D.s and papers are written by notable contributors such as C. Norman Shealy, M.D., and Elmer E. Green, Ph.D.

Polarity Therapy

Books

669. Seidman, Maruti. *A Guide to Polarity Therapy: The Gentle Art of Hands-on Healing*. Boulder, CO: Elan Press, 1991. 167 p. Illus., biblio. $16.95. ISBN: 0-9628709-00.

Based on the work of Dr. Randolph Stone, doctor of osteopathy, naturopathy and chiropractic, this metaphysical introduction to polarity therapy explains the underlying assumptions of the work, including the five elements and how they operate, the energy currents of the body, relevant anatomical information, and the basic philosophical approach of the practitioner to the work. Seidman, a long-time teacher and practitioner of polarity therapy, provides balancing techniques for each of the five elements, for various organs and parts of the body, and for the chakras or energy centers of the body. Illustrations are very helpful where provided. Many concepts from various traditions such as Ayurveda and astrology are incorporated into the text and, without a background in these areas, are difficult to understand and use. Recommendations are made on diet, exercise, herbal remedies and spiritual practices, some of which seem randomly selected, while others provide sound guidelines for practice. No index is provided but a useful though dated bibliography includes information on obtaining all of Dr. Stone's books. The book's strengths lie in its step-by-step approach to polarity release techniques, though some basic orientation to hands-on work is probably necessary to use these techniques successfully.

Reiki

Books

670. Horan, Paula. *Empowerment through Reiki: The Path to Personal and Global Transformation.* Wilmot, WI: Lotus Light Publications, 1992. 157 p. Illus., biblio., index. $14.95. ISBN: 0-941524-84-1.

Reiki, a Japanese word meaning "universal life force energy," is a method of healing which may be used for self-healing or to treat others. In this book, the author, a psychologist and Reiki master, explains what Reiki is and what it can do. A history of this healing modality is presented, and the difference between Reiki and other treatment modalities is discussed. Practical exercises are clearly explained, as is the use of Reiki in conjunction with other healing methods. Written in plain language, this book is appropriate for a general audience, but also contains sufficient information to be of interest to Reiki practitioners as well.

Therapeutic Touch

Books

671. Krieger, Dolores. *Accepting Your Power to Heal: The Personal Practice of Therapeutic Touch.* Santa Fe, NM: Bear & Co., 1993. 199 p. Illus., biblio. $10.95. ISBN: 1-879181-04-5.

Dolores Krieger, Ph.D., R.N., is a researcher, theoretician, clinical practitioner and teacher who founded Therapeutic Touch in 1972 with her colleague Dora Kunz. This widely accepted therapeutic modality is now taught at over 150 major universities throughout the world. In this highly readable account of her work, the author presents theory, detailed experiential exercises and personal accounts of her own and her students' experience with the work. Krieger first defines Therapeutic Touch, explaining its basic assumptions, what it can do, and the techniques of centering and assessing the human energy field. Exercises and visualizations to aid the reader in developing the necessary skills and awarenesses are presented throughout the book with accompanying illustrations and explanatory comments following each exercise. Krieger explains complex notions of the human energy system and how to direct, rebalance and modulate energy in a way clearly accessible to the lay person as well as the healing professional. Finally, she describes in detail specific uses of Therapeutic Touch and how to treat conditions such as pregnancy, pain, depression and headache. The book responsibly covers cautions and precautions as well as legal implications of practicing Therapeutic Touch and provides a scale for self-evaluation in the appendix. This how-to book reaches beyond technique, however, to convey the humanity, compassion and personal fulfillment inherent in this approach to healing.

CHAPTER 14: MOVEMENT THERAPIES

Alexander Technique

Books

672. Barlow, Wilfred. *The Alexander Technique: How to Use Your Body Without Stress.* Rochester, VT: Healing Arts Press, 1990. 237 p. Illus., biblio., index. $12.95. ISBN: 0-89281-385-7.

Written by one of the foremost teachers of the Alexander Technique and founder of the Alexander Institute in London, this book provides an in-depth look at the connection between good use and misuse of the body and one's mental, physical and sexual well-being. Beginning with a comprehensive overview of the principles involved, Dr. Barlow clearly explains how the way we use our bodies affects the way we function. He discusses the proper biomechanics of sitting, standing and other everyday activities, and the disorders that arise from faulty use of the body, including back pain, breathing disorders, arthritis and stress illnesses. Extensive drawings and photographs serve as effective teaching tools in demonstrating bodily distortions and comparing them to the correctly aligned and balanced body. The second part of the book covers the practice of the Alexander Technique, including a description of a typical lesson and a series of questions pupils would be likely to ask. Barlow concludes with a short biography of Alexander, a referral list, and references for further reading.

673. Leibowitz, Judith and Connington, Bill. *The Alexander Technique.* New York: HarperPerennial, 1990. 177 p. Illus., biblio., index. $14.00. ISBN: 0-06-016053-5.

Judith Leibowitz, co-founder of the American Center for the Alexander Technique, and Bill Connington, its president and chairman of the board, have written a very clear, readable introduction to the Alexander Technique. This is not a "how-to" book but an orientation to the philosophy and practice of this mind/body approach designed to increase body awareness, change habits and attitudes, and improve body movement and use. The first part of the book provides an overview of the technique, including case studies, a basic discussion of skeletal anatomy as it applies to the work, and a description of what happens in an Alexander lesson, including questions most often asked about the work. Part II describes the Leibowitz Procedures, a series of movements developed by the author designed to increase self-observation skills and "help you learn how the body moves when it is used well." Detailed guidance with illustrations in applying the Leibowitz Procedures to daily activities such as sitting, driving, lifting objects and walking, is provided as a method of increasing one's awareness of body movement and use.

Feldenkrais Method

Books

674. Feldenkrais, Moshe. *Awareness Through Movement.* New York: Harper & Row, 1992. 192 p. Illus. $11.00. ISBN: 0-06-250322-7.

Beginning with an in-depth discussion of the process of self-education, the author sets the stage for this book's movement sequences designed to improve posture and body habits, increase self-awareness, enhance self-image and expand human potential. Dr. Feldenkrais, a world-renowned teacher and founder of the Feldenkrais Institute in Israel, explains in detail how and why these changes are achieved. While the ideas presented are complex, the exercises themselves, grouped into twelve lessons, consist of simple, effortless and slow movements presented in great detail. These exercises are designed to increase awareness, overcome unconscious and restricting habitual patterns, and expand one's mental capacity through stimulating the brain's potential. Clearly described with accompanying illustrations, they include movements for various parts and functions of the body, such as breathing, the eyes, and the pelvis, and are intended to be appropriate for people of any age.

Rosen Method

Books

675. Rosen, Marion and Brenner, Sue. *The Rosen Method of Movement.* Berkeley, CA: North Atlantic Books, 1991. 97 p. Illus. $12.95. ISBN: 1-55643-117-1.

Marion Rosen, a physical therapist who worked with Carl Jung's patients in Munich in the 1930s and has practiced and taught in the United States for over fifty years, developed a system of bodywork and therapeutic movement based on relaxation, freedom of movement and breath. This down-to-earth and accessible book presents background information on Rosen's life and work, including an exploration of habit patterns, objectives, basic theory and a brief description of what occurs in each movement class. The second part of the book describes a Rosen class in more detail, including its adaptation for people with certain physical disabilities. The major portion of the work teaches the exercises, including description of each movement, simple accompanying figure drawings, and basic discussion of the anatomy involved and the benefits of each exercise. These exercises are meant to be easy and pleasurable to perform and cover the whole body from neck to feet. The last section describes sequences of movements to mobilize particular areas of the body, such as opening the chest and working the back. Instructions are clear and easy to follow. These are movements intended to be done with awareness and freedom, affecting the mind and spirit along with the body. This intent comes through in this straightforward, personal and life-affirming presentation of Rosen's work.

T'ai Chi Chuan

Books

676. Huang, Chungliang Al. *Embrace Tiger, Return to Mountain: The Essence of T'ai Ji.* Berkeley, CA: Celestial Arts, 1987. 188 p. Illus. $12.95. ISBN: 0-89087-504-0.

This classic book on T'ai Ji (the current Chinese spelling of T'ai Chi), originally published in 1973, is written by the well-known teacher Al Huang, founder of the Living Tao Foundation and director of the Lanting Institute in the People's Republic of China. After seven editions and seven foreign translations, it remains a vital and direct experience of the essence of Tao and the art of T'ai Ji. Based on actual workshop experiences, the book conveys the sense of joy and exploration in discovering the process of moving and being with the flow of the universe, of not doing, not forcing, but opening to all that is. It is a philosophy of living that is conveyed, an approach to T'ai Chi Ch'uan and to life. Written with simplicity and a feeling of immediacy, it is as if the reader is in class with the master who knows how we think and feel, our habit patterns and our resistances and knows how to lead us to a deeper awareness of self. Replete with anecdotes, history, sensory exercises and philosophy, it is an immersion into a new way of being. The book is beautifully illustrated with full-page photographs that enhance the feeling and meaning of the work.

677. Kotsias, John. *The Essential Movements of T'ai Chi.* Brookline, MA: Paradigm Publications, 1989. 169 p. Illus. $15.95. ISBN: 0-912111-04-6.

T'ai Chi Ch'uan, an ancient form of Chinese movement meditation, is designed to exercise the body, strengthen the mind, awaken the chi (life energy) and develop the chin (internal power of the body). John Kotsias, a westerner who has long studied the martial arts, has written a book in a clear and simple style that is appropriate for beginners and advanced students, young and old. The first part of the book covers the theoretical concepts of chi development including the breath, mind/body coordination, meditation and physical exercise as well as the nine basic principles of T'ai Chi movement. The main portion of the book teaches the essential movements of T'ai Chi, a series of eight basic postures that form the foundation for the solo exercises. These postures are taught through line drawings indicating body position, weight placement and direction of movement as well as through clearly written and descriptive accompanying text.

Trager[R] Psychophysical Integration

Books

678. Liskin, Jack. *Moving Medicine: The Life and Work of Milton Trager, M.D.* Barrytown, NY: Station Hill Press, 1995. 176 p. Illus., biblio., index. $24.95. ISBN: 0-88268-196-6.

Jack Liskin, Assistant Professor of Family Medicine and Director of the Physician's Assistant Education Program at the University of Southern California School of Medicine and certified Trager practitioner, speaks of his firsthand experience with Milton Trager and his work. He brings an honesty, directness and feeling of immediacy to this recounting of the development of the Trager[R] Approach, the Trager Institute, and the man. Writing with a respectful and deep understanding of his material, Liskin begins with the story of his own experience working with Dr. Trager and applying the teachings to his life. He immediately takes the reader into a class taught by Trager, conveying the feeling and essence of the man and his work. Liskin describes Trager's history from his beginnings as a child in Chicago, through his medical school experience in Mexico, his practice in Hawaii, teaching at Esalen, to the formation of the Trager Institute and his move to the Bay Area of San Francisco, charting the evolution of the Trager[R] Approach in a simple and unhurried manner that mirrors the quality of the work itself. Interspersed throughout are experiences of workshops Trager has taught that deepen the reader's understanding of the nature of this work. Finally Liskin discusses the principles of the Trager[R]

Approach in an effort to reveal "how the realm of feeling can produce positive changes in health, well being, and medical practice." Five areas are reviewed: the approach, the source of change, the source of problems, how the process works, and technique. This is a clear and helpful presentation of the underlying assumptions of the work. The Trager[R] Approach is based on a feeling experience that reaches the mind of the client. Liskin has successfully created that process for the reader as well.

679. Trager, Milton, with Cathy Hammond. *Movement as a Way to Agelessness: A Guide to Trager Mentastics.* Barrytown, NY: Station Hill Press, 1995. 176 p. Illus. $15.95. ISBN: 0-88268-167-2.

Written in the first person voice of Dr. Trager as he talks to clients or teaches a class, this book not only explains and instructs, but is itself a direct experience of the state of mind essential to the Trager[R] Approach. The simplicity, ease, and flow of the words make this an immediately accessible book for the layperson. Trager, a physician in private practice for many years and a well-known teacher and founder of the Trager Institute, weaves together the essential elements of the work through his personal history, the basic principles (hook up and effortlessness), the process (directing movements from the mind, recall and self-education), and an exploration of how the process works. Trager Mentastics[R], simple, comfortable movements that suggest to the mind "feelings of lightness, freedom, openness, grace and pleasure," can be considered a form of meditation in motion. Nine of these movement sequences are presented with accompanying illustrations and textual guidance.

Yoga

Books

680. Iyengar, Geeta S. *Yoga: A Gem for Women.* Palo Alto, CA: Timeless Books, 1990. 308 p. Illus., index. $22.95. ISBN: 0-931454-20-4.

Geeta Iyengar, daughter and long-time student of the noted yoga master B. K. S. Iyengar, focuses the study of hatha yoga on the specific needs of women. Theory, practice and experience are all discussed. Included in the section on theory is a discussion of the value of yoga for three important markers in a woman's life: menstruation, pregnancy and delivery, and menopause. The section on practice is arranged according to position (standing, forward bend, lateral, etc.), and provides step-by-step instructions for each pose. Black-and-white plates depicting each pose do not accompany the instructions but rather are found at the back of the book. The section on experience explores the use of advanced breathing techniques and meditation to achieve inner peace. Especially addressing those who are coping with the physical and mental stresses of daily life, this book provides a means for women to relieve those strains, achieving serenity and good health through the study of yoga.

681. Kent, Howard. *Yoga Made Easy: A Personal Yoga Program That Will Transform Your Daily Life.* Allentown, PA: People's Medical Society, 1994. 160 p. Illus, index. $14.95. ISBN: 1-882606-12-4.

Howard Kent, the founder of the organization Yoga for Health and author of several books on this subject, advocates balance and moderation in all aspects of one's life. In this very readable work which combines the physical and spiritual aspects of yoga, he offers a twelve-month program of instruction and practice. Beginning with very simple poses, or asanas, which stretch and relax the body, release tensions and control breathing, each month's exercises build upon poses taught in the previous months. Clear, instructive color photographs illustrate how poses should be performed. Written in plain language and offering useful tips for how to get the most out of one's practice, this is a very good book for those new to the study of yoga.

682. ***Living Yoga:*** *A Comprehensive Guide for Daily Life.* Edited by Georg Feuerstein and Stephen Bodian, with the staff of *Yoga Journal.* New York: Jeremy P. Tarcher/Perigee Books, 1993. 290 p. Illus., biblio., index. $15.95. ISBN: 0-87477-729-1.

This is a compilation of interviews, essays, illustrations and photographs which have previously appeared in Yoga Journal, and is considered by the editors to be a "Best of . . ." book. Organized according to the six primary branches of yoga—hatha, raja, bhakti, karma, tantra and jnana—the articles are written by authorities in their respective fields. Black-and-white photographs throughout the book complement the text, and are particularly helpful in the chapter on yoga postures. Beginning yoga students will find the listings of suggested readings and resource organizations helpful, while more advanced students will be attracted to the writings of noted teachers and healers such as Joan Borysenko, Ram Dass and Ken Wilber.

683. Purna, Svami. *Balanced Yoga: The 12-week Programme.* Rockport, MA: Element, 1990. 95 p. Illus. $13.95. ISBN: 1-85230-325-5.

Dr. Svami Purna, a teacher and scholar who has mastered the Eightfold Path of Yoga, has written a book on Hatha Yoga, the yoga of physical exercise. Designed as a twelve-week program, each week's lesson is focused on a guiding thought which is manifested in related yoga postures. Basic information about yoga, including postures, breathing, and preparing for practice, lay the groundwork for this program. Each lesson combines physical exercises, breathing techniques, and relaxation methods with practical concentration and meditation exercises to assist the student in overcoming stress and achieving fulfillment. Each lesson's accompanying black-and-white illustrations are appropriate for both the beginning student and the more experienced yoga practitioner.

684. Silva, Mira and Mehta, Shyam. *Yoga: The Iyengar Way.* New York: Alfred A. Knopf, 1990. 192 p. Illus., biblio., index. $18.95. ISBN: 0-679-72287-4.

Written by long-time students of the well-known spiritual leader and teacher B. K. S. Iyengar, this book provides an introduction to yoga and its practical and philosophical value in daily life. The first part of the book consists of detailed instructions accompanied by black-and-white and color photographs which instruct the reader on how to execute more than 100 yoga poses, each rated by level of difficulty. Part II covers breathing techniques and the philosophy of yoga. Part III discusses meditation and yoga's goal of inner peace. Appropriate for all levels, the book includes separate programs of yoga practice for beginners, general- , intermediate-, and advanced-level students. A brief section of yoga poses to alleviate medical conditions is also provided.

685. Singh, Ravi. *Kundalini Yoga for Strength, Success & Spirit.* New York: White Lion Press, 1991. 161 p. Illus. $15.95. ISBN: 0-961707-2-5.

Ravi Singh, well-known teacher throughout the United States for more than twenty years, has written a practical and theoretical book on kundalini yoga. The original system of yoga, kundalini yoga is a blend of breathing, movement, meditation, stretching, relaxation, rhythm and sound designed to produce a balanced, strong and aware state of being. Singh defines basic concepts clearly, including the chakras, meridians and the ten bodies, and presents the fundamental components of kundalini yoga (breath, mantras and meditation) as well as general guidelines for practicing the system. A series of warm-ups for flexibility and foundation are provided, including photographs of each exercise. Written directions contain possible modifications and the effects of each exercise on the mind/body system. Different sequences of two to five exercises each provide choice and variety. Further sections target specific areas of the body and a section called Quick Fixes teaches ten three-minute techniques for specific purposes. Various types of breathing and meditation are explained, and the book concludes with four appendices which delineate the chakras, the ten bodies, kundalini yoga mantras, and kundalini yoga teaching centers.

686. Stewart, Mary. *Yoga Over 50: The Way to Vitality, Health and Energy in the Prime of Life.* New York: Simon & Schuster, 1994. 128 p. Illus., index. $15.00. ISBN: 0-671-88510-3.

Acknowledging the need for some type of exercise in the middle and later years of life, this book emphasizes the value of yoga to meet that need. The introduction provides an overview of yoga, including philosophy, physiological and psychological benefits, a brief history of yoga, and information on how the human body works. Written in very plain language, this easy-to-read work is enhanced by clear color photographs depicting the yoga poses being discussed. Subjects in all the photos are individuals over fifty years of age, with some in their eighties. Step-by-step instructions and illustrations cover standing poses, chair poses, upside-down poses, lying flat and sitting poses. A section on relaxation introduces the spiritual aspects of yoga and provides information on breathing and meditation techniques. A final section outlines programs of exercise and relaxation for beginners, mid-level and advanced students as well as routines which address specific problems of stiffness and aches.

Journals and Newsletters

687. ***The Journal of the International Association of Yoga Therapists.*** Mill Valley, CA: International Association of Yoga Therapists. v.1, no.1, 1990. Annual. Illus., adv. Free with International Association of Yoga Therapists membership. $12.50 (subscription).

With a Board of Advisors that includes Dean Ornish, M.D., and Vasant Lad, Ph.D., as well as representatives from all over the world, this annual publication includes intelligently written pieces on all aspects of yoga therapy. Issues have included articles on yoga and the elderly, management of back pain, breathing, and cardiovascular fitness, as well as reviews of books and videotapes, and a current listing of International Association of Yoga Therapists members (see chapter 6: Yoga—Organizations). Manuscripts are accepted for consideration throughout the year. Though most appropriate for professional yoga therapists, the writing style of many of the articles also makes this journal accessible to those with a general interest in yoga.

688. ***Yoga International.*** Honesdale, PA: Yoga International, Inc. v.1, no.1, 1991. Bimonthly. Illus., adv. $18.00 (subscription). ISSN: 1055-7911.

This journal explores issues relating to physical, mental and spiritual aspects of yoga practice and holistic living. Written in a straightforward manner and aimed at anyone with an interest in this subject, its issues contain feature articles on specific philosophical aspects of yoga, interviews with or accounts of noted yoga masters, and articles on the practical aspects of yoga. Letters from readers, vegetarian recipes, and book reviews are found in each issue, as are brief articles on mind/body practices.

689. ***Yoga Journal.*** Escondido, CA: California Yoga Teachers Association. v.1, no.1, 1975. Illus., adv. Bimonthly. $21.00 (subscription). ISSN: 0191-0965.

According to its statement of purpose, *Yoga Journal* focuses on "body/mind approaches to personal and spiritual development—such as hatha yoga, holistic healing, transpersonal psychology, bodywork and massage, the martial arts, meditation, Eastern spirituality, and Western mysticism . . ." Five feature articles, often written by noted individuals in their fields, cover both practical and theoretical issues of personal and spiritual development. More than a dozen varying departments offer information on meditation, music, health and conscious living. Profiles of noted yoga personalities and reviews of recently published books of relevance to the field are also found in each issue. A down-to-earth approach to all its subjects gives this journal appeal to a broad audience.

CHAPTER 15: SELF-REGULATORY TECHNIQUES

Biofeedback

Books

690. Rosenbaum, Lilian. *Biofeedback Frontiers: Self-Regulation of Stress Reactivity.* New York: AMS Press, 1989. 268 p. Illus., biblio. $15.95. ISBN: 0-404-633266-1.

Rosenbaum, one of the early proponents of biofeedback and the founder of the Biofeedback Program at the Georgetown University Family Center, has written a book intended to provide both professionals and the general public with an overview of this subject. General introductory questions and answers are followed by information on the history of biofeedback, including its early development and applications. Also included are discussions of new research and advances in the larger field of mind-body medicine. The selection of appropriate instrumentation is outlined and "basic biofeedback training and related self-regulation techniques are described." The author discusses her biofeedback program, and addresses the issue of the cost-effectiveness of this type of treatment. A lengthy chapter is devoted to the use of biofeedback to achieve superior performance as well as for the treatment of various physical disorders. Diagrams and illustrations are used to clarify some of the more theoretical discussions.

Journals and Newsletters

691. ***Biofeedback and Self-Regulation.*** New York: Plenum Press. v.1, no.1, 1975. Quarterly. $55.00 (individual subscription), $245.00 (institutional subscription). ISSN: 0363-3586.

Published in conjunction with the Association for Applied Psychophysiology and Biofeedback (AAPB) (see chapter 7: Biofeedback—Organizations), this peer-reviewed scholarly journal covers the fields of biofeedback, basic and applied psychophysiology, physiology, and other topics in behavioral medicine. It is appropriate for a professional audience from the disciplines of psychology, psychiatry, psychosomatic and physical medicine, and cybernetics. The journal features research articles including case studies and single case experimental designs in a section entitled "Case studies and clinical replication series." Articles cover biofeedback techniques and their clinical application, self-control procedures, child development studies on self-regulation, autogenic training, progressive relaxation, and scientific studies on the alteration of consciousness. The journal stresses original research articles but also publishes review articles, position papers, case studies, abstracts from AAPB annual meetings, and book reviews. Approximately five articles per issue, ten to fifteen pages long, contain abstracts, key word descriptors, references, and relevant diagrams, charts and tabular data as well as detailed descriptions of method and results where appropriate. The journal covers varied and important aspects of the field and should be useful to the clinician and researcher working in the broad area of behavioral medicine. The large editorial board includes Edward Taub from the University of Alabama at Birmingham, Erik Peper from San Francisco State University, Paul M. Lehrer from the University of Medicine and Dentistry of New Jersey, and others from the Menninger Clinic and other well-known U.S. institutions and universities.

Hypnotherapy

Books

692. Phelps, Lynn. *Your Guide to Medical Hypnosis.* Madison, WI: Medical Physics Publishing, 1993. Illus., biblio., index. 108 p. $9.00. ISBN: 0-944838-28-6.

A family practice physician and faculty member of the University of Wisconsin Medical School, Dr. Phelps has taught medical hypnosis and used it extensively in his practice. He has written a very basic introduction to the field geared to the lay public in style, content and visual presentation. Written in simple, clear, jargon-free language, the book covers the basics: a brief history, types of health professionals using medical hypnosis, an explanation of the levels of consciousness and how the mind works, methods of producing hypnosis, and a description of the trance state. The four steps of hypnotherapy are explained, as well as the types of therapeutic suggestions, including ideosensory, ideomotor, age regression, ideonominal, ideosecretory, ideoaffective and dissociation. The remaining section discusses the practice of self-hypnosis, group hypnosis and the use of medical hypnosis for various conditions such as habit cessation, pregnancy, pain, sexual problems and cancer. Case studies are included to illustrate pertinent points and facilitate understanding. Phelps emphasizes the need to utilize a qualified, well-trained hypnotherapist and points out both the dangers and limitations of this therapeutic approach. An interesting, though dated, annotated suggested reading list is provided covering books from 1959-1984 which are appropriate for both the lay and professional audience. These include classics in the field and cover hypnosis from varying perspectives. Also included is an appendix of organizations providing information on hypnosis and referrals to qualified practitioners. This book is part of the Focus on Health Series, books for the general public covering various topics in health and medicine.

693. Yapko, Michael. *Essentials of Hypnosis.* New York: Brunner/Mazel, 1995. Biblio., index. 184 p. $19.95. ISBN: 0-87630-761-6.

Part of the Brunner/Mazel Basic Principles into Practice Series, offering fundamentals of theory and technique on different topics in psychology, this book is intended to serve as a useful tool for the professional health practitioner, as a basic text for graduate and undergraduate courses, and as an introduction to hypnosis for the informed lay public. Dr. Yapko, a clinical psychologist and Director of the Milton H. Erickson Institute of San Diego, covers both the principles and the practice of hypnosis with clarity and precision. Defining hypnosis as a "system of skilled and influential communication," Yapko first discusses the nature of hypnosis as he conceptualizes it, common misconceptions about clinical hypnosis held by both lay and professional people, and basic theories of hypnosis that are widely held. These discussions are concisely and intelligently presented and are well referenced at the end of each chapter. Further introductory sections include information on contexts in which hypnosis is used, such as medical and dental hypnosis, sports, forensic sciences and others, as well as the nature of the conscious and unconscious mind, hypnotic susceptibility and hypnotic communication. Yapko then goes on to describe the elements involved in the practice of hypnosis, including communication styles, the structures and patterns of hypnotic suggestions, hypnotic inductions, hypnotic phenomena such as age regression and dissociation, self-hypnosis, and common problems treated with hypnosis. He provides specific guidelines for communication and formulating hypnotic suggestions, all of which are referenced for further study. A sample script is provided and other pertinent issues explored, including resistance, repressed memory and ethical guidelines. This is an extremely clear, knowledgeable and well-thought-out presentation. The references provided are outstanding and make this not only a highly readable work but a scholarly endeavor useful as a starting point to further in-depth study for those interested in the subject.

Journals and Newsletters

694. ***The International Journal of Clinical and Experimental Hypnosis.*** Newbury Park, CA: Sage Publications. v.1, no.1, 1953. Quarterly. $57.00 (individual subscription), $110.00 (institutional subscription). ISSN: 0020-7144.

This professional scientific journal publishes research and clinical papers on hypnosis as applicable to the fields of psychology, psychiatry, medicine, dentistry and allied areas of science. Included are clinical and experimental studies, discussions of theory, historical and cultural topics, and questions for inclusion in a Master Class forum on problems in clinical practice. Topics covered include self-hypnosis, control of smoking, forensic uses, post-traumatic stress disorder, anxiety and pain control, the use of visual imagery, multiple personality disorder, the work of Milton Erickson, and many others. Articles include abstract and references. The journal also has a section on book reviews and conference and workshop announcements. The editor-in-chief is Fred H. Frankel of Harvard Medical School and associate and advisory editors are Ph.D.s and M.D.s from leading U.S. universities.

Imagery

Books

695. Achterberg, Jeanne. *Imagery in Healing: Shamanism and Modern Medicine.* Boston and London: Shambhala Publications, 1985. 253 p. Biblio. $16.00. ISBN: 0-87773-307-4.

Jeanne Achterberg, professor of psychology at the Institute of Transpersonal Psychology and a pioneer in the field, presents a now classic study of the practice of imagery from its spiritual aspects in shamanism to its most modern manifestations in hypnosis, biofeedback and psychoneuroimmunology. This is a basically theoretical work, exploring the nature of the imagery process, its historical and anthropological roots, and modern scientific research and practice in the medical and social sciences. The practice of imagery is conceptualized as the use of the imagination as healer. The power of this tool and how and why it works is described in an interesting, well-documented and thoughtful way. Written for both the educated lay public and professional readers, this work first places imagery in a cultural context, from analysis of shamanic practice of healing through descriptions of early Greek, Middle Ages and Renaissance imagery practices. A discussion follows on the similarities and differences in the use of imagery techniques in modern medical practice. Achterberg believes that current use of imagery must be grounded in scientific knowledge in order to be accepted by the medical community. She clearly presents the physiological and biochemical mechanisms underlying the effectiveness of imagery in health and healing as well as evidence from the behavioral and social sciences. Finally, through anecdote and scientific documentation, the link between the brain and the immune system is described, providing a further promising rationale for the harnessing of mental processes in the promotion of health. Appendices offer sample imagery scripts for various conditions and a detailed bibliography, although now dated, cites early and important works.

696. Epstein, Gerald. *Healing Visualization: Creating Health Through Imagery.* New York: Bantam Books, 1989. 226 p. Illus., index. $9.95. ISBN: 0-553-34623-7.

Drawing on scientific evidence and over fifteen years of clinical practice, Dr. Epstein, assistant clinical professor of psychiatry at Mt. Sinai Medical Center in New York, has written a handbook on the use of visual imagery for physical and emotional self-healing work. In a simple and straightforward presentation, this practical guide first discusses the nature, benefits and process of imagery therapy, including mental and physical preparation and the theoretical basis for the work. The main portion of the book offers specific prescriptions for the use of over seventy-five imagery exercises of one to five minutes in length for a wide variety of physical and mental symptoms and illnesses arranged in alphabetical order. These easy-to-follow exercises are supplemented by a section on special visualization for overall health and well-being and pointers on developing your own healing imagery.

697. Fanning, Patrick. *Visualization for Change.* 2nd ed. Oakland, CA: New Harbinger Publications, 1994. 327 p. Biblio. $13.95. ISBN: 1-879237-84-9.

Described by the author as a "toolbox," *Visualization for Change* offers a practical approach to using visualization for self-improvement and healing. Fanning, a writer and teacher for over twenty-five years, provides the historical and theoretical background of the different approaches to imagery (scientific, philosophical, psychological, religious and New Age). But his concentration is clearly on the practice. Basic skills are taught through thirteen guidelines for visualization which prepare the reader for the imagery work. The remainder of the book covers the various applications for specific problems such as weight control, stress reduction, healing of various diseases and pain control. These sections methodically analyze the situation, suggest positive affirmations appropriate to the problem, and guide the reader through specific visualizations to be utilized for change. Highly appropriate for the lay reader in both language and tone, this is a straightforward and useful primer combining technique, encouragement and a positive approach to handling life issues. A resource guide and bibliography offer information on audiotapes, music and a thorough list of books from early classics to recent publications.

698. Graham, Helen. *The Magic Shop.* York Beach, ME: Samuel Weiser, 1993. 228 p. Biblio., index. $10.95. ISBN: 0-87728-770-8.

Helen Graham, author, university lecturer and workshop leader in England, combines the teachings of modern psychology and ancient wisdom in this book on imagery and self-healing. Essentially presenting the material from her workshops in a clear and straightforward manner, eleven lengthy exercises are included. Each one is introduced with a discussion of the issue presented and its relevance to health and healing, followed by a commentary section on the exercise just performed. Often a section reflecting commonly asked questions on the topic is included. Exercises include progressive relaxation through imagery, imagining the healing process, guided fantasy imagery, communicating with pain through imagery, and inner guide visualization, Graham provides much relevant information on related topics including the subtle energies, various forms of therapies, and the history of magic and medicine. Bibliographic references and suggestions for further reading from the book and journal literature as well as a well-prepared index are included.

699. Lusk, Julie T. *Thirty Scripts for Relaxation, Imagery and Inner Healing.* v. 1. Duluth, MN: Whole Person Associates, 1992. 176 p. $19.95. ISBN: 0-938586-69-6.

In this book, twenty-seven physicians, psychologists, therapists and educators have contributed their most effective scripts for relaxation, visualization and guided meditation exercises. Compiled and edited by Julie Lusk, one of several nationally recognized experts in the field, this book serves as an introduction to practice guidelines and scripts for professionals first learning to use guided imagery as a tool, and as a source of new exercises for experienced practitioners. The scripts are appropriate for all types of settings and cover different areas of learning: relaxation, inner answers, healing and personal growth. They are simple, thoughtful, relatively short and varied, encouraging the development of visual, auditory, olfactory and kinesthetic imagery skills. This is a practical, well-rounded resource on visualization for any professional engaged in the field.

700. Naparstek, Belleruth. *Staying Well with Guided Imagery.* New York: Warner Books, 1994. 228 p. Illus., biblio, index. $19.95. ISBN: 0-446-51821-2.

The author provides a manual on the imagery process based on twenty-five years as a psychotherapist and specialist in guided imagery. In a supportive, warm and compassionate manner, Naparstek covers theory and practice, guiding the reader through the major aspects of imagery work. Her writing is lively, clear and down-to-earth, making accessible such potentially esoteric ideas as altered states and the like. Using anecdotes from her practice, workshops and personal life, she begins by explaining what imagery is and how and why it works, giving the key principles that underlie the healing abilities of imagery. The different kinds of imagery for health and well-being are described, including feeling state imagery (mood), end state, energetic, cellular, physiological and metaphoric imagery. The remainder of the book is devoted to imagery exercises with specific, clear instructions and wellness imagery scripts based on the categories noted above. Separate chapters cover imagery for emotional wellness and exercises for common physical complaints such as headache, pain, sleeplessness and fatigue. She concludes with frequently asked questions and a resource section for guided imagery audiotapes, workshops and seminars, and books. A well-thought-out index provides "See" and "See also" references to the text.

701. Rossman, Martin L. *Healing Yourself: A Step by Step Program for Better Health Through Imagery.* New York: Simon and Schuster, 1987. 220 p. Index. $8.95. ISBN: 0-671-73029-0.

Winner of the American Health book award for 1987, this is a clearly written, well-documented guide on using imagery in the process of healing illness and creating health. Dr. Rossman is a clinical associate at the University of California Medical Center at San Francisco and member of the scientific advisory council of the Institute for the Advancement of Health. He has written this practical and instructive manual based on over fifteen years of teaching imagery techniques as well as clinical research on the mind/body connection. Rossman explains what imagery is, how it works, what it can do and what conditions it can be used to treat. Beginning with basic exercises to familiarize readers with the imagery process, the book goes on to lead the reader through the entire process of developing imagery skills. Through clearly presented progressive exercises, various aspects are taught: relaxation, deepening techniques, developing your own healing imagery, and increasing inner awareness. Two appendices are included: using imagery for specific problems such as pain relief, arthritis and cancer, and a resource guide of books and audiotapes on imagery. A large type size and spacing make this very easy to read from a physical point of view.

702. Samuels, Michael. *Healing with the Mind's Eye: A Guide for Using Imagery and Visions for Personal Growth and Healing.* New York: Summit Books, 1990. 304 p. Biblio. $19.95. ISBN: 0-671-68215-6.

Author of several major books on imagery, healing and wellness, Dr. Samuels has studied the benefits and medical uses of imagery, incorporated imagery into his medical practice for more than twenty years, and developed a program of mental exercises that are the basis of workshops he conducts around the world. This book presents that program, providing step-by-step guidance in the use of imagery for healing and personal growth. Part I introduces the process of imagery and the many effects the spirit has on the mind and the mind has on the body, including enhancing the immune system, decreasing pain, lowering blood pressure and influencing emotions, attitudes and personal and spiritual growth. Part II provides direct practice in using imagery to heal the body, with each chapter covering appropriate explanatory background information, discussion about the specific exercise to be performed, and detailed guidance through mental exercises which progress from simple imagery to complex reverie states. Based on scientific, clinical and personal experience, Samuels promises "If you spend time on the exercises, you will be different at the end of this book." One gets the feeling that based on scientific, clinical and personal experience, Samuels is a man who believes in what he writes and is eager to share it. He does so convincingly in a readable, encouraging and down-to-earth way.

Meditation/Relaxation/Stress Reduction

Books

703. Benson, Herbert with Miriam Z. Klipper. *The Relaxation Response.* New York: Avon Books, 1975. 222 p. Illus., biblio., index. $5.50. ISBN: 0-380-00676-6.

In this now classic presentation of a western approach to the practice of meditation, Dr. Benson, associate professor of medicine at the Harvard Medical School and Director of the Hypertension Section of Beth Israel Hospital in Boston, brings together modern scientific information and age-old eastern and western wisdom to develop a therapeutic technique for coping with stress, fatigue, anxiety and stress-related illness. It is recommended that this easy-to-learn technique be practiced ten to twenty minutes two times a day in conjunction with more traditional medical treatment if disease is present. Benson provides the theoretical background for this approach by clearly discussing the nature of stress, the fight-or-flight response, and hypertension and its effect on the body. The process of adjusting to life's stresses through mental control or meditation is simply presented and the four basic elements identified, emphasizing the notion that the relaxation response is a universal, innate human capacity available to us all. A well-prepared index with "See" and "See also" references plus an extensive bibliography of books and journal articles provide easy access to information and lead to further writings on the subject.

704. Blumenfeld, Larry. *The Big Book of Relaxation.* Roslyn, NY: The Relaxation Co., 1994. 223 p. Illus., biblio. $14.95. ISBN: 1-55961-282-7.

A compilation of writings on ten approaches to relaxation, each chapter is prepared by acknowledged experts in their fields such as Kay Gardner on music and relaxation, Shakti Gawain on creative visualization, Ohashi on shiatsu and John Harvey on meditation. Written for the layperson with little or no background in these practices, this book offers clear, basic background information on the nature of the discipline as well as a description of how and why it works. The focus of the chapters, however, is on practical techniques to enhance relaxation. These are presented through step-by-step exercises and procedures, whether learning to meditate or preparing an aromatherapy bath. Helpful illustrations and charts accompany the text throughout. A chapter on new technologies provides interesting information on products and resources that utilize brain and mind potentials for relaxation, such as biofeedback devices for home use. The final chapter is an annotated resource guide keyed to each chapter describing books, recordings, videotapes, product sources and organizations relevant to each discipline. Despite a few graphical and typographical errors that are a bit distracting, this is a useful introduction to a variety of approaches and techniques that can easily be incorporated into one's life.

705. Borysenko, Joan. *Minding the Body, Mending the Mind.* Toronto and New York: Bantam Books, 1988. 241 p. Biblio., index. $10.95. ISBN: 0-553-34556-7.

Written by the co-founder and former director of the Mind/Body Clinic at New England Deaconess Hospital, Harvard Medical School, this book provides an overall introduction to the concept of mind/body medicine. The philosophy of this therapy is that relaxation techniques and "mindfulness" can help restore the body to physical health. Borysenko presents a scientific discussion of mind/body interactions and describes relaxation techniques taught at the clinic, focusing on how those techniques can be adapted for individual use. Instructions and detailed illustrations for various relaxation techniques are provided, as is a well-rounded bibliography covering materials ranging from meditation to popular science to fiction.

706. Dacher, Elliott. *PNI: The New Mind/Body Healing Program.* New York: Paragon House, 1991. 219 p. Illus., biblio., index. $12.95. ISBN: 1-55778-599-6.

This comprehensive look at the science of psychoneuroimmunology (PNI) introduces the reader to the basic philosophy and practice of this new medicine of the 21st century, a combination of the wisdom and knowledge of ancient healing traditions and modern scientific medicine. Dr. Dacher, a Harvard-trained practicing physician, is a well-known lecturer on wellness, PNI and self-healing. He first provides background and theory on mind/body medicine, including how it works on a physiological level and research on the relationship of stress and disease. He identifies the two major components of self-healing (mindfulness and self-regulation) and leads the reader through a mind/body healing program. This includes discussion and eighteen very clear and gentle exercises interspersed throughout the text based on the principles of meditation, imagery and biofeedback. These exercises are designed to allow the reader to experience, learn and practice the skills of awareness and self-directed change and provide the keys to this new medicine: self-healing, self-understanding and self-responsibility.

707. Dass, Ram. *Journey of Awakening: A Meditator's Handbook.* New York: Bantam Books, 1990. 426 p. Illus., biblio. $4.95. ISBN: 0-553-28572-6.

Ram Dass, a world-renowned American psychologist and spiritual teacher, has written a straightforward, simple, very human, and often humorous introduction to meditation. Speaking directly to the reader in a personal style, he presents the varied paths of meditation (mantra, visualization, movement, mindfulness), shares his understanding of it, and orients the reader on how to prepare, what to expect, the pitfalls, the benefits, and the necessary attitudes to maintain meditation practice. The second part of the book is a comprehensive published directory of groups that teach meditation, including local, national and Canadian alphabetical listings by group; retreat facilities by state, alphabetical by group name; and a bibliography of suggested readings covering thirty-five books on meditation from all disciplines and religions from the Kabbalah to Zen.

708. Fontana, David. *The Elements of Meditation.* Rockport, MA: Element, 1991. 119 p. Biblio. $8.95. ISBN: 1-85230-229-1.

This well-written introduction to the practice of meditation by psychologist Dr. David Fontana is a balanced and clear presentation of a complex art. Fontana knows both the subject and the reader well. He anticipates questions in the reader's mind, beginning with instruction on what meditation is, when to do it, for how long, how to sit, etc. Each chapter provides simple exercises for different aspects of meditation with the early exercises building the foundation for later practice. Throughout the book, Fontana uses the analogy of traveling on a journey, always keeping the focus simple while intimating the profound. The variety of forms of meditation are detailed, including focus on the breath, color, sound, visualization and other approaches to practice, and the benefits on all levels to the meditator are described. Yet it is not the goal that is emphasized in this work but the process and promise of discovery of truths and deeper states of being and knowing. This book is highly appropriate for the beginning lay reader, both in style and content. The annotated bibliography is an interesting collection of works covering both eastern and western approaches to the study of meditation.

709. Goleman, Daniel. *The Meditative Mind: The Varieties of Meditative Experience.* Los Angeles: Jeremy P. Tarcher, 1988. 214 p. Biblio., index. $8.95. ISBN: 0-87477-463-2.

This expanded version of *The Varieties of Meditative Experience,* originally published in 1977, discusses the emergence and growing acceptance of meditation in western culture. Part I explores the Visuddhimagga, part of a detailed Buddhist philosophy and psychology which Goleman offers as "a map for inner space." While Part II summarizes different traditions of meditation, among them Hindu Bhakti, Jewish Kabbalah, Christian Hesychasm, Transcendental Meditation, Tibetan Buddhism and Zen, Part III discusses commonalities among these different approaches. Part IV, which comprises close to half the book, contains the material not originally included in the 1977 work, and consists of information on the healing properties of meditation and how meditation can help deal with stress and improve the quality of one's life. This book offers something for everyone: the lay reader will find the sections on the different forms of meditation and the common traits of all forms of meditation especially useful; those who are already involved in meditation will appreciate the descriptions of rarified states of consciousness included in the book.

710. Kabat-Zinn, Jon. *Full Catastrophe Living: Using the Wisdom of Your Body and Mind to Face Stress, Pain and Illness: The Program of the Stress Reduction Clinic at the University of Massachusetts Medical Center.* New York: Dell, 1990. 467 p. Biblio., index. $12.00. ISBN: 0-385-30312-2.

Jon Kabat-Zinn, Ph.D., presents the program of the stress-reduction clinic at the University of Massachusetts Medical Center (see chapter 7: Meditation/Relaxation/Stress Reduction—Treatment Centers/Referrals), of which he is founder and director. With the goal of making meditation and mindfulness accessible to and useful for everyone, this readable and encouraging guide emphasizes the integration of meditative practice into daily life as an approach to stress reduction, health maintenance and personal growth. The book provides technique as well as theory and is grounded in both scientific and anecdotal evidence relating the state of the mind to the state of the body, one's health and level of well-being. Dr. Kabat-Zinn orients the reader to the discipline of meditation by describing the proper attitudinal approach to be taken (nonjudgment, patience, trust and nonstriving) and explaining the five main types of meditation that can be practiced. He provides instruction on how to apply a meditation plan to the six major sources of life stress (work, food, people, sleep, physical pain, time and emotional pain). This is a book that in a very concrete way is meant to open the reader's mind and change his or her approach to life.

711. ***Principles and Practice of Stress Management.*** 2nd ed. Edited by Paul M. Lehrer and Robert L. Woolfolk. New York: The Guilford Press, 1993. 621 p. Illus., index. $75.00. ISBN: 0-89862-766-4.

Writing for health professionals in the fields of behavioral medicine and psychosocial practice, Drs. Lehrer and Woolfolk have edited an authoritative, well-researched text presenting relevant findings, techniques and theoretical foundations in the area of stress management. The contributing authors represent leaders in the fields of progressive relaxation, autogenic training, music therapy, yoga-based therapy, pharmacological approaches and more. The book provides well documented background information on each approach, including history and theory, clinical assessment guidelines, adverse effects and contraindications, detailed explanation and description of the method utilized, case examples and ample relevant historical and current references. The last three chapters, written by Lehrer, Woolfolk, and others, provide an in-depth review of the literature and analysis of the factors contributing to the effectiveness of the techniques described earlier. The approaches are compared, providing guidance on their usefulness and success with various symptoms, conditions, and personality characteristics as well as data on which therapies conflict and which work well together. This empirical information offers a basis for making informed clinical decisions on the choice of therapy. The editors have succeeded admirably in presenting a cohesive analysis of the diverse field of stress management and providing clinicians with a comprehensive picture of what is currently known about effective practice.

712. Sky, Michael. *Breathing: Expanding Your Power and Energy.* Santa Fe, NM: Bear & Co, 1990. 149 p. Illus. $9.95. ISBN: 0-939680-82-3.

Michael Sky, teacher, author and holistic practitioner, presents a clearly written, simple primer on the practice of conscious breathing. Acting as a guide, the author incorporates easy, gentle and effective breathing exercises with basic information on the power and function of breath. Sky details the physical, mental, emotional and spiritual benefits of breathing with awareness. He prepares the reader well by explaining the energetic aspects of breath, the connection between feeling and breathing, and the manner in which patterns of contracted energy are formed. Circular breathing technique is then presented, and the various levels of reaction inherent in that process are clearly described. An appendix provides seven breathing exercises including the cleansing breath and the deep releasing breath. This book is written to create a direct, supportive experience of the breathing process, gently opening and transforming the reader while providing the intellectual information necessary to bring understanding to practice.

Journals and Newsletters

713. ***Annals of Behavioral Medicine.*** Rockville, MD: The Society of Behavioral Medicine. vol.1, no.1, 1991. Quarterly. $135.00 (subscription), free to members. ISSN: 0883-6612.

This peer-reviewed multidisciplinary journal for the professional reader combines the *Annals of Behavioral Medicine* and *Behavioral Medicine Abstracts,* both journals previously published separately by the Society of Behavioral Medicine. Each issue now includes a section of approximately two hundred detailed abstracts of the current literature on behavioral medicine from prominent medical journals such as *Archives of Neurology, American Journal of Epidemiology, British Heart Journal,* and many others. Complete bibliographic citations are provided as well as the reprint address for each article. This section is followed by a subject index for locating articles on the large variety of topics covered, including chronic fatigue syndrome, hypoglycemia and diabetes, arthritis, anxiety, menopause, obesity and much more. In addition, issues contain three to six substantive literature reviews presenting theory and research on psychological, social, clinical and epidemiological aspects of various health issues such as depression, coronary heart disease, stress and herpes simplex virus reactivation. These reviews are clearly written, highly relevant, and have implications for both biobehavioral treatment strategies and future research directions. They are extensively referenced (80-100 per article), and contain introductory abstracts, reprint address and useful charts and diagrams. Also variously included are articles on empirical research, book reviews, grant funding announcements, placement opportunities and continuing education events.

714. ***International Journal of Stress Management.*** New York: Human Sciences Press. v.1, no.1, 1994. Quarterly. $35.00 (individual subscription), $75.00 (institutional subscription). ISSN: 1072-5245.

The official journal of the International Stress Management Association, this peer-reviewed professional journal covers the interdisciplinary field of stress management, including medicine, dentistry, nursing, psychiatry, psychology, business and industry, and the allied health fields. Issues consist of research papers, clinical reports, reviews, and historical articles with a focus on behavioral strategies and methods for stress reduction in the workplace and interpersonal relationships. Three to five articles appear in each issue and contain initial abstracts, key words and generally very current references. The journal also publishes book reviews, letters to the editor, editorials and announcements and programs of worldwide meetings related to stress management. The international editorial board includes such well-known experts as Paul Lehrer of the University of Medicine and Dentistry of New Jersey, Neal E. Miller of Yale University, and Edward Taub of the University of Alabama.

715. ***Mind-Body Medicine:*** *A Journal of Clinical Behavioral Medicine.* Rockville, MD: The Society of Behavioral Medicine. vol. 1, no.1, 1995. Quarterly. $80.00 (individual subscription), $120.00 (institutional subscription), $35.00 (single issue). ISSN: 1195-1990.

Geared toward a professional audience of physicians, clinical psychologists, nurses and social workers with an interest in behavioral medicine, this quarterly journal is published by the Society of Behavioral Medicine and has as its co-editors-in-chief Herbert Benson, M.D., and Richard Friedman, Ph.D. Each issue contains four feature articles: the first presents original research reports on mind/body interactions; the second is a review article concentrating on the integration of behavioral approaches into clinical settings; the third is an editorial response to the earlier articles; and the fourth is a review of professional books on mind/body medicine with some coverage of popular titles. Articles begin with an abstract, are well referenced, clearly written, substantive (10-20 pages), practical, and point the way to an understanding of how and why the incorporation of mind/body concepts into everyday clinical practice can have health benefits as well as support behavioral change in the patient population.

716. ***The Newsletter of the American Institute of Stress.*** Yonkers, NY: American Institute of Stress. no.1, 1988. Monthly. $35.00 (subscription). ISSN: 1047-2517.

Appropriate for health care practitioners, this newsletter consists of articles written by contributing editors (who are also members of the American Institute of Stress' Board of Trustees) and reprints of articles on stress and stress-related topics which originally appeared in other publications such as the *Journal of Internal Medicine* and *The New York Times*. Book reviews and listings of conferences, workshops and other events of interest are also included on a regular basis.

CHAPTER 16: SENSORY THERAPIES

Aromatherapy

Books

717. Keller, Erich. *The Complete Home Guide to Aromatherapy*. Tiburon, CA: H.J. Kramer, 1991. 214 p. Biblio., index. $9.95. ISBN: 0-915811-36-7.

This guide to aromatherapy provides the lay reader with useful information on the basics of aromatherapy, including the properties of essential oils and their use in healing. The author offers a brief history of this therapy and a discussion of the sense of smell, followed by basic information on obtaining, storing and using essential oils. Of particular value is an explanation of terminology used in the labeling of essential oils and information on how to test the quality of oils. The various methods of using aromatherapy are explored and practical applications, including recipes for common ailments (colds, flu, high blood pressure, etc.) are offered. Specific chapters are devoted to the use of essential oils for women, children and to affect sexuality; a chapter on essential oils and the chakras is also included. A lengthy Index of Essential Oils describes the source, scent, properties and general uses of more than seventy oils, and an alphabetical index listing appropriate oils to use for various symptoms is especially helpful. The plain language of the text makes this book a good choice for those who are new to aromatherapy.

718. Price, Shirley. *Aromatherapy for Common Ailments.* New York: Simon & Schuster, 1991. 95 p. Illus., biblio., index. $11.95. ISBN: 0-671-73134-3.

In this practical guide, the author instructs the reader in the use of thirty different essential oils to treat more than forty common health problems including headaches, insomnia, acne, and high blood pressure. Twelve of the most versatile oils are highlighted with full-page color photos and thorough description of their properties and treatment applications. The author begins with a discussion of the nature of the production, composition, and therapeutic value of essential oils, and a two-page chart shows which oils are recommended for particular ailments. Instructions on the use of home treatments such as inhalation and baths, and helpful drawings of therapeutic massage of others and self-massage, are included. While chapter three explores the use of oils to improve hygiene and enhance health, the last section on self-help addresses the treatment of particular existing health problems. These are organized according to the mind and body systems (e.g., circulatory) for easy reference and supply clear information on dosage and treatment instructions. An index provides further access to specific complaints and oils.

719. Rose, Jeanne. *The Aromatherapy Book: Applications and Inhalations.* Berkeley, CA: North Atlantic Books, 1992. 350 p. Illus., biblio. $18.95. ISBN: 1-55643-073-6.

Jeanne Rose, a well-known practicing aromatherapist and teacher, has written a virtual encyclopedia of aromatherapy. A detailed table of contents provides access to tables of essential oils and their uses; a glossary of terms; descriptions of oils; information on how to prepare aromatics; a resource list of products, further information, journals and schools; and recipes for preparing various aromatics. The use of aromatics in rituals and dreams is explored. An extensive bibliography of sources for further reading is also included.

720. Ryman, Danielle. *Aromatherapy: The Complete Guide to Plant and Flower Essences for Health and Beauty.* New York: Bantam Books, 1991. Biblio., index. $10.95. ISBN: 0-553-37166-5.

Written for the lay public, this book presents aromatherapy as a component of modern medicine as opposed to an independent cure. The author, a practicing aromatherapist for more than twenty-five years, first offers an overview of aromatherapy, including history, current uses and possible future uses of this modality. More than eighty plants, their botanical and historical backgrounds, and the full range of their therapeutic uses are discussed, as is the preparation of plant oils from store-bought and home-grown plants. A section of more than 100 symptoms, arranged alphabetically, contains suggestions for aromatherapy treatments. Where appropriate, "See" and "See also" references to other ailments are provided. This very readable work also contains a glossary of medical terms, a list of noted physicians, scientists, herbalists and botanists, and a bibliography.

721. Tisserand, Robert. *Aromatherapy: To Heal and Tend the Body.* Wilmot, WI: Lotus Press, 1988. 224 p. Illus., biblio., index. $9.95. ISBN: 0-941524-42-6.

This book provides a solid general introduction to the subject of aromatherapy. Beginning with a discussion of its history from ancient times to the present day, it moves on to describe what aromatherapy is and how it works. Case histories on the use of aromatherapy to treat a variety of medical conditions are examined, and information is provided regarding seeking appropriate treatment. Essential oils are discussed and some simple recipes for the treatment of common, minor problems are included. The author is a leading figure in the field of aromatherapy and editor of the *International Journal of Aromatherapy.* His earlier work, *The Art of Aromatherapy,* has long been considered a standard in the field.

722. Worwood, Valerie Ann. *The Complete Book of Essential Oils & Aromatherapy.* San Rafael, CA: New World Library, 1991. 423 p. Illus., biblio., index. $18.95. ISBN: 0-931432-82-0.

Though the subject of this book is not exclusively focused on the benefits of aromatherapy for health and healing, it does contain valuable information on aromatherapy's health-related uses. The author, a well-known aromatherapist in England, first provides the reader with an overview of essential oils and their range of uses, and then describes what she considers the necessary components of aromatherapy basic care and travel kits. Chapters on work-related ailments, athletic activities, babies and children, women, men, aging, and pets discuss appropriate oils to use in every instance. Included in the appendices are charts of essential oils which indicate their uses to fight bacteria and as beauty oils for various parts of the body, and a chart which indicates the type of plant, origin and appropriate use of each oil. Also found in the appendices are information on aromamassage and a brief list of resources. This very accessible, practical work provides the general reader with a wealth of information on the medicinal uses of aromatherapy.

Journals and Newsletters

723. ***AROMAtherapy-2037.*** San Francisco, CA: the Herbal Rose Report. Quarterly plus supplements. $25.00 (subscription). ISSN: 1055-8578.

This newsletter by Jeanne Rose Aromatherapy (see chapter 8: Aromatherapy—Product Suppliers) covers herbal and aromatherapy lore, sources and uses of essential oils, herbal information, new product reviews, book reviews, articles on issues in aromatherapy, ritual dates and their essential oils, news items and a questions answered section. This is an informal, down-to- earth newsletter for the aromatherapy enthusiast.

724. ***The Aromatic "Thymes."*** Barrington, IL: Pamela Parsons. v.1, no.1, Quarterly. $7.00 (sample issue), $25.00 (subscription).

This publication is full of practical information regarding essential oils, the use of aromatherapy for healing, and the business of aromatherapy. Each issue contains an in-depth article on an essential oil as well as a calendar of events. Although the layout has a "home-made" quality to it, the content is both interesting and informative.

725. ***Beyond Scents.*** Los Angeles: Aromatherapy Seminars. v.1, no.1, 1993. Quarterly. Illus., adv. $20.00 (subscription).

The organization that offers aromatherapy classes throughout the United States publishes this quarterly newsletter which contains articles appropriate for those practicing or interested in aromatherapy. Topics covered include aromatherapy education, aromatherapy's use in healing, distillation of essential oils, information on the uses of specific oils, and aromatherapy for children. Issues contain case studies, book reviews, event reviews, and calendar listings of aromatherapy educational offerings and events.

726. ***The International Journal of Aromatherapy.*** Petaluma, CA: American Alliance of Aromatherapy. v.1, no.1, 1988. Quarterly. Illus., adv. $30.00 (subscription). ISSN: 0962-4562.

The well-known aromatherapy professional and author Robert Tisserand is the editor of this publication, which has an editorial advisory board composed of aromatherapy professionals from the United States, United Kingdom, France, Germany, Holland, Japan, and Australia. It contains information on individual essential oils, international aromatherapy news, case studies, scientific articles, research reports and book reviews. Display advertising is also included.

727. ***Scentsitivity.*** San Francisco: National Association for Holistic Aromatherapy. v.1, no.1. Quarterly. Adv. $8.00/issue, $20.00 (subscription).

Written for aromatherapy professionals, this newsletter contains articles which explore current issues in the field of aromatherapy. Also included are discussions of specific essential oils, groups of oils and their uses, as well as reviews of new products, a calendar of events, and other aromatherapy-related articles. *Scensitivity* accepts articles, classified and display advertisements, and calendar items for inclusion in the newsletter.

Color and Light Therapy

Books

728. Bassano, Mary. *Healing with Music and Color: A Beginner's Guide.* York Beach, ME: Samuel Weiser, 1992. 104 p. Illus., biblio. $9.95. ISBN: 0-87728-760-0.

This basic guide introduces the reader to the theory and practice of using various forms of sound and color for emotional, physical and mental healing. Mary Bassano, social worker and music therapist, first presents the philosophy and background of this healing work and its basic concept: positive and negative energies can cause imbalances in our energy bodies or can balance, harmonize and heal us. Her goal is to help the reader develop awareness of the properties of tones and color and learn how to use these interchangeable energies for healing. The seven major colors are explained in relation to the energy centers of the body and examples of classical and New Age music that correspond to each color/tone are provided. A detailed table for each color shows the corresponding musical, physical and energetic elements, their characteristics and applicable conditions. Further sections cover healing with crystals and techniques for various methods of applying music and color therapy for healing including visualization, colored light bulbs, solarized water, toning, records and audiotapes. This is a thorough, practical introduction from a decidedly metaphysical point of view.

729. Liberman, Jacob. *Light: Medicine of the Future.* Santa Fe, NM: Bear & Co., 1993. 288 p. Illus., index. $16.95. ISBN: 0-939680-80-7.

Dr. Liberman, O.D., Ph.D in vision science, presents an overview of the therapeutic use of light and color frequencies in physical and psychological healing. Historical and physiological information on the properties of light provide a theoretical background in the traditions of modern science and ancient wisdom. The author cites research and clinical applications for treating various ailments including cancer, depression, stress, and learning disabilities. Beautifully illustrated with lush color plates, a case is made for light therapy as part of an holistic approach to maintaining health and promoting healing. Particularly useful are listings of suggested readings, practitioners by state, full spectrum light sources and other products, and clinical investigators using phototherapy in the treatment of cancer.

730. Ott, John N. *Light, Radiation and You.* Greenwich, CT: Devon Adair, 1990. 199 p. Illus., biblio. $11.95. ISBN: 0-8159-6121-9.

This work was written by a pioneer in the field of photobiology, the biological effects of light and low levels of radiation on plants, animals and humans. Dr. Ott draws on his years of research and the work of other scientists to explain the process and effects of light, color and radiation on the living organism. He begins with background information on the basis of his methods, including the metabolic process, kinesiological testing, electrical field theory, multifrequency interaction and thermal effects. All are described in simple terms using everyday analogies, rendering scientific concepts easily understandable to the layperson. The implication of these factors for tumor growth, behavioral disturbances such as hyperactivity and aggression, viral diseases, sex drive and other conditions are analyzed and explained. A section entitled "What to Do" provides recommendations on windows, eyeglasses and contact lenses, fluorescent lights, television sets and video display terminals, colors and outdoor time. Healthful products manufactured by specific companies are mentioned where appropriate. Some of Ott's recommendations may be hard to follow (e.g., don't watch television, listen to the radio), but others are helpful guidelines for more healthy living. Ott's scientific style of intuition, openness and common sense shine through, and his conversational, grandfatherly writing style and respectful and down-to-earth approach to the lay reader make this a book that educates in the most pleasurable way. The book provides an appendix listing sources of information and lights as well as a detailed bibliography of papers and publications by the author and other scientists. Although dated, this in-depth bibliography of scientific papers from the 1930s to 1980 provides a comprehensive overview of the development of the field.

Music Therapy

Books

731. Bonny, Helen L. and Savary, Louis M. *Music & Your Mind: Listening with a New Consciousness.* Barrytown, NY: Station Hill Press, 1990. 177 p. Biblio. $10.95. ISBN: 0-88268-094-3.

Guided Imagery and Music (GIM) is a therapy which uses music to evoke imagery and explore deeper levels of human consciousness. Since the original publication of this book in 1973, GIM has become a widely-known and accepted healing modality. Techniques for reaching nonordinary levels of consciousness are described, and practical exercises for both beginning and advanced listeners, individually, in groups, or in a classroom setting, are presented. Interspersed throughout the book are quotes relating to music and consciousness by a wide range of well-known individuals including Thomas Jefferson, Plato, Ralph Waldo Emerson, Aldous Huxley, and Thomas Merton. Appendices include information on levels of consciousness and suggested pieces of music for use in GIM. All suggested musical works are readily available at major retail outlets. Co-author Helen Bonny developed the Bonny Method of Guided Imagery and Music and is the co-founder of The Bonny Foundation, a center for music-based therapies (see chapter 8: Music Therapy—Schools).

732. Dewhurst-Maddock, Olivea. *The Book of Sound Therapy: Heal Yourself with Music and Voice.* New York: Simon & Schuster, 1993. 127 p. Illus., biblio. discog., index. $14.00. ISBN: 0-671-78639-3.

Written by an experienced singer, voice teacher and music therapist, this is a well-rounded introduction to the use of music and sound for health and healing. Covering the history of healing by sound from ancient Egypt to the modern scientific tradition, the author explains the nature of sound and the voice, the process of self-exploration through sound, the various forms of music, and sounds used in conjunction with meditation. Highly readable, with a warmth and sense of humanity, the text is liberally illustrated with both explanatory drawings and color photographs. Therapeutic exercises help the reader experience the principles being discussed (resonance exercises, breathing exercises, inner voice exercises, etc.). The last section on healing with sound covers the use of voice, crystals, instruments and body movement as a way to restore inner balance on physical, emotional, mental and spiritual levels, thus disrupting patterns that lead to disease. Included are lists of resource organizations involved in sound therapy, a bibliography on sound and music, and a discography of possible musical selections for therapeutic use.

733. Gardner-Gordon, Joy. *The Healing Voice: Traditional and Contemporary Toning, Chanting and Singing.* Freedom, CA: Crossing Press, 1993. 194 p. Illus., biblio. $12.95. ISBN: 0-89594-571-1.

The aim of this book is to introduce the reader to the special power of sound to heal the emotions, the body and the spirit, emphasizing the naturalness of the process and the freedom and deep inner connection the work can bring. Joy Gardner-Gordon is an internationally known holistic healer, counselor and author. In this book she has brought together ancient uses of sound healing from various traditions with modern scientific concepts of vibrational healing in a well-researched, clearly written book. Each chapter begins with background and historical information, case histories, personal stories and theory on a particular aspect of voice healing, followed by four to five simple and well-described exercises to practice the concepts described. Examples include warming and stretching the voice, toning the internal organs, moaning and groaning, and color breathing. Included in the book are a collection of songs and chants, a glossary, listings of toning practitioners, further readings, and audiotapes and compact discs appropriate to healing work.

734. Merritt, Stephanie with Betty Deborah Ulius. *Mind, Music and Imagery: Unlocking Your Creative Potential.* New York: Plume, 1990. 240 p. Biblio., index. $8.95. ISBN: 0-452-26497-9.

The use of music as a tool for promoting health and well-being in children and adults is the subject of this book. Merritt, a teacher of creativity enhancement through music workshops around the country, presents a program which includes more than forty specially designed exercises using music to reduce stress and improve overall health. Specific suggestions are offered for using various musical pieces as a means of altering particular functions of the body, such as pulse rate and circulation. An appendix on music imaging for children which specifies objectives and identifies appropriate activities is also included.

735. *Music and Miracles.* Edited by Don Campbell. Wheaton, IL: Quest Books, 1992. 280 p. Index. $14.00. ISBN: 0-8356-0683-X.

This compendium of essays on music and vibration is compiled and edited by Don Campbell, Director of the Institute for Music, Health and Education (see chapter 8: Music Therapy—Schools, and Music Therapy—Product Suppliers). It focuses on the miraculous aspect of sound, "the unexplained mysteries of curation, healing and transformation . . ." This is a look at the mystical power of sound affecting planes of energy on the physical, mental, emotional and spiritual levels. Twenty-seven well-known contributors from the fields of medicine, psychology, religion, philosophy, music, education and research discuss various aspects of the energetic power of music. Contributors include Jeanne Achterberg, Larry Dossey, Jean Houston, Donald Epstein, Khen Rinpoche and Don Campbell. These leaders in their fields express a humanistic, inspired view of the potentialities and essence of music. The book is divided into six sections covering different perspectives on the subject: music as energy and the nature of the "miracle"; sound and music in healing; chanting and instrumentation; imaging and voice in psychotherapy; therapeutic and educational uses of sound; and music and the universal (the "upliftment of the soul"). Offering personal stories, case histories, historical information and theoretical discussion, this book opens the reader to the deep possibilities inherent in the energy carried in sound.

736. ***Music: Physician for Times to Come.*** Edited by Don Campbell. Wheaton, IL: Quest Books, 1991. 355 p. Index. $12.95. ISBN: 0-8356-0668-6.

This anthology of essays covers a wide range of theoretical issues related to the power of music and sound to therapeutically affect the body, mind and spirit. It is edited by Don Campbell, a leader in the field of healing with music. These often scholarly essays containing substantial documentation have been written by musicians, music therapists, physicians, researchers, academics, nurses, composers and spiritual teachers. Examples include an interview with Dr. Alfred A. Tomatis on chanting and the spiritual dimension of sound; Dr. Bradford S. Weeks on the physiological aspects of hearing as it relates to the mind/body and the therapeutic use of sound; Derrick de Kerchkhove, Ph.D., on the impact of culture on the nervous system and the different types of listening; and Zen master Seung Sahn on Zen chanting and universal sound. This is an exploration into an emerging field of research and practice. As stated in the introduction, "We are just beginning to realize the deep and profound scientific, medical, psychological and spiritual questions involved in the power of music." Major areas examined are the use of music for imagery in education and psychotherapy, the uses of chanting to alter physical conditions, the impact of sound vibrations according to eastern, western, Christian and esoteric traditions, and sonic entrainment.

Journals and Newsletters

737. ***Journal of the Association for Music and Imagery.*** Baltimore, MD: Association for Music and Imagery. v.1, no.1, 1991. Annual. $20.00 (individual subscription), $30.00 (institutional subscription), $15.00 (student subscription).

Written for music therapists, this scholarly journal focuses on the guided imagery and music process (GIM) and includes case studies, analysis of GIM audiotapes, and theoretical discussion. Articles are written by music therapists, psychotherapists and educators and explore a variety of issues such as the role of emotion and dreams, the use of GIM with victims of abuse, theories of music, and cross-cultural explorations. Articles are lengthy, well documented, clearly written and thought provoking, and include a 100-150 word abstract and historical as well as current references.

738. ***Music Therapy.*** Valley Forge, PA: American Association for Music Therapy. v.1, no.1, 1981. Annual. $20.00 (individual subscription), $30.00 (institutional subscription). ISSN: 0734-7367.

This professional journal for music therapists and other mental health professionals presents diverse viewpoints in the field of music therapy from a clinical and educational perspective. The journal publishes original work and perspectives including experimental research studies, theoretical papers, critical reviews of the literature, research on treatment methods, case studies, articles on education and training, professional issues, and assessment and treatment through music therapy. Also included are translations of articles not previously available in English. Examples of topics covered are pediatric applications of music therapy, music and imagery with the physically disabled elderly, acute care use and others. The editorial board consists of music therapists from well-known U.S. universities and treatment centers as well as private practitioners.

739. ***Open Ear.*** Bainbridge Island, WA: Open Ear. 1989- . Quarterly. Illus., adv. $6.00/issue, $24.00 (subscription).

This newsletter provides information on sound and music in health and education. Articles and reports of current research are accepted for consideration primarily from professionals in music- and health-related fields; a brief biography of the author follows each article. Most appropriate for professionals in the music and healing fields, each issue contains a resource section of training programs, workshops, activities and products, and a listing of music and sound and healing-related publications and services.

740. ***Tuning In.*** Valley Forge, PA: American Association for Music Therapy. Quarterly. Adv. $19.00 (subscription).

This newsletter of the American Association for Music Therapy is a good source of information about the activities of the association as well as activities in the field of music therapy generally. Each issue contains member news, reports of legislative activities, information on upcoming conferences, presentations, workshops and training programs, and listings of items on music therapy appearing in other media. Book reviews are included periodically.

APPENDIX: DIRECTORY OF PUBLISHERS

Below is an alphabetical list of publishers with current addresses and contact information for companies that publish in the area of alternative medicine and/or holistic health. For those publishers whose books are distributed by other companies, distributors are noted in parentheses next to the publisher's name. When ordering books from these companies, refer to the distributor's contact information.

American International Distribution Corp.
Box 20
Williston, VT 05495
Tel. 802-862-0095

Anchor Books
Division of Bantam Doubleday Dell
1540 Broadway
New York, NY 10036-4094
Tel. 212-354-6500

414 East Golf Road (Orders)
Des Plaines, IL 60016
Tel. 312-827-1111

Avery Publishing Group
120 Old Broadway
Garden City Park, NY 11040
Tel. 516-741-2155; 800-548-5757
FAX 516-742-1892

Avon Books
Division of Hearst Corporation
1350 Avenue of the Americas, 2nd Floor

New York, NY 10019
Tel. 212-261-6800; 800-238-0658

Ayurvedic Press
11311 Menaul N.E., Suite A (Street Address)
Albuquerque, NM 87112

Post Office Box 23445 (Mailing Address)
Albuquerque, NM 87192-1445
Tel. 505-291-9698

Bantam Books
Division of Bantam, Doubleday, Dell
1540 Broadway
New York, NY 10036-4094
Tel. 212-354-6500

414 East Golf Road (Orders)
Des Plaines, IL 60016
Tel. 312-827-1111

Bear & Company
Post Office Drawer 2860
Santa Fe, NM 87504-2860
Tel. 505-983-5968; 800-932-3277
FAX 505-989-8386

Bergner Communications
Timing Publications
4095 Jackdaw Street
San Diego, CA 92103
Tel. 619-299-1140

Berkeley Publishing Group
390 Murray Hill Parkway
Post Office Box 506
East Rutherford, NJ 07073
Tel. 201-933-9292; 800-788-6262
FAX 201-933-2316

Brunner/Mazel Publishers
19 Union Square West
New York, NY 10003
Tel. 212-924-3344; 800-825-3089

Celestial Arts Publishing Company
Subsidiary of Ten Speed Press
Post Office Box 7123
Berkeley, CA 94707
Tel. 510-559-1600; 800-841-2665

Consumer Report Books
9180 LeSaint Drive
Fairfield, OH 45014
Tel. 513-860-1178

CRC Press
2000 Corporate Boulevard N.W.
Boca Raton, FL 33431
Tel. 407-994-0555; 800-272-7737

The Crossing Press
Post Office Box 1048
Freedom, CA 95019
Tel. 408-722-0711; 800-777-1048
FAX 408-722-2749

Crown Publishing Group
201 East 50th Street
New York, NY 10022
Tel. 212-751-2600; 800-726-0600 (Customer Service);
800-733-3000 (Orders)

Devin-Adair Publishers
6 North Water Street
Greenwich, CT 06830
Tel. 203-531-7755

DeVorss & Company
Post Office Box 550
Marina del Rey, CA 90294-0550
Tel. 213-870-7478; 800-843-5743 (Bookstores only)

Elan Press (Distributed by DeVorss & Company)
Post Office Box 3175
Boulder, CO 80307
Tel. 303-499-2729

Element Books (Distributed by Penguin USA)
42 Broadway
Rockport, MA 01966
Tel. 508-546-1040
FAX: 508-546-9882

Four Walls Eight Windows
39 West 14th Street, Suite 503
New York, NY 10011
Tel. 212-206-8965; 800-626-4848
FAX 212-206-8799

Future Medicine Publishing
10124 18th Street Court East
Puyallup, WA 98371
Tel. 206-952-1130; 800-990-9499

Grove Press (Distributed by Publishers Group West)
841 Broadway, 4th Floor
New York, NY 10003-4793
Tel. 212-614-7850
FAX 212-614-7915

The Guilford Press
Division of Guilford Publications
72 Spring Street
New York, NY 10012
Tel. 212-431-9800; 800-365-7006

Halcyon Publishers
Post Office Box 4157
La Mesa, CA 91944-4157
Tel. 619-460-9030

Harmony Books
See Crown Publishing Group

HarperCollins
Subsidiary of News Corp Ltd.
10 East 53rd Street
New York, NY 10022-5299
Tel. 212-207-7000; 800-331-3761

1000 Keystone Industrial Park (Orders)
Scranton, PA 18512-4621
Tel. 717-941-1500; 800-242-7737

Harvard Health Publishers Group
164 Longwood Avenue
Boston, MA 02115
Tel. 617-432-1485
FAX 617-432-1506

Hastings House (Distributed by Publishers Group West)
Division of Eagle Publishing Corp.
141 Halstead Avenue
Mamaroneck, NY 10543
Tel. 914-835-4005

The Haworth Press
10 Alice Street
Binghamton, NY 13904-1580
Tel. 607-722-5857; 800-342-9678

Healing Arts Press (Distributed by American International Distribution Corp.)
Imprint of Inner Traditions International
1 Park Street
Rochester, VT 05767
Tel. 802-767-3174

Health Letter Associates
See Harvard Health Publishers Group

Hilltopper Publications, Inc.
320 North Larchmont Boulevard, 3rd Floor
Post Office Box 74908
Los Angeles, CA 90004
Tel. 213-469-3901
FAX 213-469-9597

Himalayan Publishers
RR 1, Box 400
Honesdale, PA 18431
Tel. 717-253-5551; 800-822-4247
FAX 717-253-9078

Houghton Mifflin
215 Park Avenue South
New York, NY 10003
Tel. 800-225-3362
FAX 800-634-7568

Human Sciences Press
Subscription Department
233 Spring Street
New York, NY 10013-1578
Tel. 212-620-8468
FAX 212-807-1047

Inner Traditions International
Sales Department
Post Office Box 388
Rochester, VT 05767
Tel. 802-767-3174
FAX 802-767-3726

InnoVision Communications
Starsong Publications
Post Office Box 7168
San Carlos, CA 94070-7168
Tel. 415-508-0314

Interface Press
4717 North Figueroa Street
Box 42211
Los Angeles, CA 90042
Tel. 213-223-2500; 800-553-6463
FAX 213-223-2519

Interweave Press
201 East 4th Street
Loveland, CO 80537
Tel. 970-669-7672; 800- 272-2193

Keats Publishing
27 Pine Street (Box 876)
New Canaan, CT 06840-0876
Tel. 203-966-8721; 800-858-7014
FAX 203-972-3991

Alfred A. Knopf (Distributed by Random House)
Subsidiary of Random House
201 East 50th Street
New York, NY 10022
Tel. 212-572-2103

Kodansha
Mail Order Department
c/o Putnam Publishing Group
390 Murray Hill Parkway
East Rutherford, NJ 07073
Tel. 800-788-6262

HJ Kramer (Distributed by New Leaf Distributing)
Post Office Box 1082
Tiburon, CA 94920
Tel. 415-435-5367

Mary Ann Liebert
2 Madison Avenue
Larchmont, NY 10538
Tel. 914-834-3100

J. P. Lippincott
12107 Insurance Way
Hagerstown, MD 21740-5184
Tel. 800-777-2295
FAX 301-824-7390

Little, Brown & Co.
200 West Street
Waltham, MA 02154
Tel. 800-759-0190

Long Mountain Press
Post Office Box 689
San Anselmo, CA 94979-0689
Tel. 415-455-9540
FAX 415-455-9541

Lotus Light Publications
Box 1008, Lotus Drive
Silver Lake, WI 53170

Tel. 414-889-8501; 800-548-3824
FAX 800-905-6887

Marlowe & Company (Distributed by Publishers Group West)
632 Broadway, Suite 7
New York, NY 10012
Tel. 212-460-5742

Measurement and Data Corp.
100 Wallace Avenue, Suite 100
Sarasota, FL 34237
Tel. 941-366-1153
FAX 941-366-5743

Medical Physics Publishing
4513 Vernon Boulevard
Madison, WI 53705-4964
Tel. 608-262-4021; 800-442-5778

Menaco Publishing Company, Inc.
Post Office Box 11280
Albuquerque, NM 87192-0280
Tel. 505-292-2225; 800-963-6225
FAX 505-275-1672

New Age Publishing
Post Office Box 53275
Boulder, CO 80321-3275
Tel. 800-234-4556

New Harbinger Publications, Inc. (Distributed by Publishers Group West)
5674 Shattuck Avenue
Oakland, CA 94609
Tel. 510-652-0215; 800-748-6273

New Leaf Distributing
5425 Tulane Drive, Southwest
Atlanta, GA 30336-2323
Tel. 401-691-6996; 800-326-2665

New World Library (Distributed by Publishers Group West)
58 Paul Drive
San Rafael, CA 94903
Tel. 415-472-2100; 800-227-3900
FAX 415-472-6131

Noah Publishing
Post Office Box 1500
Davis, CA 95617
Tel. 800-533-4263

North Atlantic Books
Post Office Box 12327
Berkeley, CA 94701
Tel. 510-559-8277
FAX 510-559-8279

Oryx Press
4041 North Central Avenue, 7th Floor
Phoenix, AZ 85012-3397
Tel. 602-265-2651; 800-279-6799

Passage Press
8188 South Highland Avenue, Suite D-5
Sandy, UT 84093
Post Office Box 21713 (Mailing Address)

Salt Lake City, UT 84121
Tel. 801-942-1440; 800-873-0075
FAX 801-943-7268

Penguin Arkana
375 Hudson Street
New York, NY 10014
Tel. 800-253-6476

Penguin USA
Post Office Box 120
Bergenfield, NJ 07621-0120
Tel. 800-442-4624
FAX 201-387-6216

People's Medical Society
462 Walnut Street
Allentown, PA 18102
Tel. 610-770-1670

Pharmaceutical Products Press
See The Haworth Press

Plenum Press
Plenum Publishing Corp.
Subscription Department
233 Spring Street
New York, NY 10013
Tel. 212-620-6468
FAX 212-807-1047

Pocket Books
Paramount Publishing
200 Old Tappan Road
Old Tappan, NJ 07675
Tel. 201-767-5937; 800-223-2348

Prentice Hall (Distributed by Paramount Publishing)
Division of Simon & Schuster
113 Sylvan Avenue, Route 9W
Englewood Cliffs, NJ 07632

Prima Publishing (Distributed by St. Martin's Press)
Post Office Box 1260
Rocklin, CA 95677-1260
Tel. 916-632-4400

Publishers Group West
Attn: Order Department
Post Office Box 8843
Emeryville, CA 94662
Tel. 510-658-3453; 800-788-3123
FAX 510-658-1834

Putnam Books
200 Madison Avenue
New York, NY 10016
Tel. 212-951-8400; 800-631-8571

Putnam Publishing Group
1 Grosset Drive
Kirkwood, NY 13795
Tel. 800-847-5515

Quest Books
306 West Geneva Road
Post Office Box 270
Wheaton, IL 60189-0270
Tel. 708-665-0130; 800-669-9425
FAX 708-665-8791

Random House
Order Department
400 Hahn Road
Westminster, MD 21157
Tel. 800-733-3000 (Orders)
FAX 800-659-2436 (Orders)
Tel. 410-857-1554; 800-726-0600 (Customer Service)
FAX 410-857-1948 (Customer Service)

RD Publications
934 Old Taos Highway
Santa Fe, NM 87501
Tel. 505-988-2425

Redwing Book Company
44 Linden Street
Brookline, MA 02146
Tel. 617-738-4664; 800-873-3946
FAX 617-738-4620

Rodale Press
Catalog Sales Department
33 East Minor Street
Emmaus, PA 18098
Tel. 610-967-8411; 800-527-8200
FAX 610-967-8962

Sage Publications
2455 Teller Road
Newburg Park, CA 91320

Tel. 805-499-0721
FAX/Order Line 805-499-0871

St. Martin's Press
175 Fifth Avenue
New York, NY 10010
Tel. 212-674-5151; 800-221-7945
FAX 800-258-2769

Shambhala Publications (Distributed by Random House)
Horticultural Hall
300 Massachusetts Avenue
Boston, MA 02115
Tel. 617-424-0030

Shooting Star
230 Fifth Avenue, Suite 1114
New York, NY 10001
Tel. 212-481-3500

Simon & Schuster
1230 Avenue of the Americas
New York, NY 10020
Tel. 212-698-7000; 800-223-2336 (Orders)

Spectrum Universal Corp.
61 Dutile Road
Belmont, NH 03220-5252
Tel. 603-528-4710

Station Hill Press
Station Hill Road
Barrytown, NY 12507
Tel. 914-758-5840
FAX 914-758-8163

Stillpoint Publishers
Post Office Box 640
Walpole, NH 03608
Tel. 800-847-4010

Jeremy P. Tarcher (Distributed by Putnam Publishing Group)
Division of Putnam Publishing Group
5858 Wilshire Boulevard, Suite 200
Los Angeles, CA 90036
Tel. 213-935-9980

Time Publishing Ventures, Inc.
301 Howard Street, Suite 1800
San Francisco, CA 94105

Post Office Box 56863 (Orders)
Boulder, CO 80322-6863
Tel. 800-274-2522

Timeless Books
Association for the Development of Human Potential
Post Office Box 3543
Spokane, WA 99220-3543
Tel. 509-838-6652

Charles E. Tuttle
153 Milk Street, 5th Floor
Boston, MA 02109
Tel. 607-951-4080

R.R. 1, Box 231-5 (Orders)
North Clarendon, VT 05759
Tel. 802-773-8930; 800-526-2778

Van Nostrand Reinhold
115 Fifth Avenue
New York, NY 10003
Tel. 212-254-3232

Visible Ink Press (Distributed by Van Nostrand Reinhold)
Division of Gale Research
835 Penobscot Building
Detroit, MI 48226
Tel. 313-961-2242; 800-877-4253

Warner Books (Distributed by Little, Brown & Co.)
1271 Avenue of the Americas
New York, NY 10020
Tel. 212-522-7200

Samuel Weiser
Post Office Box 612
York Beach, ME 03910-0612
Tel. 207-363-4383; 800-423-7087

White Lion Press
225 East 5th Street, Suite 4D
New York, NY 10003-8536
Tel. 800-243-9642

Wingbow Press
Division of Bookpeople
7900 Edgewater Drive
Oakland, CA 94621
Tel. 510-632-4700; 800-999-4650

Yoga International, Inc.
RR 1, Box 400
Honesdale, PA 18431
Tel. 717-253-5551
FAX 717-253-9078

INDEX

This is primarily a name, author, and title index. For information on the major modalities covered in this book, please refer to the table of contents. Entry numbers listed below refer to the item number of each resource described in the body of the book.

ABOUT THE AUTHORS

Francine Feuerman is a graduate of City College of New York and received her Master of Library Science degree from Queens College. She has a long-standing interest in many aspects of holistic health, particularly in the areas of homeopathy and herbal medicine. Her present position is Special Assistant to the Director of the Research Libraries of the New York Public Library, with responsibility for budget and planning. She lives with her husband and two children in Westchester County, New York.

Marsha Handel is a graduate of Columbia University and earned her degree in Library and Information Science from the City University of New York at Queens. She has studied and worked extensively in the field of holistic health and has had a private practice in movement re-education in New York City for the past eighteen years. Ms. Handel is currently a medical librarian at Beth Israel Medical Center in New York City.